Biostatistics for Epidemiology and Public Health Using R

Bertram K. C. Chan, PhD, PE, completed his secondary education in Sydney, Australia, having passed the New South Wales State Leaving Certificate (university matriculation) with excellent results in mathematics and in honors physics and honors chemistry. He then completed both a bachelor of science in chemical engineering, with first class honors (summa cum laude), and a master's in engineering science in nuclear engineering at the University of New South Wales, and a PhD in engineering at the University of Sydney. This was followed by 2 years of research work at the Australian Atomic Energy Commission Research Establishment, and 2 years of a Canadian Atomic Energy Commission postdoctoral fellowship at the University of Waterloo, Canada.

He undertook additional graduate studies at the University of New South Wales, at the American University of Beirut, and at Stanford University, in statistics, computer science, and pure and applied mathematics (abstract algebra, automata theory, numerical analysis, etc.), and in electronics, and electromagnetic engineering.

His professional career includes over 10 years of university-level teaching and research experience in several institutions, including research associate in biomedical and statistical analysis, Perinatal Biology Section, ObGyn Department, University of Southern California Medical School, Middle East University, and San Jose State University, and industrial research positions at Lockheed Missile & Space, Apple, Hewlett-Packard, and a start-up company (Foundry Networks) in the manufacture of Internet hardware and software: gigahertz switches and routers. In recent years, he supported the biostatistical work of the Adventist Health Studies II research program at the Loma Linda University (LLU) School of Medicine, California, and consulted as a forum lecturer for several years in the LLU School of Public Health (biostatistics, epidemiology, and population medicine). The LLU lectures formed part of this textbook. In these lectures, Dr. Chan introduced the use of the programming language R and designed these lectures for the biostatistical elements for courses in the MPH, MsPH, DrPH, and PhD programs, with special reference to epidemiology in particular and public health and population medicine in general.

Dr. Chan has three U.S. patents and has published over 30 research papers and authored 10 books in educational mathematics. He is a registered professional engineer (PE) in the State of California.

Biostatistics for Epidemiology and Public Health Using R

Bertram K. C. Chan, PhD, PE

SPRINGER PUBLISHING COMPANY

Springer Publishing Company, LLC
11 West 42nd Street
New York, NY 10036
www.springerpub.com

Acquisitions Editor: Nancy S. Hale
Composition: Exeter Premedia Services Private Ltd.

ISBN: 978-0-8261-1025-1
e-book ISBN: 978-0-8261-1026-8

Instructor's Manual ISBN: 978-0-8261-3279-6. Qualified instructors may request supplements by emailing textbook@springerpub.com

Student Materials: A Student Study Guide (ISBN: 978-0-8261-3278-9) and
Supplemental Chapter: Research-Level Applications of R (ISBN: 978-0-8261-3249-9) are available at springerpub .com/chan-biostatistics

15 16 17 18 / 5 4 3 2 1

The author and the publisher of this Work have made every effort to use sources believed to be reliable to provide information that is accurate and compatible with the standards generally accepted at the time of publication. The author and publisher shall not be liable for any special, consequential, or exemplary damages resulting, in whole or in part, from the readers' use of, or reliance on, the information contained in this book. The publisher has no responsibility for the persistence or accuracy of URLs for external or third-party Internet websites referred to in this publication and does not guarantee that any content on such websites is, or will remain, accurate or appropriate.

Library of Congress Cataloging-in-Publication Data

Chan, B. K. C. (Bertram Kim-Cheong), author.
 Biostatistics for epidemiology and public health using R / Bertram K.C. Chan.
    p. ; cm.
 Includes bibliographical references and index.
 ISBN 978-0-8261-1025-1 — ISBN 978-0-8261-1026-8 (e-book)
 I. Title.
 [DNLM: 1. Biostatistics—methods.   2. Epidemiology.   3. Programming Languages.
4. Public Health. WA 950]
 R853.S7
 610.1'5195—dc23

                                                                2015024102

Special discounts on bulk quantities of our books are available to corporations, professional associations, pharmaceutical companies, health care organizations, and other qualifying groups. If you are interested in a custom book, including chapters from more than one of our titles, we can provide that service as well.

For details, please contact:
Special Sales Department, Springer Publishing Company, LLC
11 West 42nd Street, 15th Floor, New York, NY 10036-8002
Phone: 877-687-7476 or 212-431-4370; Fax: 212-941-7842
E-mail: sales@springerpub.com

Contents

Preface

A national network television newscast aired the following five stories in 2006[1]:

- A report on the use of nontraditional, nonmainstream medicine, such as traditional Chinese medicine (TCM), to help people who have type 1 diabetes
- A neighborhood's concern about a sharp rise in the number of children with asthma and autism living in a western U.S. state
- A report on the latest Centers for Disease Control and Prevention (CDC) recommendations regarding who should receive the flu vaccine and when
- A discussion of the extensive infectious disease monitoring strategy being implemented in a coastal city in the southern United States that was recently hit by a massive hurricane
- A report on a study, published in a leading medical journal, of a likely association between an increased risk of cancer and workers' exposure to a particular chemical

Each of these news stories included interviews with public health officials or investigators who called themselves *epidemiologists*.

Who are these epidemiologists, and what do they do? What is *epidemiology*? This book is intended to answer these questions. In doing so, it describes what epidemiology is, how it has evolved, how it is used today, and what some of its key methods and concepts are. The focus is on epidemiology in public health practice—that is, the kind of epidemiology that is done at local, state, and national health departments.

Data analysis—the processing of information collected by observation or experimentation—is a very important part of epidemiologic investigations. Hence, the state of the art in epidemiologic studies is being steadily advanced as the capabilities and capacity of computing facilities and the computing environment in general move ahead. Today, epidemiologists around the world can choose from many commercially available and widely used biostatistical software packages.

A relatively new software package called R, developed in 1993 and freely available via the Internet, is the most promising. R has many advanced regression modeling functions, such as multilinear regression, logistic regression, survival analysis, and multilevel modeling. Supported as it is by leading biostatistical experts worldwide, R is now ubiquitous and provides everything that an epidemiologic data analyst needs.

The purpose of this book is to make R readily accessible, on a hands-on level, to all future epidemiologists for research, data processing, and presentation. This book is essentially about learning R with an emphasis on applications to epidemiology, public health, and preventive medicine. To make the best use of this text, readers

[1]U.S. Department of Health and Human Services, Centers for Disease Control and Prevention (CDC), Office of Workforce and Career Development. (2006). *Principles of epidemiology in public health practice: An introduction to applied epidemiology and biostatistics* (Self Study Course SS1000, 3rd ed.). Atlanta, GA:

should have some background in basic computer usage. With R and the supplied datasets, users should be able to work through each section, learning the techniques of data management, related biostatistical theories, and the practice of data analysis and graphical presentations. The book is systematically organized into seven chapters, each with a number of main sections covering the spectrum of applicable R codes for biostatistical applications in epidemiology and public health.

Chapters 1 and 2 introduce interactional relationships among medicine, preventive medicine, public health, epidemiology, and biostatistics in general, as well as special concepts that have been (and are being) developed to address quantitative problems in epidemiology and public health in particular. A review of the basic elements in the theory of probability is presented to introduce or reinforce readers' ability to handle this important basic concept.

Chapter 3 covers simple data handling using R programming, while Chapter 4 presents the graphics capabilities available in R. Following these initial forays into R, Chapter 5 gives an overview of the theory of probability and mathematical statistics, which is necessary because both of these areas have become integral parts of biostatistical applications in epidemiology.

Chapter 6 shows how R may be effectively used to handle classical problems in case–control studies and cohort investigations in epidemiology. Similarly, survival analysis, the backbone of much epidemiologic research, finds excellent support in the R environment, as outlined in Chapter 7.

To assist and challenge readers, a set of "review questions" appears at the end of each main section. These will help readers to recall and note the salient concepts discussed in the body of the text. Because it is primarily a quantitative subject, biostatistics may best be appreciated by undertaking appropriate, specific, and hands-on exercises involving the concepts introduced in the text. The exercises that appear at the end of most sections will guide readers through applications of these ideas to the world of real epidemiology and public health in the course of practicing their skills in computation using R. **The online Student Study Guide leads students through solutions to the exercises in the book and is available at www.springerpub.com/ chan-biostatistics. Also on www.springerpub.com/chan-biostatistics is a Supplemental Chapter entitled Research-Level Applications of R. An Instructor's Manual is also available by emailing textbook@springerpub.com.**

On November 6, 2011, Professor Tomás Aragon, MD, DrPH, of the University of California-Berkeley, in the preface to his online manual *Applied Epidemiology Using R*, made the following comment:

> We like to think of R as a set of extensible tools to implement one's analysis plan, regardless of simplicity or complexity. . . . Our hope is that more and more epidemiologists will embrace R for epidemiological applications, or at least include it in their toolbox.

The author hopes that this book will meet this need by helping to introduce R, a high-level computing language and an environment for biostatistical computing and graphical presentations, to epidemiologists and data analysts in public health and preventive medicine who are actively conducting epidemiologic investigations.

Bertram K. C. Chan, PhD, PE

## ONE

Introduction

1.1 MEDICINE, PREVENTIVE MEDICINE, PUBLIC HEALTH, AND EPIDEMIOLOGY

Medicine

The word *medicine* is derived from the Latin phrase *ars medicina*, meaning "the healing art." Thus, *medicine* refers to the art and science of healing, which uses a variety of practices evolved or developed to maintain and restore health by the treatment and prevention of diseases and injuries.

Today's medicine applies health sciences, biomedical research, and technology to diagnose and treat injury and diseases, typically through drug/medication or surgical interventions, but also through therapies as diverse as psychotherapy, prostheses (e.g., artificial limbs), and physical therapy, to name a few. Given this vast array of possible approaches and techniques, it is only natural that various specialties would arise within the medical profession as practitioners concentrated their talents and efforts on certain problems and therapies. The development of a specialty, including the specialty of preventive medicine, is often driven by new technology.

Preventive Medicine and Public Health

In the United States (as well as in the United Kingdom and many other parts of the world), *preventive medicine* is one of 24 medical specialties recognized by the American Board of Medical Specialties (ABMS). It comprises three areas of subspecialization:

1. General preventive medicine and public health (PH)
2. Aerospace medicine
3. Occupational medicine

To become board-certified in one of the preventive medicine areas of specialization, a licensed U.S. physician must successfully complete a preventive medicine medical residency program following a 1-year internship. Thereafter, the physician must complete a year of practice in that specialty area and pass the preventive medicine board examination. The residency program, which is at least 2 years in duration, includes completion of a master of public health (MPH) degree or the equivalent. (The present text is primarily directed toward the achievement of this last milestone.)

For example, in the United States, the Loma Linda University (LLU), California, offers a Family and Preventive Medicine Residency program that combines training in family medicine and preventive medicine, thus helping to fulfill LLU's mission: "To Make Man Whole." This special program includes primary care training through the LLU Family Medicine Residency program, as well as work in population-based care and health care systems through the LLU Preventive Medicine Residency program. During their 4 years in the program, all successful residents earn an MPH degree through the LLU School of Public Health and have an opportunity for unique exposure to LLU's two areas of strength: lifestyle medicine and global health.

Public Health and Epidemiology

In a major study conducted by the U.S. National Academy of Science's Institute of Medicine, the Committee for the Study of the Future of Public Health defined the mission of **public health** as "the fulfillment of society's interest in assuring the conditions in which people can be healthy" (see Centers for Disease Control and Prevention [CDC] 2006). That same study defined the substance of public health as "organized community efforts aimed at the prevention of disease and the promotion of health. [Public health] links many disciplines and rests upon the scientific core of epidemiology."

Epidemiology (EPDM), basically, is the study of the demographics of disease processes, including but not limited to the study of epidemics. The U.S. Department of Health and Human Services (DHHS), through the CDC, provides the following definition of epidemiology:

> The word *epidemiology* comes from the Greek words *epi*, meaning on or upon, *demos*, meaning people, and *logos*, meaning the study of. Thus, the word *epidemiology* has its roots in the study of what befalls a population. Many definitions have been proposed, but the following definition captures the underlying principles and public health spirit of epidemiology:
>
> Epidemiology is the study of the distribution and determinants of health-related states or events in specified populations, and the application of this study to the control of health problems. (CDC, 2006)

Review Questions for Section 1.1

1. Using Internet sources, name five medical specialties (besides preventive medicine) in the United States that are officially recognized by the ABMS.
2. (a) Do you know of any physicians practicing *only* preventive medicine?
   (b) If you were a physician, would you choose to practice only preventive medicine? Why or why not?
3. *Health research and policy (HRP)*: The Stanford University School of Medicine (Stanford, California) teaches preventive medicine within its department of HRP.

health services research (HSR). The last area, HSR, focuses on analyzing and comparing the costs, risks, and benefits of strategies for medical care, especially medical interventions. Discuss the possible benefits to preventive medicine of work in the areas of HRP.

4. *Fluoridation of drinking water:* In the United States, fluoridation of drinking water has been the subject of many court cases in which political activists have sued local governments, alleging that their rights to informed consent for medical treatment and to due process are violated by compulsory fluoridation. Individuals have sued municipalities for sicknesses that they thought were caused by the fluoridation of a town's water supply. In most of these cases, the courts have held in favor of the defendant cities or governmental entities, finding no or only a tenuous connection between health problems and widespread water fluoridation. To date, no federal court or state supreme court has found water fluoridation to be unlawful. If you were a PH provider, would you support the fluoridation of drinking water? Why or why not?

1.2   PERSONAL HEALTH AND PUBLIC HEALTH (PH)

Today, mainstream medicine is moving toward a standard of evidence-based practice, using data gathered mostly from PH research and especially from epidemiologic surveys. These data reveal trends, identify issues, and allow the evaluation of the effectiveness of various approaches for certain populations. The advantages of evidence-based health care seem obvious, in that it increases health care providers' ability to offer effective and safe treatments for any given condition.

PH data also underlie recommendations regarding personal health. According to experts, all personal health plans may be summarized simply as follows:

- Eat well and rest adequately.
- Exercise vigorously and regularly.

However, serious challenges may arise when PH generalizations are applied to an individual's personal situation.

Here is an example. Observational PH epidemiology of lifestyle has shown that eating whole-grain foods is better than eating processed foods from which many naturally occurring nutrients, vitamins, and fiber have been removed. Knowing this, one might apply these findings to one's own personal situation. A person might launch a campaign of eating only 100% whole-wheat bread, pastas, and even pizzas. This could benefit the person's nutritional status, as he or she would consume a lot more fiber and B vitamins, which are generally good for health.

But what if this person is intolerant of wheat and related products?

What if this person has the problem of gluten intolerance (gluten is found in foods containing wheat, rye, and barley)?

What if this person has an allergy to wheat?

If a person has any of these conditions, eating whole-wheat foods will make that individual ill in several possible ways. Allergic reactions can be life-threatening; celiac disease would cause serious gastrointestinal problems; wheat intolerance

intended to be beneficial. In the latter cases, eating whole-grain rice, for example, might be the best way to get the health benefits of a "whole-grain" approach without stirring up food intolerances or allergies.

This is a simple but common example in which general PH recommendations that may benefit the population at large may not necessarily benefit certain individuals personally and specifically. Each individual should decide what is right for him or her when creating an effective individualized program of health care.

Such personal health conditions and issues must be considered whenever a PH policy is being proposed or accepted. Thus, legislators considering PH care policies often face the difficult task of deciding what to do with "expert" advice based on observations and conclusions drawn from epidemiologic research and surveys. They must decide what weight to give the research findings and conclusions, the appropriateness of basing general public policy on those findings, and the utility and safety of any wide-scale PH mandates.

What happens if the evidence indicates that people generally (or even a subgroup of people who have a specific diagnosis such as diabetes) fare better or worse on a particular therapy? One may find it difficult and confusing to decide the best program: selecting a more familiar or accessible treatment for a specific health problem, rather than treatments that are less familiar and more difficult to accomplish, could keep a person from maximizing the benefits. For many people with chronic illnesses, for example, adding supplements of vitamins, minerals, and herbs to food is a way to start, but it is usually not enough. Achieving true health and healing is a complex but rewarding undertaking. A larger perspective may well clarify the path by which to reach one's objectives.

Personal Health Versus Public Health

As discussed earlier in this section, there are times when personal health and PH may conflict. In many instances, this merely means that individuals will make personal choices that deviate from general recommendations. Unfortunately, it is also quite possible for PH to be used (either as a reason or a camouflage) to enforce the will and policy of the state and override citizens' rights. PH initiatives and mandates are, in many instances, determined and administered by or under a branch of government with an objective that promotes both governmental policies and political agendas.[1] Personal interests, aspirations, individual choices, freedom, and ideals can be severely restricted by government "public health" laws and policies. Some of the numerous examples of this include:

- The one-child-only-per-married-couple policy in the People's Republic of China
- Prohibition in the United States between 1920 and 1933, which attempted (unsuccessfully) to ban alcohol, a powerful psychoactive drug that today is cheaply and widely available. Although PH data clearly show that the damage done by this drug is huge, the government legislation making its use illegal was eventually overturned.

---

[1] https://en.wikipedia.org/wiki/Public_health

■ The mandatory quarantining of a person suffering from a potentially fatal infectious disease.

■ Mandatory immunizations that involve pain, inconvenience, and risk of side effects for the entire population so that a disease may be prevented in a minority. This may be justifiable—for example, the vaccinations that led to the eradication of smallpox and polio in the United States—but there is a large, ethically gray area surrounding vaccines for which there is considerable uncertainty as to the balance of benefits versus harms.

■ An ongoing issue in the United States today is the concerns of many parents that vaccination may cause autism in children. Should these citizens have the right to refuse vaccination on behalf of their children? Similar issues exist where a person's religious beliefs forbid blood transfusions; such persons have refused blood transfusions for themselves and their dependent children, even in life-threatening medical emergencies. Although the constitutional right to freedom of religion and religious exercise has usually overridden the government's contentions in these cases, in some instances governmental authorities may declare a person a "ward of the court" and thereby take complete responsibility for both personal and public health issues.

Review Questions for Section 1.2

1. Where does personal health end and PH begin?
2. Does the Venn diagram in Figure 1.1 accurately represent personal health and PH?
   List some issues that are:
   (a) Exclusively personal health matters
   (b) Exclusively PH matters
   (c) Both personal and public health matters
   Give reasons supporting your identifications.

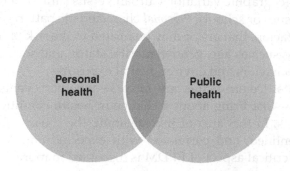

Personal health

Public health

FIGURE 1.1 Personal health and PH.

1.3   RESEARCH AND MEASUREMENTS IN EPDM AND PH

As discussed in Section 1.1, the word *epidemiology* literally means "the study of what happens to a population." Over the years, many definitions have been proposed, but the following definition captures the underlying principles and PH spirit of EPDM:

> Epidemiology is the **study** of the **distribution** and **determinants** of **health-related states or events** in **specified populations**, and the **application** of this study to the control of health problems (Broadbent, 2009).

The critical terms in this definition (in bold type here) reflect some of the important principles of EPDM:

1. **Study**. EPDM is a scientific discipline that employs established methods of scientific inquiry. It is data driven and depends on a systematic and unbiased approach to the collection, analysis, and interpretation of data. Epidemiologic methods depend on observation and use of valid comparison groups to assess whether what was observed (such as the number of cases of a disease in a certain area during a particular time period or the frequency of exposure among persons with disease) differs from what might be expected. EPDM also uses methods from other scientific fields, including BIOS and informatics, and other biologic, economic, social, and behavioral sciences. This book deals mainly with the special contribution of BIOS to EPDM.

2. **Distribution**. EPDM relates the **frequency** and **pattern** of health events and outcomes in a population of interest:
   - **Frequency** refers to the number of health events, such as the number of cases of cholera or diabetes in a population, and to the relationship of that number to the size of the population. The resulting rate allows epidemiologists to compare disease occurrence across *different* populations.
   - **Pattern** refers to the occurrence of health-related events by person, time, and place. *Time* patterns are those found in particular periods of time influencing the occurrences of injury or disease, such as annual, seasonal, weekly, daily, hourly, weekday versus weekend, and so on. *Place* patterns include geographic variations, urban versus rural differences, and location of work sites or schools. *Personal* characteristic patterns include demographic factors that are or may be related to the risk of illness, injury, or disability, such as age, gender, marital status, and socioeconomic status, as well as behaviors and environmental exposures.

3. **Determinants**. Determinants are factors—whether events, characteristics, or other things—that bring about a change in health conditions or other defined characteristics. In this area of investigation, the causes of diseases are closely studied, identified, and correlated with expected and measured health outcomes. This critical aspect of EPDM is discussed in more detail later in this section.

4. **Health-related states or events.** Originally, EPDM was concerned only with epidemics of communicable diseases (such as cholera). Subsequently, however,

to a locality or region) communicable diseases and noncommunicable infectious diseases. By the middle of the 20th century, additional epidemiologic methods had been developed and applied to injuries, chronic diseases, maternal–child health and birth defects, environmental health, and occupational health. Now epidemiologists also investigate behaviors related to health and well-being, such as lifestyle issues like the amount of exercise undertaken, and safety issues like car seat-belt use. Furthermore, with the development of biomolecular methods and the sequencing of the human genome, epidemiologists have begun examining genetic markers of diseases and disease risk factors. As a result, the term *health-related events* or *states* may be used generally to refer to any issue that affects the well-being of a population. However, in modern EPDM, the term *disease* represents the wide range of health-related states and events that are studied.

5. **Specified populations.** Even though both physicians and epidemiologists are concerned with the occurrence and control of diseases, they differ in how they view the "patient." The physician and other health care providers are primarily concerned about the health of an individual; the epidemiologist is concerned about the collective health of the people who make up a community or population. Thus, the physician and the epidemiologist have different responsibilities regarding a person who has an illness. For example, when a patient presents with diarrheal disease, both medical professionals are interested in establishing the correct diagnosis. However, the physician focuses on treating the disease and caring for the patient as an individual; the epidemiologist focuses on identifying the source or the type of exposure that caused the disease, the number of other persons who may have been similarly exposed, the potential for further spread in the community, and interventions to prevent additional cases or recurrences.

6. **Application.** EPDM is involved both in studying health in a population and in applying the knowledge gained from those studies to community-based practice. Like the practice of medicine, the practice of EPDM is both a science and an art. To make the proper diagnosis and prescribe appropriate treatment for a patient, the physician combines evidence-based scientific medical knowledge with experience, clinical judgment, and understanding of the patient. Similarly, the epidemiologist uses the scientific methods of descriptive and analytic EPDM, as well as experience, epidemiologic judgment, and understanding of local conditions, to "diagnose" the health of a community and propose appropriate, practical, and acceptable PH interventions to control and prevent disease in the community.

EPDM: The Basic Science of PH

EPDM is the basic science of PH for the following reasons:

1. EPDM is a quantitative study relying on a working knowledge of probability, BIOS, and scientific research methods.
2. EPDM is a discipline of causal reasoning in which hypotheses from various scientific fields, such as biological sciences, behavioral sciences, physical sciences,

Moreover, EPDM is not only a research discipline in itself, but also a component of PH, providing the foundation for and directing appropriate, practical PH action based on scientific, cause-and-effect reasoning. Thus, the discipline of EPDM may be described in terms of two approaches: descriptive EPDM and analytical EPDM.

DESCRIPTIVE EPDM

Descriptive EPDM covers **time**, **place**, and **person.** This approach is critically important because:

- Upon scrutinizing the data, the epidemiologist becomes familiar with its limitations based on the known variables. For example, epidemiologists often deal with large numbers of records that are missing data for each important variable. This led to the development and application of the theory of *missing-data analysis*, which allows researchers to deal with data eccentricities (for example, all cases range in age from 3 months to 4 years, plus one 19-year-old).
- The epidemiologist learns the extent and pattern of the PH problem being studied; for example, which months/neighborhoods/groups of people have the most and least cases of the phenomenon of interest.
- The epidemiologist creates a detailed description of the health of a population that can be readily communicated with graphs, tables, and maps.
- The epidemiologist can identify patterns (a difficult task, even with computers), such as areas or groups within the population that have abnormally high rates of disease. This information in turn provides clues to the causes of the disease, which inform the development of verifiable hypotheses and applicable theories.

Descriptive EPDM may be summarized in terms of the "five Ws":

- **W**hat = health issue of concern
- **W**ho = person
- **W**here = place
- **W**hen = time
- **W**hy/how = causes, risk factors, and transmission modes

ANALYTIC EPDM

Descriptive EPDM observes and identifies patterns among cases and in populations according to time, location, and person. From these observations, researchers may develop hypotheses about the causes of these patterns and about the factors that increase the risk of disease. Thus, epidemiologists use descriptive EPDM to generate hypotheses—but only rarely to test their hypotheses. For the latter, epidemiologists turn to analytic EPDM, which is characterized by the use of comparison groups.

As an illustration (White, Armstrong, & Saracci, 2008), consider the large outbreak of hepatitis A that occurred in the state of Pennsylvania in 2003. The epidemiologists found that almost all of the case patients had eaten at a particular restaurant during the previous 2 to 6 weeks (the typical incubation period for hepatitis A)

Although the researchers were able to narrow their focus to the one restaurant and were able to exclude the food preparers and servers as the source, they did not know which particular food had been contaminated. They asked the case patients which of the restaurant's foods they had eaten, but that only indicated which foods were popular. The researchers then also enrolled and interviewed a control group: a group of persons who had eaten at the restaurant during the same period but who had *not* gotten sick. Of 133 items on the restaurant's menu, the most striking difference between the case and control groups was the proportion that ate salsa (94% of case patients ate salsa, compared with only 39% of the controls).

Further investigation of the ingredients in the salsa implicated green onions as the source of infection. Shortly thereafter, the Food and Drug Administration (FDA) issued a warning to the public about green onions and the risk of hepatitis A. This action was in direct response to the convincing results of the analytic EPDM, generated by comparison of the exposure history of case patients with that of an appropriate comparison group.

When it is discovered that case patients with a particular characteristic are more likely than those without the characteristic to contract a disease, that particular characteristic is said to be **associated** with the disease. The characteristic may be a:

■ Demographic factor, such as place of residence, age, race, or gender
■ Constitutional factor, such as blood type or immune status
■ Behavior or action, such as smoking or having eaten salsa
■ Circumstance, such as living near contaminated soils or a toxic waste site or using contaminated water

Identifying the factors associated with a disease can help health officials to focus on PH control and prevention, as well as furthering research into the causes of the disease.

Main Epidemiologic Functions

Six major tasks of EPDM in PH practice have been identified:

1. PH surveillance
2. Field investigation
3. Analytic studies
4. Evaluation
5. Linkages
6. Policy development

Some of these tasks are reflected in the discussion, in Section 1.1, of the Stanford University School of Medicine's HRP departmental concentration on BIOS, data coordination, EPDM, and HSR.

Analytic EPDM concentrates on PH prevention and control activities. It also guides additional research into the causes of disease. Thus, analytic EPDM is concerned with the search for causes and effects, or the why and the how. It seeks to quantify the association between exposures and outcomes and to test hypotheses

exposure caused a particular outcome, but EPDM nevertheless provides sufficient evidence for the development and implementation of appropriate control and prevention measures.

Epidemiologic studies may be classified into two categories: experimental and observational.

EXPERIMENTAL EPDM STUDIES

In an *experimental* study, the investigator determines through a controlled process the exposure for each individual (in a clinical trial) or community (in a community trial), and then tracks the individuals or communities over time to detect the continuing effects of the exposure. The following are examples of typical experimental studies:

1. In a clinical trial of a new vaccine, the researcher usually randomly assigns some of the participants to receive the new vaccine, while others receive a placebo. (A **placebo** is an inert or innocuous substance, used especially in controlled experiments testing the efficacy of another substance as a treatment.) The researcher then tracks all participants, observing who develops the disease that the new vaccine is intended to prevent, and compares the two groups (new vaccine versus placebo) to see whether the vaccine group has a lower rate of disease.

2. In a trial to prevent the onset of diabetes among high-risk individuals, the researchers randomly assign subjects to one of three groups:
   - An antidiabetes drug
   - A placebo
   - Lifestyle intervention

   At the end of the trial period, the researchers look for the lowest incidence of diabetes and find that the lowest incidence occurred in the lifestyle intervention group, the next-lowest incidence was in the antidiabetic drug group, and the highest incidence occurred in the placebo group

OBSERVATIONAL EPDM STUDIES

In observational EPDM studies, the researcher just observes the exposure and disease status of each study participant. The classic example of an observational study is Dr. John Snow's investigation of an 1854 cholera epidemic in London.

THE CHOLERA STORY.[2] A waterborne disease known as cholera has proven to be one of the most virulent killers in history. It was through the investigation of cholera epidemics that epidemiologists discovered the link between sanitation and PH—a discovery that led to the development of the world's modern water and sewage systems.

It is now known that cholera is caused by ingesting water, food, or other material contaminated by the feces of a cholera patient or host. For example, casual contact

[2] Biographical information on Dr. John Snow, the "father" of field EPDM, and his work is available at

with a contaminated chamber pot, soiled clothing or bedding, or even an unwashed hand might be all that is required to contract cholera. The disease can be transmitted easily and acts quickly. It strikes so suddenly that a person can be in good health in the morning and be dead by the evening. From the onset of symptoms—diarrhea, muscle cramps, vomiting, and fever—death may occur within 48 hours or less. So much fluid is lost that the blood appears thick, and about 50% of patients will die, mainly of dehydration. In various parts of the world (including Europe and Asia), tens of thousands have died of this epidemic disease.

THE FATHER OF FIELD EPDM. In the mid-1800s, an anesthesiologist named Dr. John Snow conducted a series of studies in London that led to him being called the "father of field epidemiology." Dr. Snow investigated cholera outbreaks, both to discover the cause of the disease and to prevent its recurrence. His work illustrates the classic sequence from descriptive EPDM to hypothesis generation to hypothesis testing (analytic EPDM) to application:

■ In 1854, Dr. Snow conducted one of his studies when an epidemic of cholera suddenly started in the Golden Square of London. He began by determining where, in this particular area, persons with cholera lived and worked. He marked each residence on a map of the area, as shown in Figure 1.2. This type of map, showing the geographic distribution of cases, is called a *spot map*.

■ Because Dr. Snow believed that water was a carrier source of infection for cholera, he also marked the location of water pumps on the spot map, and then looked for a relationship between the distribution of households with cases of cholera and the location of the water pumps. He noticed that *more case households clustered around Pump A*, the Broad Street pump, than around Pump B or C. When he questioned residents who lived in the Golden Square area, he was told that they avoided Pump B because it was grossly contaminated, and that Pump C was located too inconveniently for most of them.

■ From this information, Dr. Snow concluded that the Broad Street pump (Pump A) was the primary source of water and the most likely source of infection for most persons with cholera in the Golden Square area.

■ He also noted that no cases of cholera had occurred in a two-block area just to the east of the Broad Street pump. Upon investigating, Snow found a brewery located there, with a deep well on the premises. Brewery workers obtained their water from this well, and also received a daily portion of malt liquor. Access to these uncontaminated rations (water and liquor) could explain why none of the brewery's employees contracted cholera.

■ To confirm that the Broad Street pump was the source of the epidemic, Dr. Snow gathered information on where persons with cholera had obtained their supply of water. *Consumption of water from the Broad Street pump was the one common factor among the cholera patients.*

■ After Dr. Snow presented his findings to municipal officials, the handle of the pump was removed—and the outbreak ended! (The site of the pump is now marked by a plaque mounted on the wall outside the appropriately named

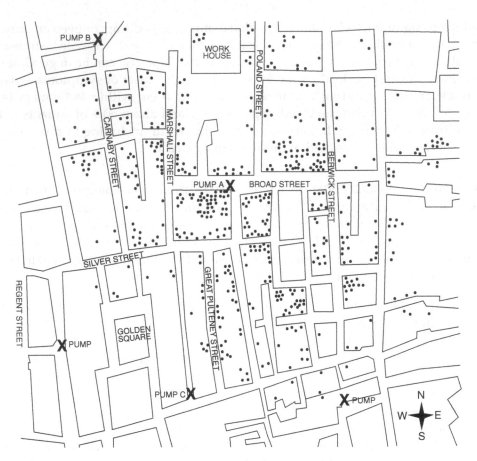

FIGURE 1.2 Spot map of deaths from cholera in the Golden Square area, London, 1854 (redrawn from original).

Source: Humphrey Milford, *Dr. John Snow on Cholera*. London: Oxford University Press, 1936.

TYPES OF OBSERVATIONAL EPDM STUDIES

The two most common types of observational studies are cohort studies and case–control studies; the third type is cross-sectional studies.

COHORT STUDIES. In a *cohort study*, whether each study participant is exposed or not:

1. The epidemiologist **records** and then **tracks** each participant to see if he or she develops the disease of interest. (This differs from an experimental study because, in a cohort study, the epidemiologist observes rather than determines the participant's exposure status.)
2. After a period of time, the epidemiologist **compares** the disease rate in the exposed group with the disease rate in the unexposed group.
3. The unexposed group serves as the comparison group, providing an estimate of the baseline or expected amount of disease occurrence in the community.
4. If the disease rate is substantively different in the exposed group compared to

The length of follow-up varies considerably. To respond quickly to a PH concern, such as an outbreak of cholera or bird flu, PH departments tend to conduct relatively brief studies. Research and academic organizations are more likely to conduct studies of cancer, cardiovascular disease, and other chronic diseases, in efforts that may last for years and even decades. For example:

- **The Framingham Health Study** is a cohort study that has followed more than 5,000 residents of Framingham, Massachusetts, since the early 1950s to establish the risk factors for cardiovascular diseases.
- **The Nurses Health Study** and **the Nurses Health Study II** are cohort studies established in 1976 and 1989, respectively, that have followed more than 100,000 nurses each and have provided useful information on oral contraceptives, diet, and lifestyle risk factors.

The Adventist Health Studies: Study 1. **The Adventist Health Study 1** (AHS-1),[3] a cohort investigation that began in 1974, had some very basic differences from earlier mortality studies. It was designed to elucidate which components of the Seventh-Day Adventist (SDA) lifestyle give protection against diseases. This study compared the rates of disease or mortality between SDAs and non-SDAs. Also, data were collected on nonfatal, as well as fatal, disease events. This study also added a more detailed investigation of diet. In the beginning, the AHS-1 was primarily a cancer investigation. In 1981, a cardiovascular component was added. The rate of return for the annual follow-up SDA questionnaires, which asked about hospitalizations and were critical to the entire research process, was in excess of 90% and usually above 95%. The final and most critical mailing saw an incredible 99.5% response.

The Adventist Health Studies: Study 2.[3] The current study, which began in 2002 and set a goal of 125,000 SDAs participating, continues to explore the links between lifestyle, diet, and disease among the broader base of Adventists in the United States and Canada. As of May 2006, Adventist Health Study-2 (AHS-2) had an enrollment of 96,741 persons. Dr. Gary E. Fraser, with a team of researchers from the School of Public Health at LLU, is conducting the study, which is funded by the U.S. National Cancer Institute. In July 2011, the National Institutes of Health (NIH) awarded AHS-2 a substantial 5-year grant to continue the study.

Cohort Study Types. The AHS-1 and AHS-2 studies are sometimes called **follow-up** or **prospective** cohort studies, because participants are enrolled when the study begins and are then followed prospectively over time to identify occurrence of the outcomes of interest.

An alternative type is a **retrospective** cohort study. In this kind of study, both the exposure and the outcomes have already occurred. Just as in a prospective cohort study, the investigator calculates and compares rates of disease in the exposed and unexposed groups. Retrospective cohort studies are commonly used

---

[3] AHS-1 and AHS-2 are available at http://publichealth.llu.edu and http://www.llu.edu/public

in investigations of disease in groups of easily identified people, such as workers at a particular factory or attendees at a wedding. For example, a retrospective cohort study was used to determine the source of infection of cyclosporiasis, a parasitic disease that broke out among members of a residential facility in Pennsylvania in 2004. The investigation implicated consumption of snow peas as the vehicle of the cyclosporiasis outbreak.

Other types of studies include case–control studies and cross-sectional studies.

CASE–CONTROL STUDIES. In a case–control study, investigators start by enrolling a group of people with disease (sometimes called *case patients* rather than *cases*, because *case* refers to an occurrence of disease, not a person). As a comparison group, the investigator then enrolls a group of people without disease (*controls*).

Investigators then compare previous exposures between the two groups. The control group provides an estimate of the baseline or expected amount of exposure in that population. If the amount of exposure among the case group is substantially higher than the amount that one would expect based on the control group, then illness is said to be associated with that exposure.

The key in a case–control study is to identify an appropriate control group—one that is comparable to the case group in most respects—to provide a reasonable estimate of the baseline or expected exposure.

CROSS-SECTIONAL STUDIES. In the cross-sectional type of observational study, a sample of persons from a population is enrolled and their exposures and health outcomes are measured simultaneously. The cross-sectional study tends to assess the presence of the health outcome at a particular point in time without regard to duration.

For example, in a cross-sectional study of diabetes, some of the enrollees with diabetes may have lived with their diabetes for many years, while others may have been recently diagnosed. From an analytic viewpoint, the cross-sectional study is weaker than either a cohort or a case–control study because a cross-sectional study usually cannot separate risk factors for occurrence of disease (incidence) from risk factors for survival with the disease.

The Cause of Diseases

"What is the cause of this disease?" is not an easy question to answer. On the cause of diseases, epidemiologists generally are of the opinion that "**Nature** loads the gun, but **nurture** pulls the trigger!" (*Nurture* is the sum of the environmental factors influencing the traits and behavior expressed by an organism.)

At this time in mainstream medicine, EPDM is facing at least two critical questions about disease causation (Broadbent, 2009):

1. How should EPDM handle certain *diseases* that appear to be etiologically more complex than the infections and deficiencies that EPDM has traditionally handled?

    Currently, chronic noncommunicable diseases (CNCDs) account for a larger proportion of deaths, at least in the industrialized world, than they did 100

not seem susceptible to definition in terms of any one causative agent. In other words, their **etiology** is complex. (*Etiology* is a branch of medical science concerned with the causes and origins of diseases.)

2. How should EPDM respond to newly identified *causes* of disease?

Although EPDM continues to discover increasingly complex and surprising environmental causes of disease, the field must now deal with the new category of causes: genetics. The depth and complexity of knowledge required to deal with both genetic and environmental determinants of health places pressure on aspects of the conceptual framework of EPDM with regard to disease causation.

MODELS OF CAUSATION

A good scientific causal model may be summarized as follows:

The requisite cause of disease D is the event E if, and only if:

(i)   An E-event is a cause of every case of D;

(ii) Given certain circumstances, an E-event is not a cause of any non-D-event (i.e., other diseases or good health).

Historically, several models of disease have been proposed and used: the monocausal model, the multifactorial model, and the contrastive model are the primary ones.

The Monocausal Model. This model says that every disease has a single cause that is necessary, and sometimes sufficient. This model is well suited to infectious diseases such as tuberculosis (TB) and cholera, along with parasitic infestations and diseases of deficiency.

However, it is unfit for CNCDs such as lung cancer or diabetes. It is possible that diabetes does have a single necessary and, in some circumstances, sufficient cause, which has not yet been discovered. But it is also a theoretical possibility that there is no cause for diabetes satisfying that description. And even if there is, it is not clear how insisting that there *must* be such a cause helps to achieve PH or any clinical goals, if one does not know what that cause is. What we have been able to identify so far are merely causal risk factors, and these are neither necessary nor sufficient. Thus, important objections may be raised regarding the monocausal model.

The Multifactorial Model. This model now dominates EPDM, but this is also not an entirely satisfactory situation because the multifactorial model fails to acknowledge what looks like a real etiological difference between diseases like cholera and conditions like lung cancer. The monocausal model has had some striking successes in the history of EPDM, and these successes are left unexplained by the mere assertion that disease causation is multifactorial. Unless one can explain the successes of the monocausal model in terms of modern multifactorial thinking, this approach is equally unsatisfactory.

The Contrastive Model. This model is defensible on the ground that it links the notions of disease and of general explanation, while avoiding the philosophical naiveties and practical difficulties of the monocausal model. For person *p* to have disease *D*, it is necessary that:

SYMPTOMS: *p* suffers from some of a set of symptoms of ill health *S*, which are

CAUSES: Among the causes of p's symptoms are events of kinds $C1, \ldots, Cn$, at least some of which are not causes of the absence of the symptoms S from each member of X.

The assumptions of the contrastive model are as follows:

1. To have a disease, p must have some symptoms of poor health. These symptoms are considered part of the definition of the disease. Not *all* the symptoms associated with that particular disease need be present, but p must have *at least* one.

   A *symptom* of ill health is an observable difference between the case subject and a contrast class, which is a just a certain set of people, some of whom may be merely hypothetical. The contrast class need not be unique (i.e., the same for everyone). The contrast class for a 59-year-old man might include some bald members, whereas the relevant contrast class for a 6-year-old child might not. This allows the analysis to cover diseases that are specific to age, gender, and other characteristics (including having another disease).

2. Having a disease requires that p's symptoms be caused by a certain cause or causes, which must not be causes of the absence of symptoms from the contrast class. These causes are also part of the definition of the disease. For example, to have cholera, one must exhibit some symptoms of poor health that a certain contrast class does not have (e.g., diarrhea); and those symptoms must be caused by a certain specified cause [viz., the active presence of *Vibrio cholerae* (*V. cholerae*) in p's small intestine].

NOTE: Having causes is not an epistemological requirement: One does not have to know about *V. cholerae* in order to count cholera as a disease. Rather, by counting cholera as a disease, one *commits* to the existence of something satisfying the CAUSES definition/requirements.

The next step is to find out what that cause is, thus making the model methodologically useful.

Some investigators also consider the concept of *illness*, or mere ill health or poor health that falls short of qualifying as a disease. For a disease, a cause or causes of certain symptoms are specified, whereas for an illness, they are not specified.

AN EXAMPLE FOR THE CONTRASTIVE MODEL

A recent example in which the contrastive model might have been useful is the discovery of the role of the bacterium *Helicobacter pylori* (*H. pylori*) in duodenal ulcers. This discovery brought tensions between the monocausal and multifactorial ways of thinking into high contrast.

Many discussions of ulcer assume that, since the discovery and implication of *H. pylori* in ulcer formation, both acid *and* stress or psychosomatic factors have been made etiologically irrelevant. Some simply considered *H. pylori* "the cause of ulcers," although epidemiologically better-informed treatments, such as a report by the NIH maintained a different stance. Critics argued that "the NIH's emphasis on multiple factors in pathogenesis reflects the extent to which multicausality is a staple of biomedical and epidemiological discourse."

However, the etiological reality clearly favors the multifactorial treatment. *H. pylori* is neither necessary nor sufficient for duodenal ulcer, nor is its elimination from a patient either necessary or sufficient for the curing of an ulcer. In effect, monocausal model thinking becomes wishful thinking, a consequence of the *desire* for treatments that work on each and every case of disease. Unfortunately, desire is not a good guide to reality. In this case, multifactorialism does not have the resources to express what the etiological reality might be, and the monocausal model is simply incorrect. In contrast, the contrastive model is helpful here.

Within the contrastive model, duodenal ulcers satisfy *symptoms*, and *H. pylori* can be made to satisfy *causes*. Cases in which duodenal ulcer is present without *H. pylori* can be handled in one of two ways: Either they are cases of a different disease with the same symptoms, or one can define the disease in terms of *H. pylori* and another cause, such as excessive hydrochloric acid in the stomach. Note that *H. pylori* infection occurs without *symptoms* in many cases. In the contrastive model, these instances are an invitation to further investigation. One can thus add precision to the claim that *H. pylori* causes stomach ulcers and acknowledge the importance of the discovery by reclassifying some cases of stomach ulcer as a distinct disease.

One should note that the contrastive model leaves a crucial component unspecified: It does not directly indicate anything about the contrast class, and especially about the concept of health.

THE BLACK SWAN STORY

We will put the discussion of the concept and definition of causation of diseases aside for a moment to consider an interesting historical incident regarding biological definitions.

"Black swan" was an expression in 16th-century England as a common statement of impossibility. It derives from the Old World presumption that all swans must be white because all historical records of swans reported that they had white feathers; hence, all swans are, *by definition*, white! Given that context, a black swan was impossible, or at least nonexistent.

In 1697, Dutch explorer Willem de Vlamingh discovered black swans (Figure 1.3) on the Swan River in Western Australia. Thereafter, the term has come to refer to a perceived impossibility that might later be disproven. The 19th-century philosopher John Stuart Mill used the *black swan* logical fallacy as a new term to identify falsification. In EPDM investigations, a "black swan" is an event with the following three attributes:

1. First, it is an *outlier* (see the discussion of probability in Section 2.3 of Chapter 2), as it lies outside the realm of regular expectations, because nothing in the past indicates its possibility.
2. It carries an extreme impact.
3. In spite of its initial outlier status, one can give plausible reasons for its occurrence after the fact.

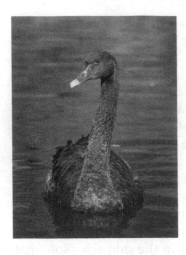

FIGURE 1.3   A black swan (*Cygnus atratus*), which remained undocumented in the West until the 18th century.

NATURE VERSUS NURTURE IN EPDM: REVERSING TYPE 1 DIABETES? (EDELMAN, OLSEN, DUDLEY, HARRIS, & ODDONE, 2004)

THE HEMOGLOBIN A1c (HBA1c) TEST FOR DIABETES MELLITUS.[4] Hemoglobin is a substance within red blood cells that carries oxygen throughout the body. In a person with poorly controlled diabetes, sugar builds up in the blood, either because the person's body does not produce sufficient insulin to transfer the sugar into the cells, or because insulin resistance hampers that transfer. The sugar in the blood, therefore, combines with hemoglobin: the hemoglobin becomes "glycated." HbA1c, or simply A1c, is the main fraction of glycosylated hemoglobin (glycohemoglobin; i.e., hemoglobin) to which glucose is bound. The glucose stays bound to hemoglobin for the life of the red blood cell (normally about 120 days), so the level of HbA1c reflects *the average blood glucose level over the past 4 months*. Thus, HbA1c is tested to monitor the long-term control of diabetes mellitus.

- The normal level for HbA1c is less than 7%. Diabetics rarely achieve such levels, but tight control aims to come close to it.
- Levels above 9% show poor control.
- Levels above 12% show very poor control.

It is commonly recommended that HbA1c be measured every 3 to 6 months in diabetics.

The Diabetes Control and Complications Trial (DCCT; Nathan, 2014) showed that diabetics who keep their HbA1c levels close to 7% have a much better chance of delaying or preventing diabetes complications that affect the eyes, kidneys, and nerves than people with levels at 8% or higher. A change in treatment is almost always needed if the level is over 8%. Lowering the level of HbA1c by any amount improves a person's chances of staying healthy.

[4] The HbA1c test for diabetes: retrieved from http://diabetes.webmd.com/guide/glycated-

TYPE 1 DIABETES. In type 1 diabetes, the patient's pancreas no longer produces the insulin that the person needs to survive, so the patient must replace the missing insulin from other (external) sources. This is why type 1 diabetes is also known as *insulin-dependent diabetes*; because the condition occurs primarily in children, it also used to be known as *juvenile diabetes* (actually a misnomer, as adult-onset cases are not unheard of).

A diagnosis of type 1 diabetes in a child can be overwhelming at first. Suddenly, the parents and the affected child must learn how to give insulin injections, count carbohydrates, and monitor blood sugar—and the child must do so for life. Although diabetes in children requires consistent care, advances in blood sugar monitoring and insulin delivery have improved the daily management of this condition.

CASE SUBJECT: A CHILD WITH TYPE 1 DIABETES. The case subject was a 14-year-old child who was clinically diagnosed as suffering from type 1 diabetes some 2 years previously. The subject was enrolled in a test in which the child orally took a prescribed medication for a period of 3 months. Interestingly, the medication was a traditional Chinese medicine (TCM; Liu et al., 2014) formulation of herbal origin.

During this period, A1c blood tests were taken to monitor the subject's progress. The progressive A1c test results were as follows:

$$9+ \rightarrow 8.4 \rightarrow 7.8 \rightarrow 7.45 \rightarrow 6.7 \, (\%)$$

Question: Did the TCM treatment influence the subject's pancreas to restart the production of the beta cells that make insulin? (Insulin processes and controls the blood glucose level.)

The following tests may be considered:

- Perhaps concomitant changes in the beta-cell level of the case subject should be measured; such a test might shed further light on the subject.
- Perhaps the case subject could be taken off the prescribed TCM medication, and the A1c levels closely checked thereafter to see if the trend is reversed or reversible.

How does this result affect the accepted medical position that type 1 diabetes is permanently irreversible? Can EPDM research help? Clearly, much EPDM investigation is called for in this situation.

Actually, a clinical trial in which the same TCM treatment was given to more than 10,000 case subjects resulted in a positive response (namely, improved stability of blood glucose control without insulin) in about 30% of the test population. Such results are strong justification for further EPDM investigations in this area!

Exposure Measurement in Epidemiology

Epidemiologic studies in PH research relate exposure to causal agents to the occurrence of a particular disease. A study may not fully explain how the disease occurred, but, by and large, it records under what circumstances one may expect the disease to occur. The accurate measurement of exposure to *mutating causes* of a disease (that is

research. There are theories, principles, and techniques that may be applied to measuring a wide range of exposures, including scientific, medical, genetic, demographic, behavioral, psychological, sociological, and environmental factors.

Techniques in epidemiologic research include:

- Use of questionnaires (often designed by the researcher)
- Personal interviews
- Abstracting information from medical records
- Use of proxy respondents
- Making biological and environmental measurements

The research may include one or more of the following:

1. A comprehensive account of measurement error and the estimation of its effects
2. The design, analysis, and interpretation of the validity and reliability of the studies
3. The ways in which validity of the measurements can be improved
4. Techniques to maximize the participation of subjects in future studies
5. Revelation of ethical issues relevant to exposure measurement
6. Some more-or-less comprehensive guidance on minimizing measurement error

Exposure measurement thus employs the methods and quality control approaches for the most commonly used data collection methods in EPDM.

Additional Issues

To achieve maximum participation of relevant subjects in an epidemiologic research, special techniques should be used. Also, consideration should be given to the ethical issues inherent in exposure measurement; in this regard, the following issues are important:

1. In reliability and validity studies that record the degree of measurement error for a specific exposure, one must establish the methods to design, interpret, and analyze the collected data. This is critical because such supporting studies are needed to understand the effects of exposure measurements on the overall epidemiologic study.
2. Methods should be chosen to maximize response rates. In this way, selection bias may be reduced. Such an approach is essential to the success of the data collection phase of the study.
3. Ethical issues in conducting the epidemiologic research overall should be considered; the benefits will be similar to those described in items 1 and 2.

Review Questions for Section 1.3

1. What are the "five Ws" of descriptive EPDM?
2. In Dr. John Snow's successful observational EPDM investigation of cholera,
   (a) What underlying assumptions did he make that led him to reach the correct conclusion regarding the cause of cholera?

3. From the black swan story, is it reasonable to suggest that there might be red/orange/yellow/green/blue/indigo/violet swans too? Why or why not?
4. (a) Given the three models for diseases, can there be overlapping areas where any two, or all three, models may fit?
   (b) Draw a Venn diagram to show the possibility (if any) of overlapping of these three models. Suggest some examples.
5. (a) What is a case-cohort health study in EPDM?
   (b) Name two U.S. health studies that enrolled more than 50,000 case subjects.
   (c) Why is such a large pool of subjects needed?
6. (a) Which factor is more important in the cause of diseases: nature or nurture? Why?
   (b) Of these two factors, which one is more readily treatable/manageable? Why?
7. (a) How can differences in genetic factors, and environmental factors be taken into account in EPDM investigations?
   (b) Of these two factors—genetic and environmental—which is more important? Why?
8. If a certain alternative or unorthodox disease management approach (such as TCM, ayurveda, acupuncture, etc.) appears to be effective in the management of certain diseases (e.g., type 1 diabetes, chronic headaches), can EPDM investigations be used to relate the "unorthodox" approach to mainstream, evidence-based medicine? Why or why not?

1.4   BIOS AND EPDM

Biostatistics—a combination word derived from *biology* and *statistics*, and also sometimes called *biometry* or *biometrics*—is the application of *statistics* to a topic in biology. BIOS includes the design of biological experiments, especially in medicine and health sciences; the collection and analysis of data from those experiments; and the interpretation of the results.

To understand the application of BIOS, let us use the example of a hypothetical community in the United States, in which an epidemiologist attempts to quantify the effect of a specific disease, such as swine flu (the common name used for the H1N1 virus, a new strain of influenza A, to distinguish it from the seasonal flu), to study the distribution of the disease among various regions. The goals are:

1. To determine the magnitude of the population affected by the disease
2. To ascertain potential causes

One should first determine the *prevalence* of the disease, defined as the fraction of subjects affected by that disease. First, one may consider the estimate of the population's prevalence under the commonly assumed condition: sampling in which one considers a randomized sample of N subjects, obtaining X cases. Also, to understand the randomness of the disease occurrence in the population, a research biostatistician often starts analyzing the data in terms of a probabilistic

which is characterized by trials that end in one of two ways: either success or failure. (*Bi* = two; hence the *"bi*nomial" name referring to the two possible outcomes of success or failure.)

Thus, to determine the prevalence of disease-infected subjects, one may take a random sample of

> N = 500 subjects in a specific community, and obtain
> X = 4 subjects with positive results from an antibody test

With these results, the biostatistician has in hand the following model:

1. A binomial model of distribution of the disease
2. A sample mean of $p = (X/N) = (4/500) = 1/125 = 0.008$, from which biostatistical predictions may be made using the well-known binomial distribution model.

(More is discussed about different probabilistic models in Chapter 5 on probability theory and inferential biostatistics.)

Thus, for a large population (under the same condition of distribution) of $n = 1,000,000$, one would use the same model (assumed to be reasonably applicable) to get the expected number of disease cases. In this example, this is given by the expected value E[X] of the binomial distribution model:

$$E[X] = np = (1,000,000)(0.008) = 8,000.$$

Clearly, major assumptions have been made. For example, it was assumed that (a) the binomial distribution model was applicable; and (b) only one sampling population was used.

In the foregoing simple example, the epidemiologic approach consisted of:

First—Hypothesizing a probability distribution for the population; in this case, the simple binomial distribution
Next—Conducting a sampling of the population and obtaining sampling parameter(s) for the population
Finally—Using the assumed probabilistic model to make predictions regarding the whole population.

These are the classic "1–2–3" steps in the application of **inferential biostatistics**, to draw conclusions by the inference approach. Of course, more appropriate biostatistical models may be used and additional sampling may have to be done, leading to more representational models and more refined biostatistical models. It is clear that concomitant to the development and use of better models are more involved computational procedures.

To support such computations, the open-source, free software R will be used in this journey of medicine, preventive medicine, public health, EPDM, and BIOS.

In addition to inferential biostatistics, an alternate and simpler approach, called *descriptive biostatistics*, is often used in epidemiologic research. The objective of descriptive biostatistics is simply to describe a dataset by summarizing all its pertinent characteristics. Both methods are fully described in Chapter 2.

Review Questions for Section 1.4

1. In EPDM investigations, quantitative sampling is taken from a target population. Does this approach call for methodologies taken from BIOS? Why or why not?
2. (a) What is the binomial distribution model in BIOS?
   (b) How does this model help in analysis of data collected in an EPDM investigation?
3. (a) Is the expected value same as the average value?
   (b) Why or why not?
4. What are the "1–2–3" steps in the application of inferential biostatistics?
5. (a) What is descriptive biostatistics?
   (b) How does descriptive biostatistics help in EPDM investigations?

REFERENCES

Broadbent, A. (2009). Causation and models of disease in epidemiology. *Studies in the History and Philosophy of the Biological and Biomedical Sciences, 40,* 302–311. Retrieved from http://www.hps.cam.ac.uk/people/broadbent/models_of_disease.pdf

Centers for Disease Control and Prevention. (2006). *Principles of epidemiology in public health practice: An introduction to applied epidemiology and biostatistics* (3rd ed.). Atlanta, GA: US Department of Health and Human Services [Self-Study Course SS1000].

Charlton, B. G. (2001). Personal freedom or public health? In M. Marinker (Ed.), *Medicine and humanity* (pp. 55–69). London: King's Fund. Retrieved from http://www.hedweb.com/bgcharlton/healthfreed.html

Edelman, D., Olsen, M. K., Dudley, T. K., Harris, A. C., & Oddone, E. Z. (2004). Utility of hemoglobin A1c in predicting diabetes risk. *Journal of General Internal Medicine (JGIM), 19*(12), 1175–1180.

Liu, X., Liu, L., Chen, P., Zhou, L., Zhang, Y., Wu, Y., . . . Yi, D. (2014). Clinical trials of traditional Chinese medicine in the treatment of diabetes nephrology—A systematic review based on a subgroup analysis. *Journal of Ethnopharmacology, 151*(2), 810–819.

Nathan, D. M. (2014). *The Diabetes Control and Complications Trial/Epidemiology of Diabetes Interventions and Complications Study at 30 years: Overview.* Retrieved from http://care.diabetesjournals.org/

White, E., Armstrong, B. K., & Saracci, R. (2008). *Principles of exposure measurement in epidemiology: Collecting, evaluating, and improving measures of disease risk factors* (2nd ed.). Oxford, UK: Oxford University Press.

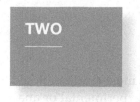

Research and Design in Epidemiology and Public Health

INTRODUCTION

Within a public health (PH) program, research and design in epidemiology (EPDM) should focus on the following aspects of the discipline (Loma Linda University, School of Public Health, 2012):

1. Conducting quality epidemiologic research, including appropriate design, biostatistical analysis of data, and interpretation and reporting of results
2. Conducting and evaluating clinical trials
3. Conducting disease surveillance as practiced in local governmental health departments
4. Critically reviewing the professional literature and identifying the strengths and weaknesses of designs, analyses, and conclusions
5. Evaluating the effects of potential confounding and interaction in a research design
6. Applying knowledge of disease mechanisms and information from the biological disciplines to interpretation of statistical findings in biomedical research
7. Collaborating with health professionals by providing technical expertise with regard to literature review, study design, data analysis, and interpretation and reporting of results
8. Maintaining a cost-effective biostatistical computation environment that can support the ever-increasing demand for and complexity of scientific computation

This book focuses on the programming language R, in support of the last of these aspects of epidemiologic research, and promotes the latest resources to encourage a computational environment built around the use of R. Several work examples are shown, using real-life research data obtained from cutting-edge epidemiologic investigations, and highlighting R programs and packages that are being developed specifically to process these datasets. Additional work examples, selected from other practical biomedical applications, are provided to illustrate the wider use of R programming in association with other high-level scientific programming languages such as FORTRAN.

The author intends for readers first to *repeat* the R computations shown herein. This is a way to gain valuable practice and develop confidence in an advanced biostatistical research computational environment.

2.1 CAUSATION AND ASSOCIATION IN EPIDEMIOLOGY AND PUBLIC HEALTH

EPDM aims to assess the cause of disease. However, because most epidemiologic studies are primarily descriptive or observational rather than experimental or analytical, a number of possible explanations for an observed association must be considered before one can validly infer that a cause–effect relationship exists. That is, an observed association may in fact be due to the effects of one or more of the following (Rothman, 1998, 2002):

- Chance (random error)
- Bias (systematic error)
- Confounding

Hence, an observed statistical association between a risk factor and a disease does not necessarily allow one to infer a causal relationship. Conversely, the absence of an association does not conclusively indicate the absence of a causal relationship. The judgment as to whether an observed statistical association represents a cause–effect relationship between exposure and disease requires investigations and inferences far beyond the data from a single study; it involves consideration of criteria that include the magnitude of the association, the consistency of findings from other studies, and biologic credibility (Loma Linda University, School of Public Health, 2012; Steiger, 2015).

In EPDM, the Bradford-Hill criteria are widely used to provide a framework within which to assess whether an observed association is likely to be causal.

The Bradford-Hill Criteria for Causation and Association in Epidemiology (Hill, 1965)[1]

The Bradford-Hill set of criteria of causation outlines the minimal conditions needed to establish a causal relationship between two items. These criteria were originally presented by Austin Bradford Hill (1897–1991), a British medical statistician, as a way of determining the causal link between a specific factor (e.g., cigarette smoking) and a disease (such as emphysema or lung cancer). While it is easy to claim that agent "A" (e.g., smoking) causes disease "B" (lung cancer), it is quite another matter to establish a meaningful, biostatistically valid connection between the two phenomena. Thus, this criterion set has formed the basis of modern epidemiologic research that establishes scientifically valid causal connections between potential disease agents and the many diseases that afflict humankind. In fact, these principles form the basis of evaluation used in *all* modern scientific research.

The **Bradford-Hill criteria** are presented here as they have been applied in epidemiologic research:

1. *Temporal relationship.* Exposure always precedes the outcome. If factor A is believed to cause a disease, then that factor A must necessarily always precede the occurrence of the disease. This is the only absolutely essential criterion.

2. *Strength of association.* This criterion is defined by the size of the association as measured by appropriate biostatistical tests. The stronger the association, the more likely it is that the relation of A to B is causal. For example, the more highly correlated hypertension (high blood pressure) is with a high-sodium diet, the stronger the relation between hypertension and sodium intake.

3. *Dose–response relationship.* As the amount of exposure increases, so does the risk. If a dose–response relationship is present, it is strong evidence of a causal relationship. However, as with specificity (see item 8 in this list), the absence of a dose–response relationship does not necessarily rule out a causal relationship; a threshold may exist above which certain specific relationships develop. At the same time, if a specific factor is the cause of a disease, the incidence of the disease should decline when exposure to the factor is reduced or eliminated. For example, in environmental epidemiology, if increasing levels of carbon dioxide in the atmosphere cause an increase in global temperatures, then—other things being equal—one should expect both a commensurate increase and a corresponding decrease in global temperatures following an increase or decrease, respectively, in carbon dioxide levels in the atmosphere.

4. *Consistency.* An association is *consistent* when results are replicated in studies in different populations using different methods. Thus, if a relationship is causal, one would expect it to appear consistently in different studies and among different populations. Hence, numerous experiments have to be undertaken before meaningful statements can be made about the causal relationship between two or more factors. For example, it required many rigorous scientific studies of the relationship between cigarette smoking and cancer before a definitive conclusion could be made that cigarette smoking increases the risk of cancer—but note that we still cannot state that "smoking causes cancer."

5. *Plausibility.* This criterion requires that the association agree with the currently accepted understanding of pathological processes. That is, there must be some theoretical basis for positing an association between a lifestyle behavior and a given disease. At the same time, research that disagrees with established theory is not necessarily false or erroneous. Rather, it may indicate that a reconsideration of currently accepted principles is warranted.

6. *Consideration of alternate explanations.* In deciding whether a reported association is causal, it is necessary to determine the extent to which investigators have taken other possible explanations into account and have effectively ruled out those alternate explanations. In other words, it is always necessary to consider multiple hypotheses before making conclusions about the causal relationship between any two items under investigation.

7. *Experiment.* The condition can be changed, weakened, or prevented by an appropriate experimental approach.

8. *Specificity.* This is established when a single commonly accepted cause produces a specific effect. This is considered by some to be the weakest of all the criteria. For example, the diseases attributed to cigarette smoking do not meet this criterion. When specificity of an association is found, it provides additional support for a causal relationship. However, the absence of specificity in no way negates a causal relationship because certain outcomes, such as the spread of a

unlikely that one will find a one-to-one cause–effect relationship between two phenomena. Causality is most often multiple; therefore, it is necessary to examine specific causal relationships within a wider perspective.

9. *Coherence*. The association should be compatible with existing theories and knowledge. That is, it is necessary to evaluate claims of causality within the context of the current state of knowledge, both within a given field and in related fields. Stated another way, what does one have to sacrifice about what one currently knows in order to accept a particular claim of causality? For example, what currently accepted theories and principles in anthropology, biology, chemistry, and physics must one reject in order to accept the creationist claim that the world was created exactly and literally as described in the Bible? Nevertheless, as with the issue of plausibility, *research results that disagree or conflict with established theory and knowledge are not automatically wrong or false*. They may force a reconsideration of accepted beliefs and principles. All currently accepted theories, including evolutionary theory, the theory of relativity, and the theory of population ecology, were at one time new ideas that challenged orthodoxy. Such changes in accepted theories are also known as *paradigm shifts*.

ROTHMAN'S COMMENTS ON BRADFIELD-HILL CRITERIA (ROTHMAN, 1998, 2002)

Critics have argued that the Bradford-Hill criteria fail to deliver on the hope of clearly distinguishing causal from noncausal relationships. For example, the second criterion, strength of association, does not take into account that not every component cause will have a strong association with the disease that it produces, nor does it recognize that strength of association often depends on the prevalence of other factors.

The third criterion, dose–response relationship, suggests that a causal association is more likely if a biological gradient or dose–response curve can be demonstrated. However, such relationships may result from confounding or other biases. According to Rothman, the only criterion that is truly a causal criterion is temporality—that is, a determination that the cause preceded the effect. (It may be difficult, however, to ascertain the time sequence of cause and effect.)

The eighth criterion, specificity, which suggests that a relationship is more likely to be causal if the exposure is related to a single outcome, may be misleading, as a cause may have many effects. For example, cigarette smoking is associated with many unpleasant effects, ranging from stained fingers and bad breath to lung cancer.

In general, the process of causal inference is complex, and arriving at a tentative identification of the causal or noncausal nature of an association is a surprisingly subjective process.

Legal Interpretation Using Epidemiology[2]

EPDM can only establish that an agent *could have* caused an effect in any particular case; it cannot prove that the agent did in fact cause the effect. This important axiom underlies all epidemiologic and biostatistical research.

EPDM is concerned with the *incidence* of disease in *populations*; it does not address the question of what caused a particular individual's disease. This question, sometimes referred to as *specific causation*, is beyond the domain of the science of epidemiology. EPDM has limits at the point where an inference or claim is made that the relationship between an agent and a disease is causal and where the magnitude of excess risk attributed to the agent has been determined. That is, EPDM addresses whether an agent *can* cause a disease, not whether an agent *did* cause a specific instance of a disease.

Nevertheless, the subdiscipline of **forensic epidemiology** is directed at the investigation of specific causation of disease or injury in an individual or a group of individuals in instances in which causation is disputed or unclear, for presentation in legal settings. Under U.S. law, EPDM alone cannot prove that a causal association does *not* exist in general. Conversely, a U.S. court in a specific, individual case can accept epidemiologic evidence to support or justify an inference that a causal association does exist, based upon a balance of probability.

Disease Occurrence (CDC, 2006)

A critical position taken in EPDM is that diseases do not occur randomly in a population, but are more likely to occur in some members of the population than others because of *risk factors* that are not distributed randomly in the population. EPDM is used to identify the factors that place some members of a population at greater risk than others.

CAUSATION

A number of models of disease causation have been proposed. Among the simplest is the epidemiologic triangle, the traditional model for infectious disease. The triangle consists of:

- An external **agent**
- A susceptible **host**
- An **environment** that brings the host and agent together

In this model, disease results from the interaction between the agent and the host in an environment that supports transmission of the agent from a source to that host.

Agent, host, and environmental factors may interrelate in many complex ways to produce diseases. Different diseases require different balances and interactions of these three components. Development of appropriate, practical, and effective PH measures to control or prevent disease usually requires assessment of all three components and their interactions.

The **agent** may be an infectious microorganism or pathogen: a virus, bacterium, parasite, or other microbes. The agent must be present for disease to occur; however, the presence of that agent alone is not always sufficient to cause disease. A variety of factors influence whether exposure to an organism will result in disease, including the organism's ability to cause disease (known as its *pathogenicity*)

The concept of the agent has been broadened to include chemical and physical causes of disease or injury, such as chemical contaminants. For example, contamination of poor-quality nutritional supplements containing L-tryptophan was deemed responsible for occurrences of eosinophilia–myalgia syndrome, an incurable and sometimes fatal flulike neurological condition. (**Tryptophan** is an essential amino acid in the human diet. Only the L-stereoisomer of tryptophan is used in structural or enzyme proteins, but the D-stereoisomer is occasionally found in naturally produced peptides.)

Although the epidemiologic triangle (or triad) serves as a useful model for many diseases, it has proven inadequate for cardiovascular disease, cancer, and other diseases that appear to have multiple contributing causes without a single necessary one.

A variety of factors intrinsic to the individual host (the human who can get the disease), sometimes called *risk factors*, can influence that individual's exposure, susceptibility, and response to a causative agent. Opportunities for exposure are often influenced by behaviors such as hygiene, sexual practices, and other personal choices, as well as by age and gender. Susceptibility and response to an agent are influenced by factors such as genetics, nutritional and immunologic status, anatomic structure, presence of other diseases or medications, and psychological makeup.

Environment refers to extrinsic factors that affect both the agent and the opportunity for exposure. Environmental factors include physical factors such as geology and climate, biologic factors such as insects that transmit the agent, and socioeconomic factors such as crowding, sanitation, and the availability of health services.

COMPONENT CAUSES AND CAUSAL PIES

Because the agent–host–environment model does not work well for many noninfectious diseases, several other models that attempt to account for the multifactorial nature of causation have been proposed. One such model, proposed by Rothman in 1976, has come to be known as the "causal pies" (Rothman, 1976).

This model is illustrated in Figure 2.1. An individual factor that contributes to causing disease is shown as a piece of a pie. After all the pieces of a pie are assembled, the pie is complete—and disease occurs. The individual factors (pieces of the pie) are called **component causes**. The complete pie, which might be considered a causal pathway, is called a **sufficient cause**. A disease may have more than one sufficient cause, with each sufficient cause being composed of several component causes that may or may not overlap. A component that appears in every pie or pathway is called a **necessary cause** because without it, disease does not occur.

The component causes may include intrinsic host factors, as well as the agent and the environmental factors in the agent–host–environment triangle. A single component cause is rarely a sufficient cause by itself. Host susceptibility and other host factors may also play a role. For example, even exposure to a highly infectious agent such as the measles virus does not invariably result in measles disease. In contrast, an agent that is usually harmless in healthy persons may cause devastating

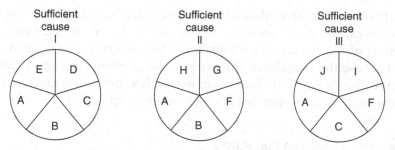

FIGURE 2.1 Rothman's causal pies.

For example, *Pneumocystis carinii* (*P. carinii*) is an organism that may colonize the respiratory tract of some healthy persons without causing any harm, but it can cause potentially lethal pneumonia in persons whose immune systems have been compromised by HIV. The presence of *P. carinii* organisms is therefore a *necessary but not sufficient* cause of pneumocystis pneumonia. In Figure 2.1, this situation is represented by component cause A. As the model indicates, a particular disease may result from a variety of different sufficient causes or pathways.

As another example, lung cancer may result from a sufficient cause that includes smoking as a component cause. However, because not all smokers develop lung cancer, smoking by itself cannot be identified as a sufficient cause. Moreover, because a small number of lung cancer patients have never smoked, smoking is also not a necessary cause.

Suppose that component cause B is smoking and component cause C is asbestos exposure:

- Sufficient cause I includes both smoking (B) and asbestos exposure (C).
- Sufficient cause II includes asbestos exposure but not smoking.
- Sufficient cause III includes smoking without asbestos exposure.

Because lung cancer can develop in persons who have never been exposed to either smoke or asbestos, a proper model for lung cancer would have to show at least one more sufficient cause pie that does not include either component B or component C.

PH action does not depend on the identification of every component cause, though. Disease prevention can be accomplished by blocking *any* single component of a sufficient cause, at least through that pathway. For example, elimination of smoking (component B) would prevent lung cancer arising from sufficient causes I and II, although some lung cancer cases would still occur through sufficient cause III.

STRENGTH OF A CAUSE

In EPDM, the **strength** of a factor may be measured by the change in disease frequency produced by introducing the factor into a population. This change may be measured in absolute or relative terms. In both cases, the strength of an effect may have important concomitant PH significance but little biological significance; this is because, given a specific causal mechanism, any of the component causes can have strong or weak effects. The actual identity of the constituent components of the

Furthermore, the strength of a factor's effect depends on the time-specific distribution of its causal complements in the population. Over a time period, the strength of the effect of a given factor with respect to the occurrence of a given disease may change because the prevalence of its causal complements in various causal mechanisms may also change. This may occur even when the causal mechanisms through which the factor and its complements act remain unchanged.

INTERACTION AMONG CAUSES

The causal pie model recognizes that several causal components may act in concert to produce an effect. However, "acting in concert" does not necessarily imply that all the factors must act at the same time.

Consider the example of a person who sustains an injury to the head that results in an equilibrium disturbance; years later, this person falls on a slippery footpath and breaks his hip. The earlier head injury and equilibrium problem played a *causal* role in the resulting hip fracture, but so did the weather conditions on the day of the fracture. If both of these factors played a causal role in the hip fracture, then they did interact with each other to cause the fracture, despite the fact that their times of action were many years apart. This allows one to conclude that *any and all of the factors in the same causal mechanism for disease interact with one another to cause disease.*

One can view each causal pie as a set of interacting causal components. In the preceding example, the earlier head injury interacted with the weather conditions, as well as with other component causes such as the type of shoes worn, the absence of a handhold, and any other conditions that were necessary to the causal mechanism of the fall and the broken hip that resulted. Thus, this model provides a biological basis for a concept of interaction among causes.

Review Questions for Section 2.1

1. Suggest aspects of the disciplines within EPDM that should be the focus for a PH program.
2. When an investigator assesses the causes of diseases, what effects might lead to a mistaken observed association that the investigator considers to indicate the existence of a cause–effect relationship?
3. (a) What are the Bradford-Hill criteria for causation and association in EPDM?
   (b) In what way are the Rothman objections to the Bradford-Hill criteria realistic regarding the following?
   - Strength of association
   - Dose–response relationship
   - Specificity
4. The legal view is that "epidemiology can only establish that an agent could have caused, but not that it did cause, an effect in any particular case." Is this a reasonable interpretation? Why or why not?
5. (a) What is the epidemiologic triangle?

6. In the context of causation of diseases, what is
   (a) a necessary cause?
   (b) a sufficient cause?
   Give an example of each.
7. Discuss the concept of Rothman's causal pies, and give some examples.
8. Within the context of disease causation, discuss the notion of a "necessary but not sufficient" cause of a disease. Give some examples.

2.2   CAUSATION AND INFERENCE IN EPIDEMIOLOGY AND PUBLIC HEALTH

In EPDM and PH (Rothman & Greenland, 2005), a **cause** of a disease is defined as an event, condition, or characteristic that *preceded* the disease, without which the disease either would not have occurred or would not have occurred until some later time. Notably, according to this definition, it may be that no specific event, condition, or characteristic is sufficient in and of itself to produce (cause) disease.

A *sufficient cause* is a complete causal mechanism that can be defined as a set of minimal conditions and events that inevitably produce disease. Here, *minimal* implies that all of the conditions or events are necessary to that occurrence. In the study of disease causation, the completion or existence of a sufficient cause may be considered equivalent to the onset of disease. (*Onset* refers to the earliest stage of the disease process rather than the actual appearance of symptoms.)

Sometimes all of the components of a sufficient cause for a given biological effect are unknown. For example, tobacco smoking is a cause of lung cancer, but by itself it is not a sufficient cause. First, the term *smoking* is too imprecise to be used in a causal description. Thus, one must specify:

- The type of smoke (e.g., cigarette, cigar, pipe)
- Whether the smoke is filtered or unfiltered
- The manner and frequency of inhalation
- The onset and duration of smoking

These *susceptibility factors* refer to and interact with other components in the various causal mechanisms through which smoking causes lung cancer.

Note also that tobacco smoking will not cause cancer in everyone who smokes. Apparently, there are some people who, by virtue of their genetic makeup or previous experience, are susceptible to the ill effects of smoking, and others who are not (they sometimes are known as the *tough rats*, in reference to laboratory-animal experiments).

Rothman's Diagrams for Sufficient Causation of Diseases (Broadbent, 2011)

A schematic diagram of sufficient causes in a disease is shown in Figure 2.2 (Rothman & Greenland, 2005). In this diagram:

- Each set of component causes represented is minimally sufficient to produce

■ Each component cause is a necessary part of that specific causal mechanism.
■ A specific component cause may play a role in one, two, or all three of the causal mechanisms shown.

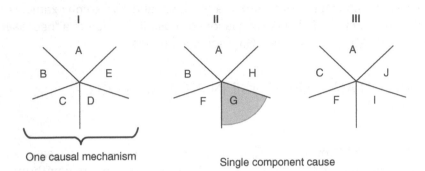

FIGURE 2.2 Rothman's diagrams for sufficient causes of diseases.

The diagram of causation shown in Figure 2.2 highlights several important principles with respect to **inference** and **causation** in human diseases. The first, and perhaps the most important, of these principles is obvious from the diagram: A given disease can have more than one cause, and every causal mechanism involves the joint action of a multitude of component causes.

■ **Example:** This harkens back to our previous example of the cause of a broken hip. John experiences a serious head injury that leads to a permanent disturbance in equilibrium. Years later, that faulty equilibrium plays a causal role in a fall that occurs while John is walking on a slippery footpath. That fall results in John breaking his hip. Other factors playing a causal role in the broken hip could include:

1. The type of shoe John was wearing
2. The lack of a handrail along the footpath
3. An unexpectedly strong gust of wind
4. Excessive body weight (John is somewhat obese)

All of these, in addition to many other factors, could play causal roles.

Thus, the complete causal mechanism involves many factors. Some factors, such as John's weight and the prior injury that resulted in his equilibrium disturbance, represent earlier events or conditions that have had lingering effects. Some genetic causal components might have affected John's weight, his way of walking, his behavior, his recovery from the earlier head injury, and so on. Other factors, such as the force of the sudden wind gust, are environmental. We can reasonably assert that there are some genetic and some environmental component causes in every causal mechanism. Thus, even an event such as a fall on a slippery footpath that results in a broken hip is part of a complicated causal mechanism that involves many component causes.

The important point about multicausality is that most identified causes are neither necessary nor sufficient to produce disease. Nevertheless, a cause need not be either necessary or sufficient for its removal to result in disease prevention. PH workers

a substantial amount of disease may still be prevented. That a cause is not necessary implies that some disease may still occur after that cause is eliminated, but that component cause will nevertheless be a necessary cause for *some* of the cases that occur. That the component cause is not sufficient implies that (a) other component causes must interact with it to produce the disease and (b) blocking any of them will result in prevention of some cases of disease. Thus, one need not identify every component cause to prevent some cases of disease. PH efforts that address only a few of the most apparently important component causes can have significant success in reducing the incidence of a disease; it is part of the job of EPDM to help identify those important causes.

SUMMING ATTRIBUTABLE FRACTIONS OF CAUSES FOR DISEASES

One can thus view each causal pie as a set of interacting causal components. This model provides a biological basis for a concept of interaction that is distinct from the usual biostatistical view of interaction (Ephron, 1984). Consider the hypothetical dataset in Table 2.1.

In the smoking-and-head/neck-cancer situation, the differences in the rates all reflect causal effects. Among those people who are cigarette smokers and also alcohol drinkers, what proportion of the cases is attributable to the effect of cigarette smoking?

In this example, it is given that the rate for these people is 15 cases per 100,000 person-years. If these same people were not cigarette smokers, we can infer that their rate of head and neck cancer would be 4 cases per 100,000 person-years. If this difference reflects the *causal role of cigarette smoking*, then we might infer that $(15 - 4) = 11$ of every 15 cases, or 73.3%, are attributable to cigarette smoking among those who *both* smoke cigarettes and drink alcohol.

If the question is what proportion of disease among these same people is attributable to alcohol drinking, we would be able to attribute $(15 - 5) = 10$ of every 15 cases, or 66.7%, to the *causal role of alcohol drinking*.

Now, can one attribute 73.3% of the cases to cigarette smoking and 66.7% to alcohol drinking among those who are exposed to both? Yes—because some cases are counted more than once.

Also, smoking and alcohol interact in some cases of head/neck cancer, and these cases are attributable both to cigarette smoking and to alcohol drinking. One consequence of interaction is that the proportions of disease attributable to various component causes seldom sum to exactly 100%.

TABLE 2.1   Hypothetical Rates of Head/Neck Cancer According to Cigarette Smoking Status and Alcohol Drinking

ALCOHOL DRINKING	NO	YES
CIGARETTE SMOKING STATUS		
Nonsmoker	1	4
Smoker	5	15

In the 1970s (Ephron, 1984), scientists at the U.S. National Institutes of Health (NIH) proposed that as much as 40% of cancer is attributable to occupational exposures. Many thought that this fraction was an overestimate. One of the arguments used in rebuttal was as follows: x% of cancer is caused by smoking, y% by diet, z% by alcohol, and so on. When all these percentages are added up, only a small percentage (much less than 40%) is left for occupational causes. However, this rebuttal is fallacious because it is based on the incorrect premise that every case of disease has a single cause and that two or more causes cannot both contribute to the same case of cancer. Today, it is accepted that because lifestyle (diet, exercise, smoking, alcohol consumption, etc.), environment (air pollution, asbestos exposure, etc.), and various occupational exposures, along with other factors, interact with one another and with genetic (hereditary) factors to cause cancer, each case of cancer can be attributed *repeatedly* to many separate component causes.

The sum of disease attributable to various component causes thus has no upper limit. A single cause or category of causes that is present in every sufficient cause of disease will have an attributable fraction of 100%.

Much research has been undertaken to develop "heritability indexes," which are supposed to measure the fraction of disease that is inherited. However, these indexes only assess the relative role of environmental and genetic causes of disease in a particular setting. For example, some genetic causes may be necessary components of every causal mechanism. If everyone in a population has an identical set of the genes that cause disease, then their effect is not included or reflected in heritability indexes, even though this gene set is a cause of the disease. If all genetic factors that determine disease are taken into account, whether or not they vary within populations, then 100% of disease can be said to be inherited. Analogously, 100% of any disease is environmentally caused, even those diseases that we often consider purely genetic.

■ **Example 1:** Phenylketonuria is considered by many to be purely genetic. Nevertheless, the mental retardation that it may cause can be prevented by appropriate dietary intervention. The treatment for phenylketonuria illustrates the interaction of genes and environment to cause a disease commonly thought to be purely genetic.

■ **Example 2:** What about an apparently purely environmental cause of death, such as death from a car accident? It is easy to conceive of genetic traits that lead to psychiatric problems, such as alcoholism, that in turn lead to drunk driving and consequent fatal car accidents. In this example, the interaction of genes and environment causes a disease commonly thought to be purely environmental.

■ **Example 3:** Consider the extreme environmental example of being killed by lightning. Partially heritable psychiatric conditions can influence whether someone will take shelter during a lightning storm; genetic traits such as athletic ability may influence the likelihood of being outdoors when a lightning storm strikes; and having an outdoor occupation or pastime that is more frequent among men (and in that sense is genetic) would also influence the probability of getting killed by a lightning strike. Furthermore, some individuals' body chemistry—a genetic factor—may actually render them more

These examples clearly show that every case of disease has both genetic and environmental causes. This mode of thinking is defensible and has important implications for research.

Causal Inferences

Causal inference is a special case of the more general process of scientific reasoning, about which there is substantial debate among scientists and philosophers.

IMPOSSIBILITY OF PROOF

The philosopher David Hume observed in the 18th century that proof is impossible in empirical science, and his observation still holds true. Epidemiologists often face the criticism that proof is impossible in EPDM—with the implication that it is possible in other scientific disciplines! Some experimental scientists hold that epidemiologic relations can only be suggestive, and that detailed laboratory study of mechanisms within a few single individuals can reveal cause–effect relations with certainty.

Unfortunately, this view overlooks the fact that all relations are suggestive in exactly the way described by Hume: Even the most careful and detailed analysis of individual events cannot provide more than associations, albeit at very detailed levels. Laboratory studies involve a degree of observer control that cannot be matched in EPDM; it is only this control, not the level of observation, that allegedly underlies the derivation of "proof" from laboratory studies.

However, such control is no guarantee against error. All the scientific work, in EPDM or any other discipline, is at best only a tentative description of nature and reality.

TESTING COMPETING EPIDEMIOLOGIC THEORIES

Biological knowledge about epidemiologic hypotheses is often scarce, and this fact occasionally results in hypotheses that appear to be little more than vague statements of causal association between exposure and disease (e.g., "smoking causes cardiovascular disease"). Though these vague hypotheses often seem intuitively correct, they can be difficult to verify empirically. To cope with this challenge, epidemiologists often focus on testing the *negation* of the causal hypothesis; in probabilistic terms, this is equivalent to the **null hypothesis** (H_0) that the exposure does *not* have a causal relation to disease. In such tests, any observed association can potentially *refute* the hypothesis, assuming that biases are absent.

If the causal mechanism is stated specifically enough, epidemiologic observations may suggest crucial tests of competing non-null causal hypotheses. However, many epidemiologic studies are not designed to test a causal hypothesis.

■ **Example:** Horwitz and Feinstein (1978) examined early epidemiologic data that appeared to indicate that women who took replacement estrogen therapy were at higher risk for endometrial cancer. These researchers then hypothesized an association that women taking estrogen will experience symptoms such as bleeding, which would then

diagnostic procedure that enabled the detection of endometrial cancer at an earlier stage in these women, as compared with women not taking estrogens in the first place.

Epidemiologic observations have been used to evaluate likely competing hypotheses:

- The causal theory predicted that the risk of endometrial cancer would tend to increase with increased use of estrogens.
- The detection bias theory predicted that women who had used estrogens for only a short while would have the greatest risk because the symptoms related to estrogen use, which led to the early medical consultation, tended to appear soon after use began.

Because the association of recent estrogen use and endometrial cancer was the same in both long-term and short-term estrogen users, the detection bias theory was refuted as an explanation for all but a small fraction of endometrial cancer cases occurring after estrogen use.

This example illustrates a critical point in understanding the process of **causal inference** in EPDM. Many of the hypotheses being evaluated through the interpretation of epidemiologic research are noncausal hypotheses; that is, they involve no causal connection between the study exposure and the disease. Thus, hypotheses explaining how specific types of bias could have led to an association between exposure and disease are the usual alternatives to the primary study hypothesis that the epidemiologist needs to consider in reaching inferences. Much of the interpretation of epidemiologic studies amounts to the testing of such noncausal explanations. The Bradford-Hill criteria, discussed in Section 2.1, are widely used in such interpretations.

Using the Causal Criteria

From the outset, the standards of epidemiologic evidence, according to the Bradford-Hill criteria, have to deal with many reservations and exceptions. Hill himself asked, "In what circumstances can we pass from this observed association to a verdict of causation?" In fact, he disagreed that there are "hard-and-fast rules of evidence" by which to judge causation (Rothman & Greenland, 2005). This conclusion accords with many others that *causal inferences cannot attain the certainty of logical deductions*.

Although some scientists continue to promote causal criteria as aids to inference, others argue that it is actually detrimental to confuse the inferential process by considering a checklist of criteria. Perhaps an intermediate approach may be found that transforms the criteria into deductive tests of causal hypotheses. If this were so, one could avoid using causal criteria to support unprovable hypotheses and theories while allowing epidemiologists to focus on evaluating competing causal theories using critical observational evidence.

Judging Scientific Evidence

Because causal criteria cannot be used to establish the validity of an inference, no criteria can be used to evaluate the validity of data as evidence. However, methods do exist by which validity may be assessed. In this spirit, one could view scientific

■ **Example:** If an epidemiologic study proposes to determine the relation between exposure to cigarette smoking and lung cancer risks, the results should be viewed as a measure of causal effect, such as the ratio of the risk of lung cancer among smokers to the risk among nonsmokers:

Risk Ratio = (Risk of lung cancer among cigarette smokers)/(Risk among nonsmokers)

The measurement of a causal effect is subject to measurement errors, just like any experiment. In addition to statistical error, measurement error may include problems relating to study design, such as subject selection and retention, information collection, uncontrolled confounding, and other sources of bias. It is not sufficient to characterize a study as having or not having any of these sources of error, as nearly every study will be subject to nearly every type of error. Nevertheless, validity of a study must be assessed. One must therefore quantify the errors. As there is no precise standard as to how much error can be tolerated before a study must be considered invalid, there is no alternative to the quantification of study errors to the extent possible.

What is required is much more than the application of a list of criteria. One must apply critical assessment to obtain a quantified evaluation of the total error inherent in the study. This type of assessment requires quantitative skill in consonance with scientific rigor. The expectation is that epidemiologic investigations will be approached through, and supported by, the application of mathematically vigorous biostatistical approaches, as described in the next section and in the remainder of this book.

Review Questions for Section 2.2

1. In EPDM investigations, whenever a disease is noted, what assumptions are usually made regarding the origin of that disease? What are the bases for those assumptions?
2. (a) What constitutes a sufficient cause of a disease? Give an example.
   (b) Given a disease, how does an epidemiologic investigation determine its sufficient cause?
3. (a) Describe Rothman's diagrams for sufficient causes of diseases.
   (b) How do these diagrams illustrate the principles with respect to inference and causation in human diseases?
4. (a) Can it be true that "one need not identify every component cause to prevent some cases of disease"? Why or why not?
   (b) Give an example of this assertion.
5. In epidemiologic investigations, what is meant by the following?
   (a) Strength of a cause
   (b) Interaction among causes
   (c) Summing attributable fractions of causes for diseases
   Give an example of each of these concepts.
6. (a) In the EPDM of disease studies, what are causal inferences?
   (b) Within the context of seeking the cause of a disease, explain the dilemma in

7. How does an epidemiologist confront the task of testing competing epidemiologic theories? Explain using an example.
8. In epidemiologic disease investigations, what is meant by the process of causal inference?
9. In epidemiologic investigations, do the Bradford-Hill criteria help in confronting the problems of causal inference? Why or why not?
10. In epidemiologic research, if the causal criteria cannot be used to establish the validity of an inference, on what basis should one judge scientific evidence? Why?

2.3   BIOSTATISTICAL BASIS OF INFERENCE

The epidemiologic approach to understanding the causation of diseases follows a causation and inference path, as discussed in Section 2.2. To support this approach, we must now delve further into the logic of inference, for which a biostatistical basis is the obvious and logical choice.

Modes of Inference

Different schools of biostatistical inference have emerged and become established. These schools, or paradigms, are not mutually exclusive; methods that work satisfactorily under one paradigm often yield attractive interpretations under other paradigms. The two main paradigms in use today are Bayesian biostatistics (BIOS) and frequentist BIOS.

In **Bayesian inference**, Bayes's theorem is used to calculate how the degree of support for (or belief in) a proposition changes according to the evidence. Bayesian inference is based on the philosophy of Bayesian probability, which asserts that degrees of belief (support) can be represented by probabilities. A typical application of Bayesian BIOS is the testing of a hypothesis.

Frequentist inference is an alternative biostatistical method in which one uses a **significance test** to arrive at a conclusion that a proposition is either true or false, or draws a conclusion that a given sample-derived **confidence interval (CI)** covers the true value. In this framework, either of these conclusions has a given probability of being correct, and this probability has either a *frequency probability* interpretation or a *pre-experiment* interpretation. A typical example of the application of frequentist BIOS is significance testing of a measured value in terms of its level within a computed CI.

Levels of Measurement

Biostatistical investigations use four levels of measurement: ratio, interval, ordinal, and nominal. Each has different degrees of usefulness in research.

- **Ratio** measurements have a specific zero value. In addition, the differences between measurements are defined, allowing flexibility in the biostatistical methods that can be used for analysis of the data.

■ **Interval** measurements show meaningful distances between measurements, with the zero value being arbitrary (as with temperature measurements using the Celsius or Fahrenheit scale).

■ **Ordinal** measurements have imprecise or uneven differences between consecutive values but have a meaningful order to those values.

■ **Nominal** measurements have no meaningful rank order among values.

Because variables applicable only to nominal or ordinal measurements cannot be measured numerically, they are sometimes grouped together as categories or categorical variables. In contrast, owing to their numerical characteristics, ratio and interval measurements are grouped together as quantitative variables, which can be either discrete or continuous.

Frequentist BIOS in EPDM

INTERVAL ESTIMATION

In most epidemiologic investigations, the sample is only a part of a population; thus, the results may not be fully representative of the whole population, and estimates obtained from the sample may only approximate the population value. **CIs** enable biostatisticians to express how closely the sample estimate matches the true value in the whole population.

Often this parameter is set at **95% CI**. Formally, a 95% CI for a value is a range in which, if the sampling and analysis were repeated under the same conditions (yielding a different dataset), the interval would include the true (population) value 95% of the time. This does *not* mean that the probability that the true value is in the CI is 95%. From the frequentist viewpoint, such a claim does not even make sense, as the true value is not a random variable. Either the true value is or is not within the given interval. However, it is true that before any data are sampled, and given a plan for how the CI will be constructed, the probability is 95% that the yet-to-be-calculated interval will cover the true value. At this point, the limits of the interval are yet-to-be-observed random variables. One approach that yields an interval that can be interpreted as having a given probability of containing the true value is to use a credible interval from Bayesian statistics. This approach depends on a different way of interpreting what is meant by "probability"; that is, as a Bayesian probability.

Note that in Bayesian BIOS, a *credible interval* is an interval in the domain of a posterior probability distribution used for interval estimation (Paoli, Haggard, & Shah, 2002). The generalization to multivariate problems is the *credible region*. Bayesian credible intervals are analogous to CIs in frequentist BIOS.

For example, in an epidemiologic investigation that determines the uncertainty distribution of a clinical parameter λ, if the probability that λ lies between 67 and 103 is 95%, then $67 \leq \lambda \leq 103$ is a 95% Bayesian credible interval of λ. Some writers call this the "Bayesian CI," but in this book, the use of the term *CI* is restricted to the frequentist confidence interval only, to avoid confusion.

THE CONCEPT OF BIOSTATISTICAL SIGNIFICANCE

Biostatistics (BIOS) seldom gives a simple yes/no answer to the question posed. Interpretation often comes down to the level of statistical significance applied to the numbers and often refers to the probability (the *p*-value) of a value accurately rejecting the null hypothesis.

A finding of *statistical* significance does not necessarily mean that the overall result is significant in real-world terms. For instance, a large drug study may show that the drug has a biostatistically significant but very small beneficial effect, such that the drug will be unlikely to help patients in a noticeable way.

Confidence Intervals in Epidemiology and Public Health[3]

When epidemiologists and PH practitioners use health BIOS, they may be interested in the actual number of health events, but more often they use BIOS to assess the true underlying risk of a health problem in the community. Observed-health BIOS (those percentages, rates, or counts that are calculated or estimated from health surveys, vital BIOS registries, or other health surveillance systems) are not always an accurate reflection of the true underlying risk in the population. Observed rates may vary from sample to sample, or year to year, even when the true underlying risk remains the same.

BIOS based on samples of a population are subject to sampling error. *Sampling error* refers to random variation that occurs because only specific subsets of the entire population are sampled and used to estimate a finding for the entire population. It is often mistakenly called "margin of error." Even health events that are based on a complete count of an entire population, such as deaths, are subject to random variation because the number of events that actually occurred may be considered as one of a large series of possible results that could have occurred under the same circumstances. In general, sampling error or random variation increases when the sample, population, or number of events is small.

Statistical sampling theory may be used to calculate a CI to provide an estimate of the potential discrepancy between the true population parameters and observed rates. Understanding the potential size of that discrepancy can provide information about how to interpret the observed statistic.

A 95% CI indicates the range of values within which a biostatistic would fall 95% of the time if the investigator were to calculate the biostatistic (e.g., a percentage or rate) from an infinite number of samples of the same size, drawn from the same population. In other words, the CI is a range of values within which the "true" value of the rate is expected to occur (with 95% probability).

Now, let us consider the most common methods for calculation of 95% CIs for some rates and estimates commonly used in EPDM and PH.

---

[3] Bayesian credible interval and frequentist CI (available at http://en.wikipedia.org/wiki/Credible_interval).

95% CI FOR A PERCENTAGE FROM A SURVEY SAMPLE

To calculate a CI for a percentage from a survey sample, one must first calculate the *standard error* of the percentage. A percentage is also known as the mean of a binomial distribution. The standard error of the mean is a measure of dispersion for the hypothetical distribution of means called the *sampling distribution of the mean*. This is a distribution of means calculated from an infinite number of samples of the same size drawn from the same population as the original sample. The *sampling distribution of the mean* has a shape that is almost identical to the normal distribution (see Figure 2.3).

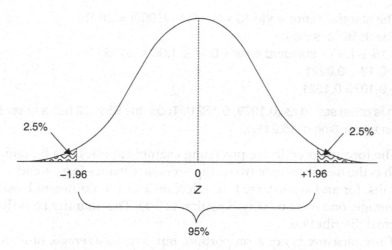

FIGURE 2.3 The sampling distribution of the mean.

After the standard error of the percentage has been calculated, one then decides how large the CI should be. The most common choice is a 95% CI. This is the width of the interval that includes the mean (the *sampling distribution of the mean*) 95% of the time. In other words, a 95% CI for a percentage is the range of values within which the percentage would be found at least 95% of the time if one were to obtain a different sample of the same size from the same population. Transforming the standard error into a 95% CI is straightforward.

A *distribution* is a tool used in BIOS to associate a biostatistic (e.g., a percentage, average, or other statistic) with its probability. When epidemiologic investigators refer to a measure as being "biostatistically significant," they have used a distribution to evaluate the probability of the biostatistic and found that it would be improbable under ordinary conditions. In most cases, one can rely on measures such as rates, averages, and proportions to have an underlying *normal distribution*, at least when the sample size is large enough.

One need only multiply the standard error by the z-score of the points in the normal distribution that exclude 2.5% of the distribution on either end (two-tailed): That z-score is 1.96.

- A z-score of 1.96 defines the 95% CI.
- A z-score of 1.65 defines the 90% CI.

For a simple random sample, the

$$\text{standard error} = \sqrt{(pq/n)} \qquad (2.3\text{-}1)$$

where:
p is the rate,
$q = 1 - p$, and
n is the sample size.

■ **Example A:** In a survey, 15% of the respondents indicated that they smoked cigarettes. The sample consisted of 1,000 persons in a simple random sample.

The standard error = $\sqrt{[0.15 \times (1 - 0.15)/1000]}$ = .0113
The 95% CI is thus:
$0.15 \pm 1.96 \times$ standard error = $0.15 \pm 1.96 \times .0113$
$= 0.13 \pm 0.0221$
$= 0.1079\ 0.1521,$

which is often stated as (0.1079, 0.1521). Thus, the 95% CI has a lower limit of 10.79% and an upper limit of 15.21%.

The formula used in the preceding example applies to a binomial distribution, which is the distribution of two complementary values (e.g., + and −, 0 and 1, heads and tails, for and against, etc.). To calculate a CI for a different biostatistic, such as an average, one must modify Equation (2.3-1). The quantity pq is the variance of a binomial distribution.

If the measure is not a proportion, but, say, an average, one must modify the formula, substituting the variance for the pq quantity.

The standard error can also be calculated as the standard deviation divided by the square root of the sample size:

$$\text{Standard error} = \sigma/\sqrt{n} \qquad (2.3\text{-}2)$$

SMALL SAMPLES

If the sample from which the percentage was calculated was small [according to the central limit theorem (CLT), one may define *small* as 29 or fewer; see Section 2.4], then the shape of the sampling distribution of the mean will *not* be the same as the shape of the normal distribution. For this case, one can use another distribution, known as the t distribution, that has a slightly different shape than the normal distribution; see Figure 2.4.

The procedures in this case are similar to those discussed for the CI, but the t-score comes from a family of distributions that depend on the *degrees of freedom* (*DFs*). The number of DFs is defined as $n - 1$, where n is the size of the sample. For a sample size of 30, the DF is equal to (30 − 1 = 29). So, for a 95% CI, one must use the t-score associated with 29 DFs. That particular t-score is 2.045. Therefore, one would multiply the standard error by 2.045 (instead of 1.96) to generate the 95% CI.

If the sample were a different size, say 20, then the DF would be (20 − 1 = 19), which is associated with a t-score of 2.093 for a 95% CI. The interval will widen as

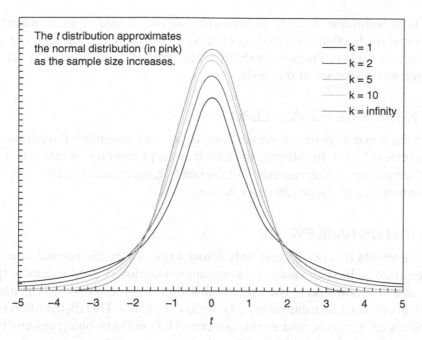

The *t* distribution approximates the normal distribution (in pink) as the sample size increases.

——— k = 1
——— k = 2
——— k = 5
——— k = 10
——— k = infinity

FIGURE 2.4 The Student's *t* distribution at varying DFs (k). The *t* distribution approximates the normal distribution (pink) as the sample size increases.

the sample size is reduced. This reflects the uncertainty in the estimate of the variance in the population. For a 95% CI with 9 DFs, the *t*-score is 2.262.

THE STUDENT'S T DISTRIBUTION AT VARYING DFs K

For a 95% CI, one would use the *t*-score that defines the points on the distribution so as to exclude the most extreme 5% of the distribution, which is 0.025 on either end of the symmetric distribution.

FINITE POPULATIONS

When the survey samples all or most of the population, using the finite population correction factor F will improve (decrease) the width of the CI. Now,

$$F = 1 - f \tag{2.3-3}$$

where *f* is the sampling fraction, and

$$f = n/N \tag{2.3-4}$$

where *n* is the size of the sample and *N* is the size of the population.

The sampling fraction *f* is the proportion of the population that was included in the sample. The standard error (SE) of the mean for a binomial distribution of a finite sample is

$$SE \text{ percentage} = \sqrt{\{(pq/n)\,(1-f)\}} \tag{2.3-5}$$

Those techniques may be conveniently accomplished using standard biostatistical software. Section 2.4 introduces the use of the R programming environment for these computations. Programs in SAS, SPSS, Stata, and other areas are also available (though not discussed in this text).

WHEN THE RATE EQUALS ZERO

When the percentage or rate equals zero, using the conventional formulas will yield an incorrect CI of 0. To estimate the CI when the percentage or rate is 0, just assume that the number on the numerator of the rate is 2, and then calculate the CI using the population size in the original calculation.

95% CIs FOR RARE EVENTS

For rare events that occur randomly across a time span, the normal distribution no longer applies. In such cases, the Poisson distribution is used to model the events, such as a 100-year flood. The Poisson distribution is also used to calculate CIs for health events such as infant mortality or cancer deaths. This distribution is not symmetric about its mean, and so the associated CIs will not be symmetric (the upper limit is farther from the estimate than the lower limit IS).

The Poisson distribution assumes the shape of a normal distribution when there are 20 or more events in the numerator. Hence, use a Poisson distribution for rare events (i.e., when the number of events is less than 20), but use the normal distribution when the number of events is 20 or more.

POISSON DISTRIBUTION

To calculate the CI using a Poisson distribution, multiply the estimated rate by the confidence factor associated with the number of events on which the rate is based.

■ **Example B:** In a given geographic area, there were 853 births in a single year and 8 infant deaths in that same year. The infant mortality rate was therefore 9.4 per 1,000 live births, calculated as [(8/853) × 1,000]. The lower and upper confidence limits are calculated using the confidence factors found in Appendix B of the online ancillary. The factors for seven events are 0.4317 and 1.9704 for the lower and upper limits of the CI, respectively.

Hence,
the lower limit of the CI = 9.4 × 0.4317 = 4.05, and
the upper limit of the CI = 9.4 × 1.9704 = 18.52
for an infant mortality rate of 9.7 per 1,000 live births, with a 95% CI from 4.05 to 18.52.

DIRECTLY AGE-ADJUSTED DEATH RATE (DAADR)

When comparing across geographic areas, some method of age adjustment is typically used to control for area-to-area differences in health events that can be explained by differing ages of the area populations. For example, an area that has an older population will have higher crude (not age-adjusted) rates for cancer, even though its exposure levels and cancer rates for specific age groups are the same as those of other areas. One might incorrectly attribute the high cancer rates to some characteristic of the area other than age. Age-adjusted rates control for age effects, allowing better comparability of rates across areas. Direct standardization adjusts the age-specific rates observed in the small area to the age distribution of a standard population. The directly age-adjusted death rate (DAADR) is a weighted average of the age-specific death rates, where the age-specific weights represent the relative age distribution of the standard population:

$$\text{Directly age-adjusted death rate (DAADR)} = \Sigma W_{si} \times D_i / P_i = \Sigma W_{si} \times R_i$$

where W_{si} = the weight for the ith age group in the standard population (the proportion of the standard population in the ith age group):

$$= P_{si} / \Sigma P_{si}$$

P_{si} = the population in age group i in the standard population
D_i = number of deaths (or other event) in age group i of the study population
P_i = the population in age group i in the study population
R_i = the age-specific rate in the ith age group.

Using the properties of the Poisson distribution, the variance of the age-specific death rate is given by

$$\text{var}(R_i) = \text{var}(D_i / P_i) = 1 / P_i^2 \, \text{var}(D_i) = D_i / P_i^2 = R_i^2 / D_i$$

The variance of a DAADR can then be computed as follows:

$$\text{var(DAADR)} = \Sigma W_{si}^2 \times \text{var}(R_i) = \Sigma W_{si}^2 \times R_i^2 / D_i$$

$$\text{SE(DAADR)} = \sqrt{\{\text{var(DAADR)}\}}$$

where:

var(DAADR) = the variance of the directly standardized rate
W_{si} = the weight for the ith age group in the standard population
R_i = the age-specific rate in the ith age group
var(R_i) = the variance of the age-specific death rate in the ith age group of the study population

$$= R_i^2 / D_i$$

Di = number of deaths (or other events) in age group i of the study population
SE(DAADR) = standard error of the directly standardized rate.

The age-adjusted death rate is a linear combination of independent Poisson random variables and therefore is not itself a Poisson random variable. It can be placed in the more general family of gamma distributions of which the Poisson is a member.

Most biostatistical software packages have a function to calculate factors that may be applied to age-adjusted death rates to calculate 95% CIs. These factors are derived from a standard gamma distribution.

INDIRECTLY AGE-ADJUSTED RATES

The direct method can present problems when population sizes are particularly small. Direct calculation of standardized rates requires calculating age-specific rates, and for small areas, these age-specific rates may be based on only one or two events. The general rule of thumb is that if there are fewer than 20 to 25 cases in the index population, indirect standardization of rates should be used.

Indirectly standardized rates are based on the standardized mortality ratio (SMR) and the crude rate for a standard population. Indirect standardization adjusts the overall standard population rate to the age distribution of the small area. It is valid to compare indirectly standardized rates only with the rate in the standard population; they cannot be compared with each other.

An indirectly standardized death or disease rate (ISR) can be computed as

$$ISR = SMR * Rs$$

SMR = observed deaths/disease in the small area = $D/e = D/\Sigma (R_{si} \times n_i)$ expected deaths/disease in the small area, where:

SMR = observed deaths in the small area/expected deaths in the small area

   D = observed number of deaths in the small area

   $e = \Sigma(R_{si} \times n_i)$ = expected number of deaths in the small area

   R_s = the crude death rate in the standard population

   R_{si} = the age-specific death rate in age group i of the standard population

      = # deaths/population count, before applying the constant

   n_i = the population count in age group i of the small area.

When the ratio of events to total population is small (<0.3) and the sample size is large, the following two methods can be used to calculate the CI.

(1)   When the number of events ≥ 20:

$$CI_{ISR} = \pm1.96 \sqrt{(SMR/e)} \times R_s \times K$$

where:

   SMR = observed deaths in the small area/expected deaths in the small area

      e = expected deaths in the small area = $\Sigma(R_{si} \times n_i)$

      R_s = the crude death rate in the standard population

      R_{si} = the age-specific death rate in age group i of the standard population

         (# deaths/population count)

      n_i = the population count in age group i of the small area

      K = a constant (e.g., 100,000) that is being used to communicate the rate.

(2)   When the number of events ≤ 20:

   LLISR = (lower limit for parameter estimate from Poisson table/e) $\times R_s \times K$

   ULISR = (upper limit for parameter estimate from Poisson table/e) $\times R_s \times K$

   where LL is the lower CI limit, and UL is the upper CI limit.

Bayesian Credible Interval[3]

In Bayesian statistics, a **credible interval** (or Bayesian credible interval) is an

the size of an interval. The generalization to multivariate problems is the **credible region**. Credible intervals are analogous to CIs in frequentist BIOS. For example, in an experiment that determines the uncertainty distribution of parameter t, if the probability that t lies between 35 and 45 is 90%, then $34 \leq t \leq 45$ is a 90% credible interval.

A BAYESIAN CREDIBLE INTERVAL VERSUS A FREQUENTIST CI

A frequentist 90% CI of 35 to 45 means that with a large number of repeated samples, 90% of the calculated CIs would include the true value of the parameter. The probability that the parameter is inside the given interval (say, 35–45) is either 0 or 1 (the nonrandom unknown parameter is either there or not). In frequentist terms, the parameter is *fixed* (cannot be considered to have a distribution of possible values) and the CI is *random* (as it depends on the random sample). Thus, a CI is an interval generated by a procedure that will give correct intervals 90% of the time.

In general, Bayesian credible intervals do not coincide with frequentist CIs, for two reasons:

1. Credible intervals incorporate problem-specific contextual information from the prior distribution, whereas CIs are based only on the data.
2. Credible intervals and CIs treat nuisance parameters in radically different ways.

Many professional biostatisticians and decision scientists, as well as nonstatisticians, intuitively interpret CIs in the Bayesian credible interval sense, and thus credible intervals are sometimes also called CIs. It is widely accepted, especially in the decision sciences, that credible interval is merely the subjective subset of CIs. In fact, much research in calibrated probability assessments never uses the term *credible interval*; it is common to simply use *CI*.

Review Questions for Section 2.3

1. (a) What are the two main modes of statistical inferences used in BIOS?
   (b) What are their similarities and differences? Give examples.
2. (a) In BIOS data analysis, what is a CI?
   (b) What is meant by a statement such as "I am 95% confident that X is between (this) and (that)"?
3. As an epidemiologic investigator, how should one respond to the following questions?
   (a) If the smoking rate among teens decreases from 12% to 10%, should we celebrate that as a significant decrease? Why or why not?
   (b) If the state infant death rate of 6.75 increases to 7.05 in a 1-year interval, should we be concerned about that increase? Why or why not?
4. (a) What is the normal distribution?
   (b) What is the Student's t distribution?
   (c) How are these two related?
5. Explain what is meant by "confidence intervals in epidemiology and public health"

2.4   BIOS IN EPDM AND PH

By definition, *biostatistics (BIOS)* is the application of statistics to a topic in biology. In medicine and health sciences, these applications include the design of biological experiments, the collection and analysis of data from those experiments, and the interpretation of the results. Biostatisticians who professionally communicate concerning their activities, work, and results can help build a wider appreciation of BIOS.

Applications of BIOS[4]

BIOS typically finds application in:

- PH, including EPDM, health services research, nutrition, and environmental health.
- Design and analysis of clinical trials in medicine.
- Population genetics and statistical genetics, often in order to link a variation in genotype with a variation in phenotype. This has been done in agriculture to improve crops and farm animals (through selective animal breeding). In biomedical research, this work can assist in finding candidates for gene alleles that can cause or influence predisposition to disease in human genetics.
- Analysis of genomics data (for example, from microarray or proteomics experiments, which often concern diseases or disease stages).
- Ecology and ecological forecasting.
- Biological sequence analysis.
- Systems biology, for gene network inference or pathway analysis.

Statistical methods are beginning to be integrated into medical informatics, PH informatics, bioinformatics, and computational biology. Professional work in these areas is often published in **BIOS journals** such as the following:

Biometrics
Biometrika
Biostatistics
Canadian Journal of Epidemiology and Biostatistics
International Journal of Biostatistics
Journal of Agricultural, Biological, and Environmental Statistics
Journal of Biometrics & Biostatistics
Journal of Biopharmaceutical Statistics
Pharmaceutical Statistics
Statistical Applications in Genetics and Molecular Biology
Statistics in Biopharmaceutical Research
Statistics in Medicine
Turkiye Klinikleri Journal of Biostatistics

BIOS shares several methods with quantitative fields, including:

- Computational biology
- Computer science
- Operations research
- Psychometrics
- Statistics
- Econometrics
- Mathematical demography

BIOS in EPDM and PH

Within the fields of EPDM and PH, BIOS takes a pivotal position in data analysis to provide useful and meaningful inferences and conclusions upon which critical and useful PH decisions and policies can be based. These activities include:

- Generating descriptive analyses to display and summarize data
- Applying concepts underlying statistical inference
- Using biostatistical methods for the analysis of continuous and binary data
- Applying biostatistical aspects of study design, such as sampling, probability distributions, and sampling distribution of the mean; CI and significance tests for one sample, two paired samples, and two independent samples for continuous data as well as binary data
- Seeking correlation and simple linear regression
- Considering distribution-free methods for two paired samples, two independent samples and correlation, and power and sample size estimation for simple studies
- Introducing statistical aspects of study design and analysis

LEARNING OBJECTIVES (UNIVERSITY OF SYDNEY, 2012)

The student who successfully reads and learns from this book will be able to:

1. Summarize biostatistical data using tables, graphs, and appropriate summary BIOS.
2. Interpret significance tests and CIs.
3. Compare two samples using the Student's t-test for continuous variables and the chi-squared test for categorical data, in both paired and unpaired cases; calculate CIs for the main results; and summarize the conclusions from such analyses.
4. Compare two samples using nonparametric tests, in both paired and unpaired cases, and summarize the conclusions from such analyses.
5. Analyze the association between two variables using scatter plots, parametric and nonparametric measures of correlation, and simple linear regression.
6. Calculate the sample size required for simple studies.
7. Create a statistical analysis plan, detailing the major steps in the statistical design and analysis of a study.
8. Use the statistical software R to process, analyze, and present data.

Students will be required to perform analyses using sample data and will be

APPLYING BIOS IN EPDM (CDC, 2006; VIRASAKDI, 2011; ARAGON, 2011)

Many variables used by epidemiologists are categorical variables. Some of these have only two categories:

- Exposed: YES or NO
- Tested: + or −, case or control, and so on

These variables have to be summarized with frequency measures such as rates, ratios, and proportions. Three frequency measures that are used to characterize the occurrence of health events in a population are incidence, prevalence, and mortality rates.

To begin, we consider these concepts by calculating and interpreting the following epidemiologic measures:

- Ratio
- Proportion
- Incidence proportion (attack rate)
- Incidence rate
- Prevalence
- Mortality rate

Processing and Analyzing Basic Epidemiologic Data

Basic data in epidemiologic investigations may be analyzed in terms of the following parameters and approaches.

FREQUENCY MEASURES

A measure of central location provides a single value that summarizes an entire distribution of data. In contrast, a frequency measure characterizes only part of the distribution. Frequency measures compare one part of the distribution to another part of the distribution or to the entire distribution. Common frequency measures are **ratios**, **proportions**, and **rates**. All three **frequency measures** have the same basic form:

$$(\text{Numerator}/\text{Denominator}) \times 10^n$$

where $n = \ldots, 3, 2, 1, 0, 1, 2, 3, \ldots$.

RATIO

A **ratio** is the relative magnitude of two quantities or a comparison of any two values. It is calculated by dividing one interval- or ratio-scale variable by the other. The numerator and denominator need not be related. Therefore, one could compare apples with oranges (or apples with the number of clinical visits).

The method for calculating a ratio uses the number or rate of events, items, persons, and so on in one group divided by the number or rate of events, items, persons,

TABLE 2.2 Epidemiologic Measures of Occurrence and Association

TYPE	MEASURES[a]	DESCRIPTION
Measures of occurrence	Time incidence[b]	Average time in a state ("survival") Number of new cases
	Prevalence[c]	Number of existing cases
	Rate	New cases per person-time at risk
	Risk[d]	Probability of becoming a case
	Odds	Odds of becoming a case
Measures of association	Rate ratio	Comparison of two rates
	Risk ratio (RR)	Comparison of two risks
	Odds ratio (OR)	Comparison of two odds

[a] All measures have a time element that must be specified.
[b] Sometimes expressed as a proportion by dividing by "total population."
[c] Commonly expressed as a proportion by dividing by "total population."
[d] Sometimes estimated using a proportion (binomial model).

the result is expressed in the form "[number] to [number]" (e.g., "3 to 1") or as "[number]:[number]" (e.g., "3:1").

Tables 2.2 and 2.3 display the measures of occurrence and measures of association commonly used in EPDM. Among these parameters, researchers focus first on incidence, prevalence, rate, risk, odds, and the ratio of rates (rate ratio), risks (risk ratio [RR]), and odds (odds ratio [OR]). The incidence and rates are determined by the numbers of new cases occurring over a time period. These processes may be represented by Poisson probability models.

TABLE 2.3 Epidemiologic Measures: Ratios, Proportions, and Rates

CONDITION	RATIO	PROPORTION	RATE
Morbidity (disease)	Risk ratio (RR; relative risk) Rate ratio Odds ratio (OR) Period prevalence	Attack rate (incidence proportion) Secondary attack rate Point prevalence Attributable proportion	Person-time incidence rate
Mortality (death)	Death-to-case ratio	Proportionate mortality	Crude mortality rate Case-fatality rate Cause-specific mortality rate Age-specific mortality rate Maternal mortality rate Infant mortality rate
Natality (birth)			Crude birth rate

TABLE 2.4   Estimation Methods Commonly Used for Epidemiologic Measures

MEASURE	LARGE SAMPLE	SMALL SAMPLE
One-sample	UMLE	MUE
Two-sample	UMLE	MUE, CMLE, SSAE

Abbreviations: CMLE = conditional maximum likelihood estimation; MUE = median unbiased estimation; SSAE = small-sample adjustment estimation; UMLE = unconditional maximum likelihood estimation.

Prevalence and risk may be estimated using proportions, represented by binomial probability models. The choice of the point estimation method depends on whether one estimates a one- or two-sample measure, on the sample size, and on the choice of methods (summarized in Table 2.4).

The odds ratio from a 2 × 2 table provides an example of unconditional maximum likelihood estimation (UMLE), conditional maximum likelihood estimation (CMLE), median unbiased estimation (MUE), and small-sample adjustment estimation (SSAE). Using the notation for a 2 × 2 table (Table 2.5), the UMLE odds ratio is the ratio of the disease odds for a cohort study, or the ratio of the exposure odds for a case–control study:

$$\text{Disease odds ratio} \equiv \text{DOR} = (A_1/B_1)/(A_0/B_0) = A_1 B_0/A_0 B_1 \tag{2.4-1}$$

$$\text{Exposure odds ratio} \equiv \text{EOR} = (A_1/A_0)/(B_1/B_0) = A_1 B_0/A_0 B_1 \tag{2.4-2}$$

$$\text{Hence, DOR} = \text{EOR} \tag{2.4-3}$$

Table 2.6 shows data from a cohort study of diarrhea in breast-fed infants infected with a strand of cholera bacteria. The occurrence of diarrhea was assessed by comparing infants whose conditions are indicated by lows versus highs of the sample dilutions of the antibody detected.

The UMLE disease odds ratio may then be calculated as follows:

$$\text{OR}_{\text{UMLE}} = (12/2)/(7/9) = (12)(9)/(7)(2) = 108/14 = 7.7143$$

This reveals that the odds of developing diarrhea were 7.7 times higher in infants with low-antibody titers compared to infants with high-antibody titers.

TABLE 2.5   Notations for a Crude 2 × 2 Table

	EXPOSED	UNEXPOSED	TOTAL
Cases	A_1	A_0	M_1
Noncases	B_1	B_0	M_0

TABLE 2.6 Comparison of Diarrhea in 30 Breast-Fed Infants Colonized With *Vibrio cholerae*, by Antibody Titers in Mother's Breast Milk

	ANTIBODY LEVEL		
	LOW	HIGH	TOTAL
Diarrhea	12	7	19
No diarrhea	2	9	11
Total	14	16	30

The CMLE OR calculation is obtained using the hypergeometric distribution for tables with small numbers, such as Table 2.5. In this case, one may treat the margins as fixed and model the distribution of A_1. The hypergeometric equation (Equation 2.4-4) is the basis of Fisher's exact test:

$$\Pr(A_1 = a_1 \mid m_1, m_0, n_1, n_0) = \frac{\binom{n_1}{a_1}\binom{n_0}{m_1 - k}OR^{a_1}}{\sum_k \binom{n_1}{k}\binom{n_0}{m_1 - k}OR^k} \qquad (2.4\text{-}4)$$

where k ranges over all possible values of A_1. The solution to the OR in Equation (2.4-4) is the CMLE OR.

In the R computation environment, one may use the special function fisher.test to calculate the CMLE OR with the result: $OR_{CMLE} = 7.17$.

The MUE OR is based on calculating exact lower and upper p-values. Using this hypergeometric example, the MUE OR satisfies Equation (2.4-4) when:

$$P_{lower} = P_{upper} = 0.5$$

or

$$0 = P_{lower} - P_{upper} \qquad (2.4\text{-}5)$$

With Equation (2.4-5), one can use the uniroot and fisher.test functions in R to compute the MUE OR, with the result: $OR_{MUE} = 6.88$.

Moreover, for both small and large samples, one may use simple functions in R to calculate an OR for a crude 2×2 table (Table 2.7).

TABLE 2.7 Summary of Odds Ratio Estimation Using Data From Table 2.5

METHOD	ODDS RATIO	COMMENT
Unconditional MLE	7.7	Large sample
Conditional MLE	7.2	Small sample
Median Unbiased Estimate	6.9	Small sample

NOTE:

(1) If the observed or expected number in any cell < 5, then use one of the small-sample methods for estimation (Rothman, 1976).
(2) If there is a zero in the denominator of a UMLE, then use Jewell's small-sample adjustment or similar mathematical treatments since division by zero is impossible (Rothman, 1976).

Analyzing Epidemiologic Data

An evening newscast reported a series of health-related items:

1. The increasing level of smog in an inner-city neighborhood was blamed for the increase in asthma attacks among the child and elderly populations.
2. A youth who had previously been diagnosed with type I diabetes (the insulin-dependent kind) had a significantly improved level of blood glucose control after undergoing a course of nonstandard medical treatment using traditional Chinese medicine.
3. The revised Federal Health Department recommendations for who should receive the flu vaccine this year.
4. A report on the extensive disease-monitoring strategies being implemented in a southern city recently affected by a massive hurricane.
5. A description of a finding recently published in a leading medical journal of an association between exposure to certain chemicals and an increased risk of cancer.

Each of these news stories included interviews with PH officials called *epidemiologists*. Their work, and the way EPDM is applied, are the main subjects of this book.

To begin with, epidemiologic investigations consider various health-related events, and take various measurements with the objectives of quantitatively relating causes and effects. To study any such cause–effect relations, one may begin by analyzing:

- One-sample measurements (measuring occurrence: rate, risk, and prevalence)
- Two-sample measurements (measuring associations: rate ratio, RR, and OR)

To analyze the events, one may consider:

1. The point estimate:
   - Measures of occurrence are one-sample measures.
   - Measures of association are two-sample measures.
2. The variability and precision of this estimate, using CIs
3. The reference value, calculating *p*-values and Type I errors
4. The differences from the references (effect size, power, and Type II errors)
5. The effective sample sizes:
   - To achieve a desired confidence interval width
   - To detect whether a one-sample measure differs from a reference value
   - To detect whether a two-sample measure differs from a reference value

The point estimate enables epidemiologic inferences, such as:

■ The risk of disease occurrence or the prevalence of a condition
■ The RR for development of disease among exposed persons compared to unexposed persons

The CI provides information on:

■ The variance of the estimate; the variance depends on the natural variability of the measure (e.g., weight and height in various populations)
■ Measurement random error (e.g., instrument, technician)
■ Sample size (increasing the sample size improves estimation precision and reduces the CI)

Often BIOS is used to determine whether a point estimate is consistent with a reference value. Assuming that the estimate comes from a distribution with the mean equal to the reference value (the null hypothesis), we can calculate the probability (two-sided p-value) of getting the test biostatistic value or more extreme values. If the null hypothesis is true, but it is incorrectly rejected because the p-value is lower than the arbitrarily chosen .05, then one has a Type I error.

If the point estimate is "consistent" ($p > \alpha$), one must then ask whether the sample size was sufficient to detect a meaningful difference, if one existed. One should avoid the mistake of inferring that there was no difference when the sample size was too small to support such a conclusion.

This requires defining what we mean by *meaningful difference*, and then calculating the probability of detecting the effective size (or larger), if it exists. This probability is the **biostatistical power** $(1 - \beta)$. An effective size implies an alternative hypothesis. The probability of failing to detect the effective size under the alternative hypothesis is designated as β. It is a Type II error.

If one decides to sample a population to estimate epidemiologic measures, the required sample size depends on whether the biostatistic is a one-sample measure (measures of occurrence) or a two-sample measure (measures of association). For a one-sample measure, one may use the following:

■ A sample size to achieve a desired CI width (used for descriptive studies).
■ A sample size for hypothesis testing (meaningful difference from some reference value). This requires setting Type I errors (α) and Type II errors (β).

ESTIMATION

This procedure was discussed earlier in this section. Additional features and methodologies are presented in the discussion of the R computational environment.

CONFIDENCE INTERVALS

The very useful concept of CIs was discussed in Section 2.3. Additional features and methodologies are presented in the discussion of the R computational environment.

HYPOTHESIS TESTING AND P-VALUES

A reasonable question in evaluating an epidemiologic measure is: "How compatible is the estimate r compared to some reference value?"

■ **Example:** If r proportion of patients suffered a serious relapse last year, and the future goal is to have not more than r_0 proportion experiencing a similar complication, how compatible is the experience r with a reference value of r_0?

To answer this, one may specify the null hypothesis:

$$r = r_0$$

For a given sample population, one may calculate the probability p of observing a value of r or greater under the null hypothesis:

$$p = P(r \geq r \mid r = r_0)$$

Because one is interested only in an *increase* in complications, a one-sided p-value is appropriate and adequate. If this p-value is high, then the estimate (r) is more compatible with the null hypothesis. This result means that values of r or more extreme are likely to occur by chance alone (a random error). However, if this p-value is low, then the estimate is less compatible with the null hypothesis; that is, values of r or more extreme are unlikely to occur by chance alone. High p-values (p-values more compatible with the null hypothesis) can occur because the null hypothesis is true, or because the sample size is too small to detect an alternative hypothesis (i.e., insufficient statistical power).

As with CIs, to calculate the p-value, one must either know or make assumptions about the relevant distribution. For example, suppose that 5% of hospital admissions resulted in serious relapses and the goal was to stay at or below a reference value of 2%. One should make certain that the observed 5% is compatible with the reference goal of 2% or lower. The one-sided p-value depends on the magnitude of the difference (5% vs. 2%) and number of hospitalizations:

(a) Calculate the binomial probability of the reference goal of 2%.
(b) Say that 5 out of 100 hospital admissions (5%) resulted in a serious relapse. Are 5 relapses compatible with the reference goal of 2% or less?

$$k = 5$$

$$n = 100$$

$$r = k/n = 5/100 = 0.05$$

$$r_0 = 2\% = 0.02$$

The required binomial probability is given by

$$p = P(r \geq r \mid r_0) = P (r \geq 0.05 \mid r_0 = 0.02) \tag{2.4-6}$$

To find probabilities from a binomial distribution, one may calculate them directly or use a binomial distribution calculator. To assess the compatibility, one may use a computer with the appropriate software—in this case, the R environment. Here, all

DIRECT CALCULATION. In general, if the random variable K follows the binomial distribution $B(n, p)$ with parameters n and p, one may write $K \sim B(n, p)$. The probability of getting exactly k successes in n trials is given by the probability mass function

$$f(k; n, p) = \Pr(K = k) = \binom{n}{k} p^k (1 - p)^{n-k} \tag{2.4-7}$$

for $k = 0, 1, 2, \ldots, n$, where

$$\binom{n}{k} = \frac{n!}{k!(n-k)!} \tag{2.4-8}$$

$$= {}_nC_k \tag{2.4-9}$$

Hence, using a handheld calculator and working to four decimal places,

$$\begin{aligned}
\Pr(k = 2) = f(2; 100, 0.05) &= {}_nC_k\, p^k (1 - p)^{n-k} \\
&= {}_{100}C_2\, (0.05)^2\, (1 - 0.05)^{100-2} \\
&= \{(100)(99)/(2)(1)\}(0.05)^2(0.95)^{98} \\
&= (4{,}950)\, (0.0025)\, (0.0066) \\
&= 0.0812
\end{aligned}$$

USING A BINOMIAL DISTRIBUTION CALCULATOR. The online binomial distribution calculator (available at http://stattrek.com/tables/binomial.aspx) may be used to compute individual and cumulative binomial probabilities:

▪ Enter a value in each of the first three text boxes.
▪ Click the **Calculate** button.
▪ The calculator will compute binomial and cumulative probabilities.

Probability of success on a single trial	0.05
Number of trials	100
Number of successes (x)	2
Binomial probability: P(X = 2)	0.08118177185776542
Cumulative probability: P(X < 2)	0.0370812093273546
Cumulative probability: P(X ≤ 2)	0.11826298118512
Cumulative probability: P(X > 2)	0.88173701881488
Cumulative probability: P(X ≥ 2)	0.88173701881488

Binomial probability $\Pr(k = 2) = 0.081181771\ldots$

When you reach Chapter 3 of this book, you may enter the R computing environment and use the R function binom.test() to obtain the following results:
> binom.test(5, 100, p = 0.02, alternative = "greater",
+ conf.level=0.05) # *Outputting:*

EXACT BINOMIAL TEST
data: 5 and 100,
number of successes = 5,
number of trials = 100,
p-value = .05083,
alternative hypothesis: true probability of success is greater than .02,
5% CIs [0.08919625, 1.00000000],
sample estimates: probability of success .05.

Also, the computer output shows that there is a 5.083% probability of observing five or more severe complications with 100 admissions. Is this compatible with 2%? There is no definitive answer, but if one had selected a significance level $\alpha = 0.05$, then one would conclude that "yes, it is compatible," because $p > .05$, and one does not reject the null hypothesis.

With the approach of merely increasing the sample size (i.e., the number of hospitalizations), the p-value becomes significant (less than .05), even if the magnitude of the difference remains the same (5% vs. 2%).

Later, by explicitly specifying what differences matter, one may handle this type of problem differently.

POWER

If β = the probability of failing to reject a false null hypothesis (i.e., a Type II error), then $(1 - \beta)$ is the probability of rejecting a false null hypothesis. Biostatisticians call this probability, $(1 - \beta)$, the **power** of the test. It is used to indicate the effectiveness of a test, reflecting that the null hypothesis is falsified.

In epidemiologic research design, it is common to plan experiments such that the expected power is 80% or greater, or the power 0.80 or greater, so that the investigation will be effective in rejecting a false null hypothesis.

SAMPLE SIZE CALCULATIONS FOR ANALYTIC STUDIES (TRIOLA & TRIOLA, 2006)

In hypothesis testing with sample data consisting of only a few observations, the power will be low. The power can be increased by:

- Increasing the sample size, with other factors remaining unchanged
- Increasing the significance level
- Increasing the standard deviation
- Using extreme values for the population parameters

Here are some examples on sample size calculations.

■ **Example 1:** In a given population, a sample is to be taken to allow accurate estima-

Solution:
The required sample size n may be estimated from

$$n = (z_{\alpha/2}\,\sigma/E)^2 \tag{2.4-10}$$

where:

$z_{\alpha/2}$ = critical z-score based on the desired confidence level,
σ = population standard deviation,
E = desired margin of error.

Remarks:
To arrive at the result given by Equation (2.4-10), the steps shown in the following subsections were taken.

STEP 1: STARTING WITH THE CLT[5]

In probability theory, the **CLT** states conditions under which the mean of a sufficiently large number of independent random variables, each with finite mean and variance, will be approximately normally distributed.

A simple example of the CLT is rolling a large number of identical, biased dice. The distribution of the sum (or average) of the rolled numbers will be well approximated by a normal distribution. Because real-world quantities are often the balanced sum of many unobserved random events, the CLT also provides a partial explanation for the prevalence of the normal probability distribution. It also justifies the approximation of large-sample BIOS to the normal distribution in controlled experiments.

The CLT has a number of variants. In its common form, the random variables must be identically distributed. In variants, convergence of the mean to the normal distribution also occurs for nonidentical distributions, given that they comply with conditions.

The CLT may be expressed in various forms, depending on the applicable situation. Two common forms are the classical CLT and the Lyapunov CLT.

CLASSICAL CLT. Let $X_1, X_2, X_3, ..., X_n$ be a random sample of size n—that is, a sequence of independent and identically distributed random variables with expected values μ and variances σ^2. Suppose that one is interested in the behavior of the sample average of these random variables: $S_n = (X_1 + X_2 + X_3, ..., + X_n)/n$. In this instance, the CLT says that as n gets larger, the *distribution* of S_n approaches the normal with mean μ and variance σ^2/n. The true strength of the theorem is its recognition that S_n approaches normality regardless of the shapes of the distributions of individual X_is.

LYAPUNOV CLT.[6] Let X_n, $n \in N$ = the set of natural numbers {1, 2, 3, ...}, be a sequence of independent random variables. Suppose that each X_n has a finite expected value

$$E[X_n] = \mu_n \tag{2.4-11}$$

[5] The CLT (retrieved from http://en.wikipedia.org/wiki/Central_limit_theorem).
[6] Lyapunov's CLT (retrieved from http://www.enotes.com/topic/Lyapunov's central limit

and finite variance

$$\text{Var}\,[X_n] = \sigma_n^{\,2} \tag{2.4-12}$$

Also, let

$$S_N^2 \equiv \sum_{n=1}^{N} \sigma_n^2 \tag{2.4-13}$$

If for *some* $\delta > 0$, the expected values $E[\,|\,Xk\,|^{2+\delta}]$ are finite for every $k \in N$, and the **Lyapunov's condition**

$$\lim_{n \to \infty} \frac{1}{S_n^{2+\delta}} \sum_{i=1}^{n} E\left[\left|X_i - \mu_i\right|^{2+\delta}\right] = 0 \tag{2.4-14}$$

is satisfied, then the CLT holds. That is, the random variable

$$Z_N := \frac{\sum_{n=1}^{N} (X_n - \mu_n)}{S_N} \tag{2.4-15}$$

converges in distribution to a standard normal random variable as $N \to \infty$ [i.e., $Z_N \to N(0, 1)$].

A useful special case of Lyapunov's condition is when $\delta = 1$.

Note: A vigorous proof of the CLT may be found in many classical texts on the theory of mathematical statistics. It is believed that the earliest discovery of CLT dates back to the scientist Laplace in 1776.

STEP 2: ESTIMATING A PROPORTION (LARGE SAMPLE)[7]

This method aims to construct a CI for a sample proportion p. The approach described here is valid under the following conditions:

- The sampling method is simple random sampling.
- The sample includes at least 5 to 10 successes and 5 to 10 failures.

THE VARIABILITY OF THE SAMPLE PROPORTION. To construct a CI for a sample proportion, one needs to know the variability of the sample proportion. This allows one to compute the *standard deviation and/or the standard error of the sampling distribution*.

Suppose that k possible samples of size n can be selected from the population. The standard deviation of the sampling distribution is the "average" deviation between the k sample proportions and the true population proportion, P. The standard deviation of the sample proportion σ_p is

$$\sigma_p = [\surd\{P(1 - P)/n\}] \times [\surd\{(N - n)/(N - 1)\}] \tag{2.4-16}$$

where P is the population proportion, n is the sample size, and N is the population size. When the population size is much larger (at least 10 times larger) than the sample size:

$$[\surd\{(N - n)/(N - 1)\}] \approx 1$$

7 Standard deviation of sample proportions (retrieved from http://stattrek.com/lesson4/proportion

the standard deviation can be approximated by

$$\sigma_p = \sqrt{\{P(1-P)/n\}} \qquad (2.4\text{-}17)$$

When the true population proportion P is *not* known, the standard deviation of the sampling distribution cannot be calculated. Under these circumstances, use the *standard error*. The standard error (SE) provides an unbiased estimate of the standard deviation. It can be calculated from Equation 2.4-18:

$$SE_p = [\sqrt{\{p(1-p)/n\}}] \times [\sqrt{\{(N-n)/(N-1)\}}] \qquad (2.4\text{-}18)$$

where p is the sample proportion, n is the sample size, and N is the population size.

When the population size is at least 10 times larger than the sample size, again $[\sqrt{\{(N-n)/(N-1)\}}] \approx 1$, and the standard error can be approximated by

$$SE_p = \sqrt{\{p(1-p)/n\}} = \sqrt{(pq/n)} \qquad (2.4\text{-}19)$$

where $q = 1 - p$.

STEP 3: THE CONCEPT OF THE CRITICAL VALUE (TRIOLA & TRIOLA, 2006)

Consider the use of a standard z-score that can be used to distinguish between sample BIOS that are likely to occur and those that are less likely or unlikely. This z-score is called a **critical value**, and is based on the following assumptions:

(a) Under certain conditions, the sampling distribution of sample proportions can be approximated by a normal distribution (whenever the CLT applies).

(b) Sample proportions have a relatively equal chance, with probability of α, of falling in one of the tails of the normal curve.

(c) Denoting each of the two tail areas by $\alpha/2$, it is seen that there is a total probability of $2(\alpha/2) = \alpha$ that a sample proportion will belong to one of these two tail areas.

(d) As their complements, there is therefore a probability of $(1 - \alpha)$ that a sample proportion will belong to the main (nontail) area.

(e) The z-score separating the right-tail region is denoted by $z_{\alpha/2}$ and is called its *critical value* because it marks the borderline separating sample proportions that are likely to occur from those that are not likely to occur.

Hence, one may define the critical value as follows: A **critical value** is the number on the borderline that separates sample BIOS that are likely to occur from those that are not likely to occur.

The number $z_{\alpha/2}$ is a critical value, which is a z-score such that it separates an area of $\alpha/2$ in the right tail of the standard normal distribution.

■ **Example:** The Critical Value $z_{\alpha/2}$ Using the z-Table

Corresponding to any confidence level, the critical value z may be obtained using the z-table.

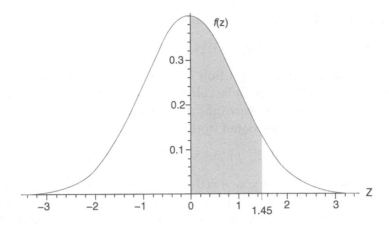

FIGURE 2.5 The standard normal curve and the critical value $z = 1.45$.

In the standard normal curve shown in Figure 2.5, the mean is 0 and the standard deviation is 1. In the diagram, the gray-shaded area represents the area that is within 1.45 standard deviations from the mean. The area of this shaded portion is 0.4265 (or 42.65% of the total area under the curve).

To get this area of 0.4265:

1. Read down the left side of the table for the standard deviation's first two digits (the whole number and the first number after the decimal point, in this case 1.4).
2. Read across the table for the "0.05" part (the top row represents the second decimal place of the standard deviation of interest).

z	0.00	0.01	0.02	0.03	0.04	0.05	0.06
1.4	0.4192	0.4207	0.4222	0.4236	0.4251	0.4265	0.4279

3. The result is (left column) 1.4 + (top row) 0.05 = 1.45 standard deviations.

The area represented by 1.45 standard deviations to the right of the mean is shaded in green in the standard normal curve in Figure 2.5.

The table in the appendix at the end of this chapter shows how to find the value of 0.4265 in the full z-table: Follow the "1.4" row across and the "0.05" column down until they meet at 0.4265.

■ **Example:** Using the z-Table to Find the Critical Value $z_{\alpha/2}$

In this example, we use the z-table to find the critical value $z_{\alpha/2}$ corresponding to a 95% confidence level.

A 95% confidence level corresponds to

$$\alpha = 1 - (95\%/100\%) = 1 - 0.95 = 0.05$$

and

$$\alpha/2 = 0.05/2 = 0.0250$$

corresponds to the critical value of $z_{\alpha/2}$—a half-area under the standard normal distribution curve of

$$0.0500 - 0.0250 = 0.4750.$$

STEP 4: THE CONCEPT OF THE MARGIN OF ERROR (TRIOLA & TRIOLA, 2006)

When data collected from a random sample are used to estimate a population proportion p, the **margin of error** E is the maximum likely difference between the observed sample proportion $\underline{p}$ and the true population proportion p, with probability $(1 - \alpha)$. E may be obtained by multiplying the critical value and the standard deviation of sample proportions:

$$E = z\alpha/2\,\sqrt{(\underline{pq}/n)} \qquad (2.4\text{-}20)$$

This is based upon the following assumptions.

Assumption 1: Since both the conditions $np \geq 5$ and $nq \geq 5$ are satisfied, the sampling distribution of proportions is approximately normal. Thus, one may use results from another assumption regarding the normal distribution (again for these conditions, when working with binomial distributions): namely, that the binomial random variable has a probability distribution that can be approximated as a normal distribution with the mean μ and standard deviation σ given by

$$\mu = np \qquad (2.4\text{-}21)$$

and

$$\sigma = \sqrt{(npq)} \qquad (2.4\text{-}22)$$

Both these parameters are based on n trials. Thus, their values on a per-trial basis may be obtained, by dividing by n, as follows:

$$\text{Mean of sample proportions } \mu = (\mu \text{ for } n \text{ trials})/n = np/n = p \qquad (2.4\text{-}23)$$

This is the *standard deviation of sample proportions:*

$$\sigma = (\sigma \text{ for } n \text{ trials})/n = [\sqrt{(npq)}]/n = \sqrt{(pq/n)} \qquad (2.4\text{-}24)$$

STEP 5: USING THE MARGIN OF ERROR RULE

Using the margin of error rule, Equation (2.4-20), with the further assumption of
$p = $ **Population** probability to be approximated by **Sample** probability $= \underline{p}$

$$p \approx \underline{p}, \text{ and } q \approx \underline{q}$$

so that Equation (2.4-24) becomes

$$\sqrt{(\underline{pq})} \approx \sigma\,\sqrt{(n)} \qquad (2.4\text{-}25)$$

and Equation (2.4-20) becomes

$$E = z_{\alpha/2}\,\sqrt{(\underline{pq}/n)} \qquad (2.4\text{-}26)$$

$$E = z_{\alpha/2}\,\sqrt{(\underline{pq})}/\sqrt{n}$$

$$= z_{\alpha/2}\,\sigma\,\sqrt{(n)}/n$$

$$E = z_{\alpha/2}\,\sigma/\sqrt{(n)} \qquad (2.4\text{-}27)$$

STEP (6) FINDING THE REQUIRED SAMPLE SIZE

Finally, Equation (2.4-27) shows that the required sample size

$$n = (z_{\alpha/2}\, \sigma/E)^2 \tag{2.4-28}$$

depends on:

- The critical score $z_{\alpha/2}$, which is based on the required confidence level
- The population standard deviation σ
- The required margin of error E

Remarks:

1. Equation (2.4-28) may not yield a whole number for n, in which case, apply the following **round-off rule**: *Always increase the value of the sample size n to the next larger whole number.*
2. When using Equation (2.4-28), note that it requires the value of the population standard deviation σ, which is usually unknown. The following methods may be used to overcome this problem:
   (a) Estimate the standard deviation σ using the range rule of thumb as follows: $\sigma \approx \text{range}/4$.
   (b) Conduct a pilot study by starting the sampling process. From the first collection of 30 or more randomly selected sample values, calculate the sample standard deviation s, and then use s in place of σ. As more sample data are collected, the estimated value of σ may be improved.
3. Use the results of other studies to estimate the value of σ.
4. When calculating the sample size n, errors should be conservative; having n too large will give more accurate results than having it too small. For example, doubling the margin of error results in decreasing the sample size to one quarter of its original value. Conversely, halving the margin of error increases the sample-size value fourfold.

■ **Example:** The Epidemiology of Epidemiologists

It should be obvious by now that epidemiologists are highly intelligent professionals, each with a high IQ. IQ tests are designed so that the mean is 100 and the standard deviation is 15. Therefore, it is expected that epidemiologists will have IQ scores with mean greater than 100 and standard deviation less than 15, as they are a more intellectually homogeneous group than the average population. To determine the mean IQ for the population of epidemiologists, one would like to know:

How many epidemiologists must be randomly chosen for IQ testing, if one wants 90%, 95%, or 99% confidence that the sample mean is within 5 IQ points of the population mean?

Solution:
Using Equation (2.4-28),

$$n = (z_{\alpha/2}\, \sigma/E)^2$$

the values required for calculating the sample size n are determined as follows:

These are found by converting the 90/95/99% confidence levels to α = 0.10/0.05/0.01, respectively, and then finding the critical value $z_{\alpha/2}$, as shown in Step 3.

Set $E = 2$. This is chosen so that the sample mean will be within 2 IQ units of the mean μ, and makes the required margin of error 2.

$\sigma = 15$. This is specified in the statement of the problem.

With these values, one can now use Equation (2.4-28) to calculate n:

$$n = (z_{\alpha/2} \, \sigma/E)^2 = \{(1.645 \text{ or } 1.960 \text{ or } 2.575)(15)/2\}^2$$

$$= 152.21/216.09/372.97$$

which round off to 153, 217, or 373, respectively.

So, if one can find a random sample of 217 epidemiologists, and obtain the IQ of each, one may have a 95% confidence level that the sample mean $\underline{x}$ will be within 2 IQ units of the true population mean. If only 153 epidemiologists can be located, settle for the 90% confidence level. But if 373 epidemiologists can be found, then go all out for the 99% confidence level. (Care to try any of that?)

Using R

Of course, one can use the R environment to run this computation as follows:
```
>
> # IQ Testing of Epidemiologists
> # 90/95/99 % Confidence Levels Computation
> # Computing n = the required Sample Sizes of Case-subjects
>
> z <- c(1.645, 1.960, 2.575) # z is being entered as a 3-vector
> E <- 2
> s <- 15
> n <- (z*s/E)**2
> n # Outputting the 3 corresponding Sample Sizes:
[1] 152.2139 216.0900 372.9727
>
```
Using R, you can obtain the same results in a single run.

■ **Example:** Using an Online Sample Size Table or Calculator

Numerous computing tools are available online. Some examples are:

Using tables: www.itl.nist.gov/div898/handbook/prc/section2/prc222.htm
Using a calculator: http://statisticslectures.com/topics/samplesizepopulationmean

Evaluating a Single Measure of Occurrence (Virasakdi, 2011)

Generally, the probability of encountering a significant epidemiologic event is very small. Therefore, instead of probability, measurement is focused on **density**, which means incidence or the number of occurrences over a period of time. Time is only one dimension: the same concept applies to the density of counts of small objects in

When events are independent from another, the occurrence is at random. Mathematically, it can be proven that under this condition, the densities in different units of time vary with a variance equal to the average density. When the probability of having an event is affected by some factors, a model may be used to explain, analyze, and predict the density. Variation among different strata is explained by the factors. Within each stratum, the distribution is random.

Poisson Count (Incidence) and Rate Data

Poisson regression deals with outcome variables that are counts in nature (whole numbers or integers). Independent covariates are similar to those encountered in linear and logistic regression.

In EPDM, Poisson regression is used for analyzing grouped cohort data, looking at incidence density among person-time contributed by subjects of similar characteristics of interest. It is one of three commonly used generalized linear models (GLMs):

- Poisson regression
- Linear regression
- Logistic regression

There are two main assumptions for Poisson regression:

First, risk is homogeneous among person-times contributed by different subjects who have the same characteristics of interest (e.g., gender, age group, etc.) and the same period.

Second, asymptotically (i.e., as the sample size increases), the mean of the counts is equal to the variance.

The Poisson distribution is a discrete probability distribution with the following density function:

$$P(X = x) = \frac{x^{-\lambda} \lambda^x}{x!} \tag{2.4-29}$$

where X is the random variable, x is the observed count, and λ is the *expected count*. The distribution function is

$$P(X \le x) = \sum_{k=0}^{x} \frac{K^{-\lambda} \lambda^k}{k!} \tag{2.4-30}$$

Binomial Risk and Prevalence Data (Lachin, 2011)

BINOMIAL RISK

In epidemiologic research, a typical data structure consists of n independent and identically distributed (iid) observations $\{x_i\}$ from a sample of n case subjects ($i = 1, 2, 3, \ldots, n$) drawn at random from a population with probability p of a characteristic

Thus, X is a binary variable such that:

$$x_i = I\{\text{positive response for the } i\text{th observation}\}$$

where I{.} is the indicator function: I{.} = 1, if true, or = 0 if not.

The total number of case subjects in the sample with a positive response is $y = \sum_i x_i$, and the simple proportion with a positive response in the sample is $p = y/n$. In such cases, the binomial distribution probability model is usually the model of choice for analysis of the data; hence, **binomial risk** is introduced.

PREVALENCE DATA

The **prevalence** of a characteristic is the probability P that the characteristic appears in the population, or the proportion p in a sample, with that characteristic present in a cross-section of the population at a specific time. For example, the prevalence of adult-onset type 2 diabetes as of 1980 was estimated to be about 6.8% of the U.S. population based on the National Health and Nutrition Examination Survey. Half of those who met the criteria for diabetes on an oral glucose tolerance test (3.4%) were previously undiagnosed. In that study, n is the total sample size of which y have the positive characteristic, in this instance type 2 diabetes.

The **incidence** of an event (the positive characteristic) is the probability P in the population, or the proportion p in a sample, that acquire the positive characteristic or experience an event over an interval of time among those who were free of the characteristic at baseline. In this case, n is the sample size at risk in a prospective longitudinal follow-up study of whom y experience the event over a period of time. For example, from the annual National Health Interview survey, it was estimated that the incidence of a new diagnosis of diabetes among adults in the U.S. population is 2.42 new cases per 1,000 in the population per year.

Such estimates of the prevalence of a characteristic, or the incidence of an event of interest, are generally simple proportions based on a sample of n iid observations.

Evaluating Two Measures of Occurrence—Comparison of Risk: Risk Ratio and Attributable Risk

To compare the risk of disease in different exposure groups, two methods may be used:

1. **Risk ratio (RR;** also called **relative risk)** is the *ratio* of the risk of getting the disease among the exposed compared with that among the unexposed. It indicates how many times the risk would increase if the subject changed his or her status from unexposed to exposed. The increment is considered in multiples or "-fold," and therefore RR is a multiplicative model.
2. **Risk difference (RD)** measures the *amount* of risk gained or lost if the subject changes from unexposed to exposed. The increase is absolute, and therefore RD is an *additive* model.

RR is an important indicator for causation. An RR greater than or equal to 10 strongly suggests a causal relationship. However, RD has more public health implications than the RR. A high RR may not be of public health importance if the disease is very rare. However, the RD measures direct health burden and the need for health services.

For example, the risk of developing lung cancer among the exposed (e.g., smokers) is l higher than that among the unexposed (e.g., nonsmokers). In this situation, the RD changes sign from positive to negative. The RR reciprocates to a small value.

The RR increases as the dose (time) of exposure to smoking increases.

DOSE–RESPONSE RELATIONSHIP

A criterion for causation is evidence of a dose–response relationship. If a higher dose of exposure is associated in a linear fashion with a higher level of risk, then the exposure is likely to be the cause.

Comparing Two Rate Estimates: Rate Ratio *rr*

Suppose that we have a cohort study that yields binomial data in the format shown in Table 2.8.

The corresponding rate ratio *rr* relations are

$$\text{rate ratio } rr \equiv r_1/r_0 = (a/PT_1)/(b/PT_0) \tag{2.4-31}$$

Comparing Two Risk Estimates: Risk Ratio *RR* and Disease (Morbidity) Odds Ratio *DOR*

A cohort study yields binomial data in the format shown in Table 2.9.

The corresponding risk ratio *RR* relations are

$$\text{Risk ratio } RR \equiv R_1/R_0 = (a/N_1)/(b/N_0) \tag{2.4-32}$$

$$\text{Disease Odds Ratio } DOR \equiv \frac{R_1 / (1 - R_1)}{R_0 / (1 - R_0)}$$

$$= \frac{(a / N_1) / (1 - a / N_1)}{(b / N_0) / (1 - b / N_0)}$$

$$= \frac{a(N_0 - b)}{b(N_1 - a)} \tag{2.4-33}$$

TABLE 2.8   **Table Notation for Cohort Study, Person-Time Data**

	EXPOSED	UNEXPOSED	TOTAL
Number of new cases	*a*	B	M
Person-time at risk	PT_1	PT_0	T

TABLE 2.9   Cohort Study, Binomial Data

	EXPOSED	UNEXPOSED
Number of new cases	a	b
Person at risk	N_1	N_0

ODDS AND OR

The concept of odds is related to probability: If p is the probability, then $p/(1\ p)$ is the **odds**. Conversely, the probability p would be equal to *odds/(odds + 1)*.

DISEASE (MORBIDITY) OR/RATES

In PH studies, rates are used to describe the likelihood of an event, to monitor the health status of a population, and so on. Usually, a time interval of 1 year is used to describe these rates.

A *rate* is the frequency of occurrence of a significant event. It is the relative frequency of the event multiplied by some number, typically a value such as 1,000 or 100,000. The rate is expressed as $(x/y)k$, where:

x = frequency count of the number of subjects for whom the event occurred,
y = total number of people exposed to the risk of the occurring event,
k = a number such as 1,000 or 100,000.

This definition may be applied to measures of, for example, mortality (deaths), morbidity (diseases), and fertility (births). In these instances, k is usually taken as 1,000.

■ **Example of Mortality Rate:** In the United States in a particular year, there were 2,416,000 deaths in a population of 285,318,000. What is the crude mortality rate?

Solution: The crude mortality rate = $(2,416,000/285,318,100) \times 1,000 = 8.4677$. This is rounded off to a mortality rate of 8.5 deaths for each 1,000 people in the population.

■ **Example of Infant Mortality Rate:** In a recent year, in the United States there were 4,026,000 live births and 27,500 deaths of infants under 1 year of age. What is the infant mortality rate?

Solution: The infant mortality rate = $(27,500/4,026,000) \times 1,000 = 6.8306$. This is rounded off to an infant mortality rate of 6.8 per 1,000 infants under 1 year of age. This is substantially lower than the infant mortality rate of more than 35 per 1,000 in some countries.

Comparing Two Odds Estimates From Case–Control: The Salk Polio Vaccine Epidemiologic Study

In one of the most renowned epidemiologic investigations (Triola & Triola, 2006), it was found that of 200,745 children receiving the Salk vaccine, 33 developed paralyzing poliomyelitis. Hence, for this treatment group:

$$P(\text{polio}) = 33/200{,}745 = 0.000{,}163{,}9$$

This single measure does not tell the whole story, because this measure carries no information about the rate of polio for those who were given a placebo shot. *The risk of polio for children treated with the Salk vaccine should be compared to the risk of polio for those given a placebo.* Now consider the data for that investigation summarized in Table 2.10.

Based on Table 2.10, one can calculate the following probabilities:

Polio rate for treatment group = $P(\text{polio}/\text{vaccine})$
= $33/200{,}745 = 0.000{,}163{,}9 = p_1$

Polio rate for placebo group = $P(\text{polio}/\text{placebo})$
= $115/200{,}229 = 0.000{,}574{,}3 = p_2$

The RR, or the relative risk, is

$$p_1/p_2 = 0.000{,}163{,}9/0.000{,}574{,}3 = 0.285{,}4$$

The **reciprocal risk ratio** = $1/0.285{,}4 = 3.504$, which means that the placebo group is 3.504 times more likely to suffer polio.

Review Questions for Section 2.4

1. (a) Name five areas of epidemiologic investigation in which BIOS is used for data analyses.
   (b) Research epidemiologists frequently publish their findings in professional journals. List five journals in which their work is often found.
2. (a) Name five epidemiologic measures of occurrence and association.
   (b) How does one obtain these measures in PH investigations?
3. (a) In epidemiologic research, what are one-sample measurements? Give an example of each.
   (b) What are two-sample measurements? Give examples.
4. (a) What are the following epidemiologic measures: ratios, proportions, and rates? Give examples of each.
   (b) What are the commonly used estimation methods for epidemiologic measures? Give examples.

TABLE 2.10 **Epidemiologic Investigation of Poliomyelitis and the Salk Vaccine**

TREATMENT	POLIO	NO POLIO	TOTAL
Salk vaccine	33	200,712	200,745

5. (a) What are the CIs in epidemiologic estimation of sample sizes? Give an example.
    (b) Using null hypothesis testing, how may one determine the CIs corresponding to a prescribed confidence level?
6. (a) What is biostatistical power?
    (b) How is this power related to the sample size of an epidemiologic investigation? Give an example.
7. (a) What is the central limit theorem (CLT) in mathematical statistics?
    (b) How does it contribute to the process for estimating the required sample size in an epidemiologic investigation? Give an example.
8. (a) Briefly explain the concepts of binomial risk and prevalence, and give an example of each.
    (b) Contrast the concepts of RR and risk difference, and give an example of each.
9. (a) Describe the use of odds and OR, giving an example of each.
    (b) In the comparison of risks, what are an attributable risk and its RR?
10. (a) What is meant by mortality rate, infant mortality rate, and fertility rate? Give an example of each.
    (b) In a case–control epidemiologic investigation, what is the RR (or the relative risk) and the reciprocal risk ratio? Give an example.

EXERCISES FOR CHAPTER 2 (CDC, 2006; BROADBENT, 2011)

Using Probability Theory

1. In each of the following situations, express the indicated degree of likelihood as a probability value:
    (a) The weather forecast says there is a 25% chance of snow tomorrow.
    (b) In guessing the answer for the five options in a multiple-choice test question, one has less than a 50-50 chance of success.
    (c) One has no more than 1 chance in 10 million of winning the lottery.
    (d) The sun will rise tomorrow morning.
    (e) In rolling two dice (each die is six-sided), there is 1 chance in 36 to get a pair of sixes.
2. A married couple has four children. What is the probability of each of the following outcomes?
    (a) All four are girls.
    (b) All four are boys.
    (c) Three girls and a boy.
    (d) One girl and three boys.
    (e) Two girls and two boys.

Disease Symptoms in Clinical Drug Trials

3. A group of 937 case subjects was given a trial drug in a clinical treatment of obesi-

     (a) What is the probability that a case subject taking the test drug will have the symptom of fever?

     (b) Would it be considered normal for an individual taking the same drug to experience fever? Why or why not?

Risks and Odds in Epidemiology

4. Use the data summarized in Table 2.10 (Epidemiologic Investigation of Poliomyelitis and the Salk Vaccine) to calculate:

     (a) the absolute risk reduction that may be used to assess the effectiveness of the Salk vaccine

     (b) the relative risk

     Explain in words what is meant by each calculated result.

Case–Control Epidemiologic Study

5. In a case–control study of the effectiveness of bicycle safety helmets for the prevention of facial injuries, the data are summarized in the following table:

	HELMET WORN	HELMET NOT WORN
Facial injuries received	30	182
All nonfacial injuries	83	236

     (a) Calculate the value of absolute risk reduction for facial injuries in the two groups.

     (b) For those not wearing helmets, what are the odds for facial injuries?

     (c) What is the OR for facial injuries in the group that did not wear helmets compared to the group that wore helmets? What does this ratio mean?

     (d) Does wearing a helmet decrease the risk of facial injuries? How do you know?

     (e) What is the risk ratio of facial injuries for those wearing helmets? What is the risk ratio for those not wearing helmets? Is it reasonable to make helmet wearing a legal requirement? Why or why not?

Mortality, Morbidity, and Fertility Rates

7. In a certain year in the United States, the following epidemiologic BIOS were taken:

Population: 285,318,000   Deaths: 2,416,000
Live births: 4,026,000   Infant deaths: 27,500
Women aged 15–44: 61,811,000   HIV-infected persons: 900,000
Deaths from HIV infection: 17,402   Motor vehicle deaths: 43,900

     (a) What is the infant mortality rate?

     (b) What is the birth rate?

     (c) What is the HIV mortality rate for HIV-infected persons?

(d) What is the general fertility rate?
(e) Using $k = 100,000$, calculate the motor vehicle death incidence rate.

Incidence Rates in Case-Cohort Survival Analysis

8. A team of epidemiologic investigators enrolled 4,200 women in a study and followed them annually for 4 years to determine the incidence rate of heart disease.
   - After 1 year, none had a new diagnosis of heart disease, but 200 had been lost to follow-up.
   - After 2 years, 1 had a new diagnosis of heart disease, and another 198 had been lost to follow-up.
   - After 3 years, another 7 had new diagnoses of heart disease, and 1,586 had been lost to follow-up.
   - After 4 years, another 8 had new diagnoses of heart disease, and 784 more had been lost to follow-up.

   Calculate the incidence rate of heart disease among this cohort. Assume that persons with new diagnoses of heart disease and those lost to follow-up were disease-free for half the year, and thus contribute ½ year to the denominator.

9. A diabetes follow-up study included 218 diabetic women and 3,823 nondiabetic women. By the end of the study, 72 of the diabetic women and 511 of the nondiabetic women had died. The diabetic women were observed for a total of 1,862 person-years; the nondiabetic women were observed for a total of 36,653 person-years. Calculate the incidence rates of death for the diabetic and nondiabetic women.

Prevalence

10. In a study of 1,150 women who gave birth, a total of 468 reported taking a prescribed dose of vitamins at least 4 times a week during the month before becoming pregnant. Calculate the prevalence of frequent vitamin use in this group.

Mortality Rates

11. Table 2.11 provides the number of deaths from all causes and from accidents (unintentional injuries) by age group in 2002 in the United States.
    (a) Calculate the following mortality rates:
        (i) The unintentional-injury-specific mortality rate for the entire population
        (ii) The all-cause mortality among males
        (iii) The all-cause mortality rate for 25- to 34-year-olds
        (iv) The unintentional-injury-specific mortality among 25- to 34-year-old males
    (b) Suggest what to call each mortality rate.

TABLE 2.11 All-Cause and Unintentional Injury Mortality and Estimated Population by Age Group, for Both Genders and for Males Alone, United States, 2002

AGE GROUP (YEARS)	ALL RACES, BOTH SEXES			ALL RACES, MALES		
	ALL CAUSES	UNINTENTION-AL INJURIES	ESTIMATED POP. (X 1000)	ALL CAUSES	UNINTEN-TIONAL INJURIES	ESTIMATED POP. (X 1000)
0–4	32,892	2,587	19,597	18,523	1,577	10,020
5–14	7,150	2,718	41,037	4,198	1,713	21,013
15–24	33,046	15,412	40,590	24,416	11,438	20,821
25–34	41,355	12,569	39,928	28,736	9,635	20,203
35–44	91,140	16,710	44,917	57,593	12,012	22,367
45–54	172,385	14,675	40,084	107,722	10,492	19,676
55–64	253,342	8,345	26,602	151,363	5,781	12,784
65+	1,811,720	33,641	35,602	806,431	16,535	14,772
Not Stated	357	85	0	282	74	0
Total	2,443,387	106,742	288,357	1,199,264	69,257	141,656

Source: Web-based Injury Statistics Query and Reporting System (WISQARS) [online database] Atlanta; National Center for Injury Prevention and Control. Available from: http://www.cdc.gov./ncipc/wisqars.

Estimating Sample Sizes

12. Finite Population Correction Factor for CI:
For an **infinite** population, the standard error of the mean = $\sigma/\sqrt{n}$
For a **finite** population N, one must apply the correction factor $\sqrt{\{(N - n)/(n - 1)\}}$, whenever n > 0.05N. This factor should be applied in Equation (2.4-27):

$$E = z_{\alpha/2}\, \sigma /\sqrt{(n)} \tag{2.4-27}$$

so that the margin of error will be given by

$$E = \{z_{\alpha/2}\, \sigma /\sqrt{(n)}\} \sqrt{\{(N - n)/(n - 1)\}} \tag{2.4-34}$$

Find the 95% CI for the mean of the IQ scores taken for 1,000 epidemiologists, if 40 of these scores produced a mean of 120. Assume that $\sigma = 15$.

13. Finite Population Correction Factor for Sample Size:
In Equation (2.4-27), it was assumed that the population is infinite or very large, and that the sampling was undertaken *with replacement*. However, if the population is small, and the sampling was undertaken *without replacement*, one should modify the margin of error E to include a finite population correction factor so that E is to be given by Equation (2.4-34). Solving this equation for *n*, one obtains:

Repeat the preceding Example: The Epidemiology of Epidemiologists, assuming that the epidemiologists are randomly selected *without replacement* from a population of *N* = 300 reputable epidemiologists.

REFERENCES

Aragon, T. J. (2011). *Applied epidemiology using R* (epir). Berkeley, CA: University of California, Berkeley, School of Public Health & San Francisco Department of Public Health.

Broadbent, A. (2011). Inferring causation in epidemiology: Mechanisms, black boxes, and contrasts. In P.M. Illari, F. Russo, & J. Williamson (Eds.), *Causality in the sciences.* Oxford, UK: Oxford University Press. Retrieved from http://www.hps.cam.ac.uk/people/broadbent/epidemiology_mechanisms_inference.pdf

Ephron, E. (1984). *Apocalyptics: Cancer and the big lie—How environmental politics controls what we know about cancer.* New York, NY: Simon & Schuster.

Hill, A. B. (1965). The environment and disease: Association or causation. *Proceedings of the Royal Society of Medicine, 58,* 295–300.

Horwitz, R. I., & Feinstein, A. R. (1978). Alternative analytic methods for case-control studies of estrogens and endometrial cancer. *New England Journal of Medicine, 299,* 1089–1094.

Lachin, J. M. (2011). *Biostatistical methods: The assessment of relative risks* (Wiley Series in Probability and Statistics). Hoboken, NJ: John Wiley & Sons.

Loma Linda University, School of Public Health. (2012). *Programs in EPDM.* Retrieved from http://www.llu.edu/public-health/programs/mph-epdm-track2-research.page

Paoli, B., Haggard, L., & Shah, G. (2002). *Confidence intervals in public health.* Utah, UT: Utah Office of Public Health Assessment. Retrieved from http://health.utah.gov/opha/IBIShelp/ConfInts.pdf

Rothman, K. J. (1976). Causes. *American Journal of Epidemiology, 104,* 587–592.

Rothman, K. J. (1998). *Modern epidemiology.* Boston, MA: Lippincott Williams & Wilkins.

Rothman, K. J. (2002). *Epidemiology: An introduction.* New York, NY: Oxford University Press.

Rothman, K. J., & Greenland, S. (2005). Causation and causal inference in epidemiology. *American Journal of Public Health, 95*(Supp. 1), S1, S144–S150.

Steiger, J. H. (2015). *A basic introduction to statistical inference.* Retrieved from http://www.stat-power.net/Content/310/A Basic Introduction to Statistical Inference.pdf

Triola, M. M., & Triola, M. F. (2006). *Biostatistics for the biological and health sciences.* Boston, MA: Pearson/Addison Wesley.

U.S. Department of Health and Human Services, Centers for Disease Control and Prevention (CDC), Office of Workforce and Career Development. (2006). *Principles of epidemiology in public health practice: An introduction to applied epidemiology and biostatistics* (Self-Study Course SS1000, 3rd ed.). Atlanta, GA: Author.

University of Sydney, Australia, School of Public Health Program. (2012). Retrieved from http://sydney.edu.au/medicine/public-health/future-student/study-program/coursework-degrees/clinical-epidemiology-structure.php

Virasakdi, C. (2011). *Analysis of epidemiological data using R and Epicalc.* Epidemiology Unit, Prince of Songkla University, Thailand. Retrieved from cvirasak@medicine.psu.ac.th

APPENDIX

The z-Table for a Standard Normal Distribution

z	0.00	0.01	0.02	0.03	0.04	0.05	0.06	0.07	0.08	0.09
0.0	0.0000	0.0040	0.0080	0.0120	0.0160	0.0199	0.0239	0.0279	0.0319	0.0359
0.1	0.0398	0.0438	0.0478	0.0517	0.0557	0.0596	0.0636	0.0675	0.0714	0.0753
0.2	0.0793	0.0832	0.0871	0.0910	0.0948	0.0987	0.1026	0.1064	0.1103	0.1141
0.3	0.1179	0.1217	0.1255	0.1293	0.1331	0.1368	0.1406	0.1443	0.1480	0.1517
0.4	0.1554	0.1591	0.1628	0.1664	0.1700	0.1736	0.1772	0.1808	0.1844	0.1879
0.5	0.1915	0.1950	0.1985	0.2019	0.2054	0.2088	0.2123	0.2157	0.2190	0.2224
0.6	0.2257	0.2291	0.2324	0.2357	0.2389	0.2422	0.2454	0.2486	0.2517	0.2549
0.7	0.2580	0.2611	0.2642	0.2673	0.2704	0.2734	0.2764	0.2794	0.2823	0.2852
0.8	0.2881	0.2910	0.2939	0.2967	0.2995	0.3023	0.3051	0.3078	0.3106	0.3133
0.9	0.3159	0.3186	0.3212	0.3238	0.3264	0.3289	0.3315	0.3304	0.3365	0.3389
1.0	0.3413	0.3438	0.3461	0.3485	0.3508	0.3531	0.3554	0.3577	0.3599	0.3621
1.1	0.3643	0.3665	0.3686	0.3708	0.3729	0.3749	0.3770	0.3790	0.3810	0.3830
1.2	0.3849	0.3869	0.3888	0.3907	0.3925	0.3944	0.3962	0.3980	0.3997	0.4015
1.3	0.4032	0.4049	0.4066	0.4082	0.4099	0.4115	0.4131	0.4147	0.4162	0.4177
1.4	0.4192	0.4207	0.4222	0.4236	0.4251	0.4265	0.4279	0.4292	0.4306	0.4319
1.5	0.4332	0.4345	0.4357	0.4370	0.4382	0.4394	0.4406	0.4418	0.4429	0.4441
1.6	0.4452	0.4463	0.4474	0.4484	0.4495	0.4505	0.4515	0.4525	0.4535	0.4545
1.7	0.4554	0.4564	0.4573	0.4582	0.4591	0.4599	0.4608	0.4616	0.4625	0.4633
1.8	0.4641	0.4649	0.4656	0.4664	0.4671	0.4678	0.4686	0.4693	0.4699	0.4706
1.9	0.4713	0.4719	0.4726	0.4732	0.4738	0.4744	0.4750	0.4756	0.4761	0.4767
2.0	0.4772	0.4778	0.4783	0.4788	0.4793	0.4798	0.4803	0.4808	0.4812	0.4817
2.1	0.4821	0.4826	0.4830	0.4834	0.4838	0.4842	0.4846	0.4850	0.4854	0.4857
2.2	0.4861	0.4864	0.4868	0.4871	0.4875	0.4878	0.4881	0.4884	0.4887	0.4890
2.3	0.4893	0.4896	0.4898	0.4901	0.4904	0.4906	0.4909	0.4911	0.4913	0.4916
2.4	0.4918	0.4920	0.4922	0.4925	0.4927	0.4929	0.4931	0.4932	0.4934	0.4936
2.5	0.4938	0.4940	0.4941	0.4943	0.4945	0.4946	0.4948	0.4949	0.4951	0.4952
2.6	0.4953	0.4955	0.4956	0.4957	0.4959	0.4960	0.4961	0.4962	0.4963	0.4964

2.7	0.4965	0.4966	0.4967	0.4968	0.4969	0.4970	0.4971	0.4972	0.4973	0.4974
2.8	0.4974	0.4975	0.4976	0.4977	0.4977	0.4978	0.4979	0.4979	0.4980	0.4981
2.9	0.4981	0.4982	0.4982	0.4983	0.4984	0.4984	0.4985	0.4985	0.4986	0.4986
3.0	0.4987	0.4987	0.4987	0.4988	0.4988	0.4989	0.4989	0.4989	0.4990	0.4990
3.1	0.4990	0.4991	0.4991	0.4991	0.4992	0.4992	0.4992	0.4992	0.4993	0.4993
3.2	0.4993	0.4993	0.4994	0.4994	0.4994	0.4994	0.4994	0.4995	0.4995	0.4995
3.3	0.4995	0.4995	0.4995	0.4996	0.4996	0.4996	0.4996	0.4996	0.4996	0.4997
3.4	0.4997	0.4997	0.4997	0.4997	0.4997	0.4997	0.4997	0.4997	0.4997	0.4998
3.5	0.4998	0.4998	0.4998	0.4998	0.4998	0.4998	0.4998	0.4998	0.4998	0.4998
3.6	0.4998	0.4998	0.4999	0.4999	0.4999	0.4999	0.4999	0.4999	0.4999	0.4999
3.7	0.4999	0.4999	0.4999	0.4999	0.4999	0.4999	0.4999	0.4999	0.4999	0.4999
3.8	0.4999	0.4999	0.4999	0.4999	0.4999	0.4999	0.4999	0.4999	0.4999	0.4999

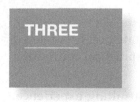

Data Analysis Using R Programming

THREE

INTRODUCTION

A job vacancy advertisement on the Internet for a biostatistician reads as follows:

Job Summary: Biostatistician I

Salary: Open

Employer: XYZ Research and Biostatistics

Location: City X, State Y

Type: Full Time—Entry Level

Category: Biometrics/biostatistics, Data analysis/processing, Statistical organization and administration

Required Education: Master's degree
XYZ Research and Biostatistics is a national leader in designing, managing, and analyzing cancer clinical trials. XYZ partners with clinical investigators to offer respected biostatistical expertise supported by sophisticated web-based data management systems. XYZ services assure timely and secure implementation of trials and reliable data analyses.

Job Description:
Position Summary: An exciting opportunity is available for a biostatistician to join a small but growing group focused on cancer clinical trials and related translational research. XYZ, which is located in downtown City XX, is responsible for the design, management, and analysis of a variety of phase I, phase II, and phase III cancer clinical trials, as well as the analysis of associated laboratory data, including microarray, SNP, and proteomics data. The successful candidate will collaborate with fellow biostatistics staff and clinical investigators to design, evaluate, and interpret clinical studies.

Primary Duties and Responsibilities: Analyzes clinical trials and associated ancillary studies in collaboration with fellow statisticians and other scientists. Prepares tables, figures, and written summaries of study results; interprets results in collaboration with other scientists; and assists in preparation of manuscripts. Provides statistical consultation with collaborating staff. Performs other job-related duties as assigned.

Requirements:

Required Qualifications: Master's degree in statistics, biostatistics, or a related field. Sound knowledge of applied statistics. Proficiency in statistical computing in SAS.

Preferred Responsibilities/Qualifications: Biostatistical consulting experience. S-Plus or R programming language experience. Experience with analysis of high-dimensional data. Ability to communicate well orally and in writing. Excellent interpersonal/teamwork skills for effective collaboration. Spanish-language skills a plus.

*In your cover letter, describe how your skills and experience match the qualifications for the position.

To learn more about XYZ, visit www.XYZ.org (American Statistical Association, n.d.).

Clearly, anyone planning a career in biostatistics should be cognizant of the overt requirement of an acceptable level of professional proficiency in data analysis using the R programming environment. Even if one is not a biostatistician working in the fields of epidemiology, public health, and preventive medicine, a skill set that includes R programming would be helpful.

3.1 DATA AND DATA PROCESSING

Data are facts or figures from which conclusions can be drawn. When the data have been recorded, classified and organized, related, and interpreted within a framework so that meaning emerges, they become **information**. There are several steps involved in turning data into information, and these steps are known as **data processing**. This section describes data processing and how computers perform these steps efficiently and effectively. Many of these processing activities may be undertaken using R programming or performed in an R environment with the aid of available R packages where R functions and datasets are stored.

The simplified flowchart that follows shows how raw data are transformed into information (Statistics Canada, 2013):

Data → Collection → Processing → Information

Data processing takes place once all of the relevant data have been collected. They are gathered from various sources and entered into a computer where they can be processed to produce **information**—the output.

Data processing includes the following steps, each of which will be discussed in the next sections:

- Data coding
- Data capture
- Editing
- Imputation
- Quality control

Data Coding

Before raw data can be entered into a computer, they must first be coded. To do this, survey responses must be labeled; usually simple, numerical codes are used. Labeling may be done by the interviewer in the field or by an office employee. The data-coding step is important because it makes data entry and data processing easier. Surveys use two types of questions: *closed* and *open*. The responses to these questions affect the type of coding performed. With a **closed question**, only a fixed number of predetermined survey responses are permitted. These responses already will have been coded. The following, drawn from a survey on sporting activities, is an example of a closed question:

> **To what degree are sports important in providing you with the following benefits?**
> <1/> Very important
> <2/> Somewhat important
> <3/> Not important

When **open questions** are used, any response is allowed, making subsequent coding more difficult. To code an open question, the processor must sample a number of responses and then design a code structure that includes all possible answers.

The following code structure is an example of an open question:

> **What sports do you participate in?**
> Specify (28 characters) _____

In the U.S. Census and almost all other surveys, the codes for each question field are premarked on the questionnaire. When the questionnaire is processed, the codes are entered directly into the database and prepared for data capturing. The following is an example of premarked coding:

> **What language does this person speak most often at home?**
> <18/> English
> <19/> French
> <20/> Other—Specify _____

AUTOMATED CODING SYSTEMS

Programs are available to automate repetitive and routine tasks. Some of the advantages of an automated coding system are that the process increasingly becomes faster, more consistent, and more economical.

The next step in data processing is inputting the coded data into a computer

Data Capture

Data capture is the process by which data are transferred from paper, such as questionnaires and survey responses, to an electronic file in a computer. Before this procedure takes place, the questionnaires must be *groomed* (prepared) for data capture. In this processing step, each questionnaire is reviewed to ensure that all of the minimum required data have been reported and that they are decipherable. Grooming is usually performed through extensive automated edits.

Several methods are used for capturing data:

- **Tally charts** are used to record data such as the number of occurrences of a particular event and to develop frequency distribution tables.
- **Batch keying** is one of the oldest methods of data capture; the data are input through a computer keyboard. This process is very practical for high-volume entry, where fast production is a requirement. No editing procedures are necessary, but there must be a high degree of confidence in the editing program.
- **Interactive capture** is often referred to as *intelligent keying*. Usually, captured data are edited before they are input. However, interactive capture combines data capture and data editing in one function.
- **Optical character readers** or **bar-code scanners** are able to recognize alpha or numeric characters or bar codes. These readers scan lines and translate them into the program. Bar-code scanners are quite common and often used in stores. They can take the shape of a handheld gun or a wand, as well as "pass-over" glass plates.
- **Magnetic recordings** have both reading and writing capabilities. Magnetic recording may be used in areas where data security is important. An important application for this type of data capture is the magnetic strip found on debit and credit cards.

A computer keyboard is one of the best-known input (or data entry) devices in current use. In the past, people performed data entry using punch cards or paper tape. Some other examples of modern data-input devices are:

- Optical mark reader
- Bar-code reader
- Scanner used in desktop publishing
- Light pen
- Trackball
- Mouse

Once data have been entered into a computer database, the next step is to ensure that all of the responses are accurate; this requires **data editing**.

Data Editing

Data should be edited before being presented as information. This action ensures that the information provided is accurate, complete, and consistent. There are two

Microediting corrects the data at the record level. This process detects errors in data through checks of the individual data records. The intent at this point is to determine the consistency of the data and correct the individual data records.

Macroediting also detects errors in data, but does so through the analysis of aggregate data (totals). The data are compared with data from other surveys, administrative files, or earlier versions of the same data. This process determines the compatibility of data.

Imputations

Editing adds little value to the overall improvement of the actual survey results if no corrective action is taken when items fail to follow the rules set out during the editing process. When all of the data have been edited using the applied rules and a file is found to have missing data, then **imputation** is usually done as a separate step.

Nonresponse and invalid data definitely affect the quality of the survey results. Imputation resolves the problems of missing, invalid, or incomplete responses identified during editing, as well as any editing errors that might have occurred. At this stage, all of the data are screened for errors because respondents are not the only ones capable of making mistakes; errors can also occur during coding and editing.

Some other types of imputation methods include the following:

- **Hot deck** uses other records as "donors" to answer the question (or a set of questions) that requires imputation.
- **Cold deck** uses a fixed set of values that cover all of the data items. These values can be constructed using historical data, subject-matter expertise, and so on.
- **Substitution** relies on the availability of comparable data. Imputed data can be extracted from the respondent's record from a previous cycle of the survey, or they can be taken from an alternative source file (e.g., administrative files or other survey files for the same respondent).
- **Estimator** uses information from other questions or from other answers (from the current cycle or a previous cycle), and through mathematical operations, it derives a plausible value for the missing or incorrect field.

Donor data can also be found through a method called **nearest neighbor imputation**. In this case, some sort of criterion must be developed to determine, in accordance with predetermined characteristics, which responding unit is "most like" the unit with the missing value. The closest unit to the missing value is then used as the donor.

Imputation methods can be performed automatically, manually, or in combination.

Data Quality

Quality is an essential element at all levels of processing. To ensure the quality of a product or service in survey development activities, both *quality assurance* and

QUALITY ASSURANCE

Quality assurance refers to all planned activities necessary to provide confidence that a product or service will satisfy its purpose and the users' needs. In the context of survey-conduct activities, quality assurance activities and checks may take place at any of the major stages of survey development: planning, design, implementation, processing, evaluation, and dissemination.

Quality assurance:

- Anticipates problems before they occur
- Uses all available information to generate improvements
- Is not tied to a specific quality standard
- Is applicable mostly at the planning stage
- Is all-encompassing in its activities

QUALITY CONTROL

Quality control is a regulatory procedure through which one:

- Measures quality
- Compares quality with preset standards
- Acts on the differences

Some examples of this include controlling the quality of the coding operation, the quality of the survey interviewing, and the quality of the data capture.

Quality control:

- Responds to observed problems
- Uses ongoing measurements to make decisions on the processes or products
- Requires a prespecified quality standard for comparison
- Is applicable mostly at the processing stage
- Is a set procedure that is a subset of quality assurance

QUALITY MANAGEMENT IN STATISTICAL AGENCIES

The quality of the data must be defined and assured in the context of being "fit for use"; this fitness will depend on the intended function of the data and the fundamental characteristics of quality. It also depends on the users' expectations and what they consider to be useful information.

There is no standard definition among statistical agencies for the term *official statistics*. There is a generally accepted, but evolving, range of quality issues underlying the concept of fitness for use. These elements of quality must be considered and balanced in the design and implementation of an agency's statistical program.

The following is a list of the elements of *quality*:

- Relevance
- Accuracy
- Timeliness
- Accessibility
- Interpretability

These elements of quality tend to overlap. Just as there is no single measure of accuracy, there is no effective statistical model for bringing together all these characteristics of quality into a single indicator. Also, except in simple or one-dimensional (1D) cases, there is no general statistical model for determining whether one particular set of quality elements provides higher overall quality than another.

Producing Results

After editing, data may be processed further to produce a desired output. The computer software used to process the data will depend on the form of output required. Software applications for word processing, desktop publishing, graphics (including graphing and drawing), programming, databases, and spreadsheets are commonly used. The following are some examples of ways that software can produce data:

- **Spreadsheets** are programs that automatically add columns and rows of figures, calculate means, and perform statistical analyses.
- **Databases** are electronic filing cabinets. They systematically store data for easy access and can produce summaries, aggregates, or reports. Relational databases make it easier to view and compare selected subsets of data.
- **Specialized programs** can be developed to edit, clean, impute, and process the final output.

Review Questions for Section 3.1

1. What basic statistical computing languages were noted as being important in the sample job description for an entry-level biostatistician? Why?
2. In a typical school of public health or school of medicine, should the core curriculum for a typical Master of Public Health program in epidemiology and public health, or for a degree in preventive medicine, include the development of proficiency in the use of R programming for biostatistics? Why or why not?
3. (a) Contrast the concepts of data and information.
   (b) How are data converted into information?
4. In the steps that convert data into information, how are statistics and computing applied to the various data processing steps?
5. (a) Describe and delineate quality assurance and quality control in computer data processing.
   (b) In what way does statistics feature in these phases of data processing?

3.2   BEGINNING R

R is an open-source, freely available, integrated software environment for data manipulation, computation, analysis, and graphical display. The R environment consists of:

- A data handling and storage facility

- A collection of tools for data analysis
- Graphical capabilities for analysis and display
- An efficient and continuously developing, algebra-like programming language that consists of loops, conditionals, user-defined functions, and input and output capabilities

The term *environment* is used to show that R is indeed a planned and coherent system (Aragon, 2011; Venables et al., 2004).

R and Biostatistics

R was initially written by **R**obert Gentleman and **R**oss Ihaka* of the Statistics Department of the University of Auckland, New Zealand, in 1997. Since then, an R development core group of about 20 people has write-access to the R source code.

The original R environment, evolved from the S/S-PLUS languages, was *not* primarily directed toward statistics and biostatistics. However, since its development in the 1990s, it has been become the preferred tool of many working in the areas of classical and modern statistical techniques, including many who apply it in biostatistics with respect to epidemiology, public health, and preventive medicine (Aragon, 2011; Dalgaard, 2002; Everitt & Hothorn, 2006; Mittal, 2011; Murrell, 2006; Peng & Domonici, 2008; Teetor, 2011; Venable et al., 2004; Virasakdi, 2011; Verzani, 2005). These latter applications are the *raison d'être* for this book.

As of this writing, the latest version of R is R-2.14.1, officially released on December 22, 2011. The primary source of R packages is the Comprehensive R Archive Network (CRAN), at http://cran.r-project.org.

R packages may also be found in numerous publications, such as the *Journal of Statistical Software*. That journal's 45th volume is available at www.jstatsoft.org/v45.

We will now get started with the R-2.9.1 version environment by downloading it from the Internet and taking a first look at the R computing environment. Recall from Chapter 1 that the R environment was obtained as follows:

Access the Internet at the website of CRAN (http://cran.r-project.org).

To install R: **R-2.9.1-win32.exe**
http://www.r-project.org/
=> download R
=> Select: USA
http://cran.cnr.Berkeley.edu <http://cran.cnr.berkeley.edu/>
University of California, Berkeley, CA
=> http://cran.cnr.berkeley.edu/
=> Windows (95 and later)
=> base
=> R-2.9.1-win32.exe
AFTER the download completes:
=> Double-click on: R-2.9.1-win32.exe
(on the desktop) to unzip and install R

=> An icon (Script R 2.9.1) will appear on your computer desktop as shown in Figure 3.1.

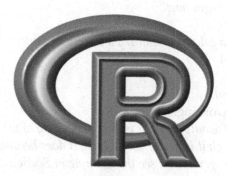

FIGURE 3.1 The R icon on the computer desktop.

In this book, the following scheme is used for all statements during the computational activities in the R environment to clarify the various inputs to and outputs from the computational process:

1. Regular book text
2. Line input in R code
3. **Line output in R code**
4. *Line comment statements in R code*

Note: The # sign is the comment character: All text in a line following this sign is treated as a comment by the R program, and no computational action will be taken regarding such a statement. That is, the computational activities will ignore the comments and proceed as though the comment statements did not exist. These comment statements help the programmer and user by providing some clarification of the purposes of the rest of the R environment. However, the computations will proceed even if these comment statements are eliminated.

To use R with a Microsoft Windows operating system, double-click on the R 2.9.1 icon.

After you select and click on R, the R window opens, with the following declaration:

R **version 2.9.1 (2009-06-26)**
Copyright (C) 2009 The R Foundation for Statistical Computing ISBN 3-900051-07-0
R **is free software and comes with ABSOLUTELY NO WARRANTY.**
You are welcome to redistribute it under certain conditions.
Type 'license()' or 'licence()' for distribution details.
R **is a collaborative project with many contributors.**
Type 'contributors()' for more information and 'citation()' on how to cite R **or** R
   packages in publications.
Type 'demo()' for some demos, 'help()' for on-line help, or 'help.start()' for an
   HTML browser interface to help.

Type 'q()' to quit R.
[Previously saved workspace restored]
> # *This is the R computing environment.*
> # *Computations may begin now!*
>
> # *First, let's use R as a calculator and try a simple arithmetic*
> # *operation, say:* 1 + 1
> 1+1
[1] 2 # *This is the output!*
> # WOW! It's really working!
> # *The* **[1]** *in front of the output result is part of R's way of printing numbers*
> # *and vectors. Although it is not so useful here, it does become so when the*
> # *output result is a longer vector: see the example in Section 3.5.*
>

From this point on, this book is most beneficially read with the R environment at hand. It will be a most effective learning experience if you practice each R command as you go through the textual materials.

A First Session Using R

This subsection introduces some important and practical features of the R environment (Venables et al., 2004).

Log in and start an R session in the Windows system of the computer:
>
> # *This is the R environment.*
> help.start()   # *This outputs a page that lists the various online help manuals*
>   # *and materials available, such as*
>   # *Statistical Data Analysis Manuals,*
>   # **"An Introduction to** R" (Venables et al., 2004)
starting httpd help server ... done
If nothing happens, you should open
'http://127.0.0.1:28103/doc/html/index.html' yourself

At this point, explore the Hypertext Markup Language (HTML) interface for online help right from the desktop, using the mouse pointer to note the various features of this facility available within the R environment.

One may now access each of these R program packages and use them for further applications as needed.

Returning to the R environment:
> x <- rnorm(100)
> # *Generating a pseudo-random 100-vector x*
> y <- rnorm(x)
> # *Generating another pseudo-random 100-vector y*
> plot (x, y)
> # *Plotting x vs. y in the plane, resulting in a graphic window* (Figure 3.2).

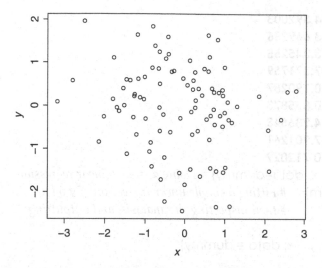

FIGURE 3.2 Graphical output for plot (x, y).

Remark: For reference, the appendix at the end of this chapter contains the CRAN documentation of the R function plot(), available for graphic outputting, which may be found by the R code segment:

```
> ?plot
```

CRAN has documentation for many R functions and packages.
Again returning to the R workspace, enter:

```
>
> ls()    # (This is a lowercase "L" followed by "s"; it is the "list" command.)
>         # (NOT 1 = "ONE" followed by "s")
>         # This command will list all the R objects now in the R workspace.
>         # Outputting:
[1] "E" "n" "s" "x" "y" "z"
```

Return to the R workspace and enter:

```
>
> rm (x, y)  # Removing all x and all y from the R workspace
> x          # Calling for x
Error: object 'x' not found # Of course, the xs have just been removed!
> y          # Calling for y
Error: object 'y' not found # Because the ys have been removed too!
>
> x <- 1:10 # Let x = (1, 2, 3, 4, 5, 6, 7, 8, 9, 10)
> x # Outputting x (just checking!)
[1] 1 2 3 4 5 6 7 8 9 10
> w <- 1 + sqrt(x)/2 # w is a weighting vector of standard deviations
> dummy <- data.frame (x = x, y = x + rnorm(x)*w)
> # Making a data frame of two columns, x and y, for inspection
> dummy # Outputting the data frame dummy
      x           y
```

```
2    2     4.392003
3    3     3.669256
4    4     3.345255
5    5     7.371759
6    6    -0.190287
7    7    10.835873
8    8     4.936543
9    9     7.901261
10   10    10.712029
```

> fm <- lm(y~x, data=dummy) # *Doing a simple linear regression*
> summary(fm)   # *Fitting a simple linear regression of y on x,*
>   # *then inspecting the analysis, and outputting:*
Call:
lm(formula = y ~ x, data = dummy)

Residuals:

Min	1Q	Median	3Q	Max
-6.0140	-0.8133	-0.0385	1.7291	4.2218

Coefficients:

	Estimate	Std. Error	t value	Pr(>|t|)
(Intercept)	1.0814	2.0604	0.525	0.6139
x	0.7904	0.3321	2.380	0.0445 *

Signif. codes: 0 '*' 0.001 '**' 0.01 '*' 0.05 '.' 0.1 ' ' 1**

Residual standard error: 3.016 on 8 degrees of freedom
Multiple R-squared: 0.4146, Adjusted R-squared: 0.3414
F-statistic: 5.665 on 1 and 8 DF, p-value: 0.04453

> fm1 <- lm(y~x, data=dummy, weight=1/w^2)
> summary(fm1)   # *Knowing the standard deviation, then doing a weighted*
>   # *regression and outputting:*
Call:
lm(formula=y ~ x, data=dummy, weight=1/w^2)

Residuals:

Min	1Q	Median	3Q	Max
-2.69867	-0.46190	-0.00072	0.90031	1.83202

Coefficients:

	Estimate	Std. Error	t value	Pr(>|t|)
(Intercept)	1.0814	2.0604	0.525	0.6139
x	0.7904	0.3321	2.380	0.0445 *

Signif. codes: 0 '*' 0.001 '**' 0.01 '*' 0.05 '.' 0.1 ' ' 1**

Residual standard error: 1.356 on 8 degrees of freedom
Multiple R-squared: 0.4424, Adjusted R-squared: 0.3728
F-statistic: 6.348 on 1 and 8 DF, p-value: 0.03583

The following object(s) are masked _by_ '.GlobalEnv':
x
> lrf <- lowess(x, y) # *A nonparametric local regression function lrf*
> plot (x, y) # *Making a standard point plot, outputting* Figure 3.3.

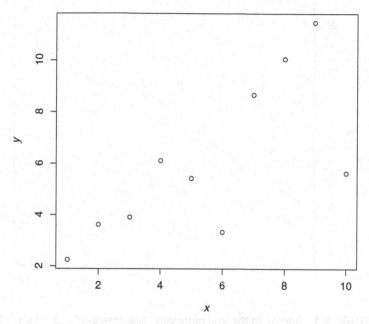

FIGURE 3.3 A standard point plot.

> lines(x, lrf$y)   # *Adding in the local regression line*
>   # *outputting* Figure 3.4.

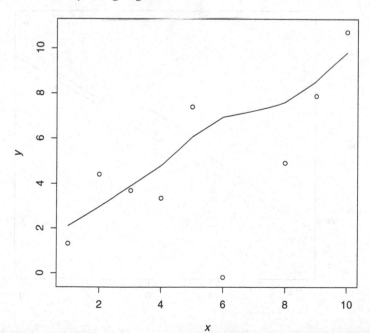

```
> abline(0, 1, lty = 3)    # adding in the true regression line:
>                          # (Intercept = 0, Slope = 1)
>                          # outputting Figure 3.5.
```

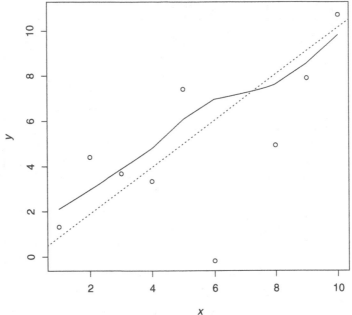

FIGURE 3.5 Adding in the true regression line (intercept = 0, slope = 1).

```
> abline(coef(fm))    # adding in the unweighted regression line
>                     # outputting Figure 3.6.
```

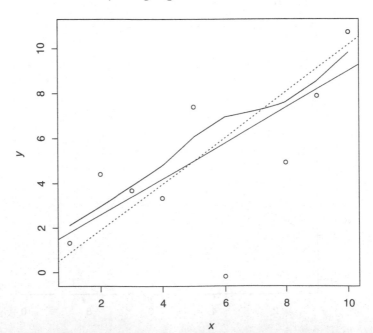

```
> abline(coef(fm1), col="red")   # adding in the weighted regression line
>                                # outputting Figure 3.7.
```

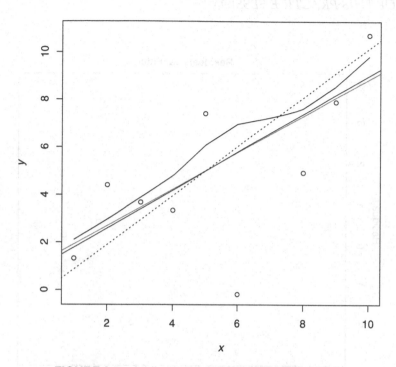

FIGURE 3.7   Adding in the weighted regression line.

```
> detach() # Removing data frame from the search path
> plot(fitted(fm), resid(fm),    # Doing a standard diagnostic plot
+ xlab="Fitted values",          # to check for heteroscedasticity*,
+ ylab="residuals",              # checking for differing variance
+ main="Residuals vs. Fitted")   # outputting Figure 3.8.
```

Heteroscedasticity occurs when the variance of the error terms differs across observations.

```
> qqnorm(resid(fm), main="Residuals Rankit Plot")
> # Doing a normal scores plot to check for skewness, kurtosis, and outliers.
> # (Not very useful here.) Outputting Figure 3.9.

>
> rm(fm, fm1, lrf, x, dummy)     # Removing these 5 objects
> fm
Error: object 'fm' not found     # Checked!
> fm1
Error: object 'fm1' not found    # Checked!
> lrf
Error: object 'lrf' not found    # Checked!
> x
```

```
> dummy
Error: object 'dummy' not found    # Checked!
# END OF THIS PRACTICE SESSION
```

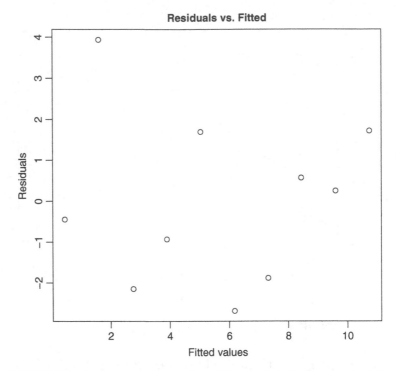

FIGURE 3.8 A standard diagnostic plot to check for heteroscedasticity.

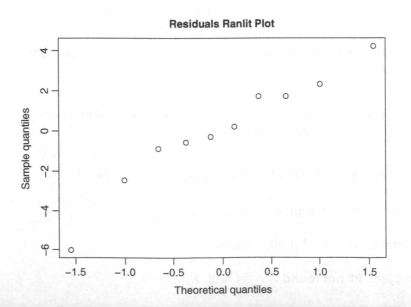

The R Environment

Getting through the first session (in the previous section) shows that:

■ Technically, R is an expression language with a simple syntax that is almost self-explanatory. It is case sensitive: thus, x and X are different symbols and refer to different variables. All alphanumeric symbols are allowed, plus "." and "-", with the restriction that a name must start with "." or a letter. If it starts with ".", the second character must *not* be a digit. The command prompt > indicates when R is ready for input. This is where you type commands to be processed by R; processing will start when you hit the ENTER key.

■ Commands consist of either expressions or assignments. When an expression is given as a command, it is immediately evaluated and printed, and the value is discarded. An assignment evaluates an expression and passes the value to a variable—but the value is *not* automatically printed. To print the computed value, simply enter the variable again at the next command.

■ Commands are separated either by a new line or by a semicolon (";"). Several elementary commands may be grouped together into one compound expression by braces ("{" and "}").

■ Comments, which start with a hash mark/number sign ("#"), may be put almost anywhere. Everything to the end of the line following this sign is a comment. Comments may not be used in an argument list of a function definition or inside strings. If a command is not complete at the end of a line, by default R will give a different prompt (a "+" sign) on the second and subsequent lines, and continue to read input until the command is completed syntactically.

■ The result of a command is printed to the output device. If the result is an array, such as a vector or a matrix, then the elements are formatted with line breaks (wherever necessary) with the indices of the *leading* entries labeled in square brackets: [index]. For example, an array of 15 elements may be outputted as follows:

```
> array(8, 15)
[1]  8 8 8 8 8  8 8 8 8 8
[11] 8 8 8 8 8
```

The labels [1] and [11] indicate the first and eleventh elements in the output. These labels are *not* part of the data itself.

Similarly, the labels for a matrix are placed at the start of each row and column in the output. For example, for the 3 × 5 matrix M, it is outputted as follows:

```
>
> M <- matrix(1:15, nrow=3)
> M
     [,1]  [,2]  [,3]  [,4]  [,5]
[1,]   1    4    7    10    13
[2,]   2    5    8    11    14
[3,]   3    6    9    12    15
```

Note that the storage is a *column-major*; that is, the elements of the first column are printed out first, followed by those of the second column, and so on. To cause a matrix to be filled in a row-wise manner rather than the default column-wise fashion, use the additional switch byrow=T; this will cause the matrix to be filled row-wise rather than column-wise:

```
>
> M <- matrix(1:15, nrow=3, byrow=T)
> M
      [,1]   [,2]   [,3]   [,4]   [,5]
[1,]    1      2      3      4      5
[2,]    6      7      8      9     10
[3,]   11     12     13     14     15
>
```

The first session (completed in the preceding subsection) also shows that a host of helpful resources are embedded in the R environment that you can readily access, using the online help provided by CRAN.

Review Questions for Section 3.2

1. Follow the step-by-step instructions given in the opening paragraphs of the first session to set up an R environment. The R window should look like this:
   ```
   >
   ```
   Now enter the following arithmetic operations; remember to press ENTER after each entry:
   (a) 2 + 3 <Enter>
   (b) 13 – 7 <Enter>
   (c) 17 * 23 <Enter>
   (d) 100/25 <Enter>10/25
   (e) Did you obtain the following results: 5, 6, 391, 4?

2. Here are a few more. (The <Enter> prompt will be omitted from now on.)
   (a) 2^4
   (b) sqrt(3)
   (c) 1i [1i is used for the complex unit i, where $i^2 = 1$.]
   (d) (2 + 3i) + (4 + 5i)
   (e) (2 + 3i) * (4 + 5i)

3. Here is a short session on using R to do complex arithmetic. Just enter the following commands into the R environment and report the results:
   ```
   > th <- seq(-pi, pi, len=20)
   > th (a) How many numbers are printed out?
   > z <- exp(1i*th)
   > z (b) How many complex numbers are printed out?
   > par(pty="s")
   ```
   (c) Along the menu bar at the top of the R environment:
   ▪ Select and left-click on "Window".
   ▪ Move downward and select the second option:

■   Go to the "R Graphic Device 2 (ACTIVE)" window.

(d) What is there?

> plot(z)

(e) Describe what is in the Graphic Device 2 window.

3.3   R AS A CALCULATOR (ARAGON, 2011; DALGAARD, 2002)

Mathematical Operations Using R

To learn to do biostatistical analysis and computations, start by considering the R programming language as a simple calculator. Begin here: Just enter an arithmetic expression, press the ENTER key, and look for the answer from the machine on the next line.

```
>
> 2 + 3
[1] 5
>
```

What about other calculations? For example, $13 - 7$, 3×5, $12/4$, 7^2, $\sqrt{2}$, e^3, $e^{i\pi}$, $\ln 5 = \log_e 5$, $(4 + \sqrt{3})(4 - \sqrt{3})$, $(4 + i\sqrt{3})(4 - i\sqrt{3})$, ... and so on. Just try:

```
>
> 13 - 7
[1] 6
> 3*5
[1] 15
> 12/4
[1] 3
> 7^2
[1] 49
> sqrt(2)
[1] 1.414214
>
> exp(3)
[1] 20.08554
>
> exp(1i*pi) [1i is used for the complex number i = √−1.]
[1] −1 − 0i [This is the famous Euler's identity equation: eⁱᵖ + 1 = 0.]
> log(5)
[1] 1.609438
> (4+sqrt(3))*(4-sqrt(3))
[1] 13 [Checking: (4 + √3)(4 − √3) = 4² − (√3)² = 16 − 3 = 13 (Checked!)]
> (4 + 1i*sqrt(3))*(4 − 1i*sqrt(3))
[1] 19+0i [Checking: (4 + i√3)(4 − i√3) = 4² − (i√3)² = 16 − (−3) = 19 (Checked!)]
```

Remark: Remember, the [1] in front of the computed result is R's way of output-

enclosed in brackets [N] is the index of the first number on that line. For example, if you generate 23 random numbers from a normal distribution, the following result is obtained:

```
>
> x <- rnorm(23)
> x
 [1] -0.5561324   0.2478934  -0.8243522   1.0697415   1.5681899
 [6] -0.3396776  -0.7356282   0.7781117   1.2822569  -0.5413498
[11]  0.3348587  -0.6711245  -0.7789205  -1.1138432  -1.9582234
[16] -0.3193033  -0.1942829   0.4973501  -1.5363843  -0.3729301
[21]  0.5741554  -0.4651683  -0.2317168
>
```

Remark: After the random numbers have been generated, there is no output until you call for x; then x becomes a vector with 23 elements, so we call it a 23-vector.

The [11] on the third line of the output indicates that 0.3348587 (highlighted in gray here for emphasis) is the eleventh element in the 23-vector x. The number of outputs per line depends on the length of each element, as well as the width of the page.

Assignment of Values in R and Computations Using Vectors and Matrices

R is designed to be a *dynamically typed language*; that is, at any time, one may change the data type of any variable. For example, you can first set x to be numeric, as has been done so far; say, $x = 7$. You may also set x to be a vector; say, $x = c (1, 2, 3, 4)$. Then again, you may set x to be a word object, such as "Hi!" Just watch the following R environment:

```
>
> x <- 7
> x
[1] 7
> x <- c(1, 2, 3, 4) # x is assigned to be a 4-vector.
> x
[1] 1 2 3 4
> x <- c("Hi!") # x is assigned to be a character string.
> x
[1] "Hi!"
> x <- c("Greetings & Salutations!")
> x
[1] "Greetings & Salutations!"
> x <- c("The rain in Spain falls mainly on the plain.")
[1] "The rain in Spain falls mainly on the plain."
> x <- c("Biostatistics", "Epidemiology", "Public Health")
> x
[1] "Biostatistics" "Epidemiology" "Public Health"
```

Computations in Vectors and Simple Graphics

The use of arrays and matrices was introduced in the preceding subsection. In finite mathematics, a *matrix* is a two-dimensional (2D) array of elements, which are usually numbers. In R, the use of the matrix extends to elements of any type, such as a matrix of character strings. Arrays and matrices may be represented as vectors with dimensions.

In biostatistics, most variables carry multiple values, so computations are usually performed between vectors of many elements. These operations among multivariates result in large matrices. To demonstrate the results, often graphical representations are useful. The following simple example illustrates these operations being readily accomplished in the R environment:

```
>
> weight <- c(73, 59, 97)
> height <- c(1.79, 1.64, 1.73)
> bmi <- weight/height^2
> bmi # Read the notes on BMI after the example.
[1] 22.78331 21.93635 32.41004
> # To summarize the results, proceed to compute as follows:
> cbind(weight, height, bmi)
     weight  height      bmi
[1,]     73    1.79  22.78331
[2,]     59    1.64  21.93635
[3,]     97    1.73  32.41004
>
> rbind(weight, height, bmi)
               [,1]        [,2]        [,3]
weight  73.00000   59.00000   97.00000
height   1.79000    1.64000    1.73000
bmi     22.78331   21.93635   32.41004
>
```

Clearly, the functions cbind and rbind bind (join, link, glue, concatenate) the vectors by column and by row, respectively, to form new vectors or matrices.

Use of Factors in R Programming

In the analysis of epidemiologic datasets, categorical variables are often needed. These categorical variables indicate subdivisions of the original dataset into various classes (for example, age, gender, disease stages, degrees of diagnosis, etc.). Input of the original dataset is generally delineated into several categories using a numeric code: 1 = age, 2 = gender, 3 = disease stage, and so on. Such variables are specified as *factors* in R, resulting in a data structure that enables one to assign specific names to the various categories. In certain analyses, it is necessary for R to distinguish among categorical codes and variables whose values have direct

A factor has four levels, consisting of two items:

1. A vector of integers between 1 and 4
2. A character vector of length four containing strings that describe the four levels

Consider the following example:

- A certain type of cancer is being categorized into four levels: stages 1, 2, 3, and 4.
- The corresponding pain levels consistent with these diagnoses are none, mild, moderate, and severe, respectively.
- In the dataset, five case subjects have been diagnosed in terms of their respective stages.

The following R code segment delineates the dataset:

```
> cancerpain <- c(1, 4, 3, 3, 2, 4)
> fcancerpain <- factor(cancerpain, level=1:4)
> levels(fcancerpain) <- c("none", "mild", "moderate", "severe")
```

The first statement creates a numerical vector cancerpain that encodes the pain levels of six case subjects. This is considered a categorical variable for which, using the factor function, a factor fcancerpain is created. This may be called with one argument in addition to cancerpain (namely, levels = 1 to 4), which indicates that the input coding uses the values 1–4. In the final line, the pain level names are changed to the four specified character strings. The result is:

```
> fcancerpain
[1] none severe moderate moderate mild severe
Levels: none mild moderate severe
> as.numeric(fcancerpain)
[1] 1 4 3 3 2 4
> levels(fcancerpain)
[1] "none" "mild" "moderate" "severe"
```

Remark: The function as.numeric outputs the numerical coding as numbers 1 to 4, and the function levels outputs the names of the respective levels. The original input coding in terms of the numbers 1 to 4 is no longer needed, There is an additional option to use the function ordered, which is similar to the function factor used here.

BMI (BMI NOTES, 2012)

Body mass index (BMI) is a useful measure for human body fat based on an individual's weight and height, although it does *not* actually measure the percentage of fat in the body. Invented in the early 19th century, BMI is defined as a person's body weight (in kilograms) divided by the square of the person's height (in meters). The formula universally used in medicine produces a unit of measure of kg/m^2:

$$BMI = body\ mass\ (kg)/\{Height\ (m)\}^2 \qquad (3.3\text{-}1)$$

A BMI chart may be used to display BMI as a function of weight (horizontal axis) and height (vertical axis), with contour lines for different values of BMI or colors for different BMI categories (see Figure 3.10).

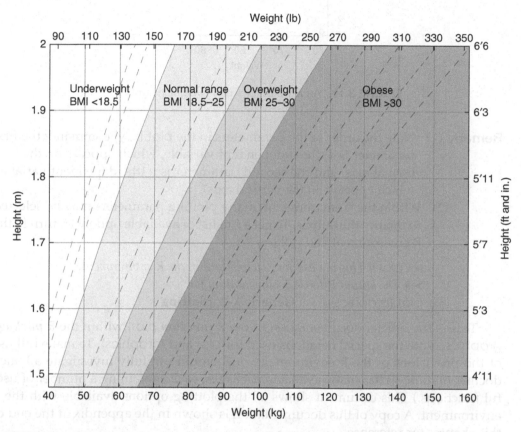

FIGURE 3.10   A graph of BMI. The dashed lines represent subdivisions within a major class; the "Underweight" classification is further divided into "severe," "moderate," and "mild" subclasses.
Source: World Health Organization data (BMI Notes, 2012).

Simple Graphics

Generating graphical presentations is an important aspect of biostatistical data analysis. Within the R environment, one may construct plots that allow production of graphics and control of the graphical features. Using the previous example, the relationship between body weight and height may be considered by first plotting one versus the other, using the following R code segments:

```
>
> plot (weight, height)
> # Outputting Figure 3.11.
>
```

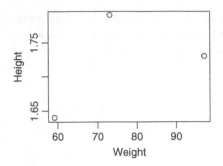

FIGURE 3.11 An x-y plot for > plot (weight, height).

Remark: (1) Note the order of the parameters in the plot (x, y) command: the first parameter is *x* (the independent variable, which appears on the horizontal axis) and the second parameter is *y* (the dependent variable, which appears on the vertical axis).

(2) Within the R environment, many plotting parameters may be selected to modify the output. To get a full list of available options, return to the R environment and call for:

> ?plot # *This is a call for "Help!" within the* R *environment.*
> # *The output is the* R *documentation for:*
plot {graphics}   **Generic X–Y plotting**

This is the official documentation of the R *function* plot, within the R *package* graphics. Note the special notations used for plot and {graphics}. To make full use of the provisions of the R environment, one should carefully investigate all such documentation. (R has many available packages, each containing a number of useful functions.) This document shows all the plotting options available with the R environment. A copy of this documentation is shown in the appendix at the end of this chapter for reference.

For example, to change the plotting symbol, you may use the keyword pch (for "plotting character") in the following R command:

> plot (weight, height, pch=8)
> # *Outputting* Figure 3.12.

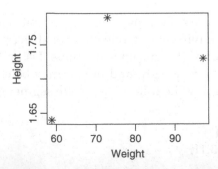

FIGURE 3.12 An x-y plot for plot (weight, height, pch = 8).

Note that the output is the same as that shown in Figure 3.11, except that the points are marked with little asterisks, corresponding to Plotting Character pch = 8.

In the documentation for pch, a total of 26 options are available, providing different plotting characteristics for points in R graphics. They are shown in Figure 3.13.

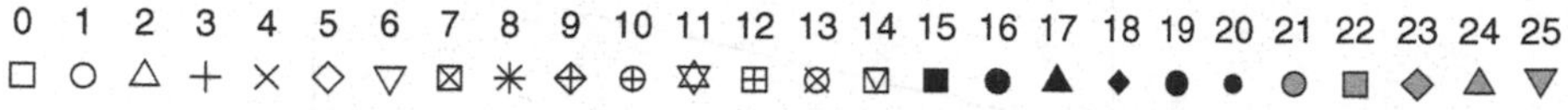

0   1   2   3   4   5   6   7   8   9   10   11   12   13   14   15   16   17   18   19   20   21   22   23   24   25
□   ○   △   +   ×   ◇   ▽   ⊠   ✳   ⊕   ⊕   ✡   ⊞   ⊠   ▽   ■   ●   ▲   ◆   ●   ●   ●   ■   ◆   ▲   ▽

FIGURE 3.13   Plotting symbols in R: pch = n, n = 0, 1, 2, ..., 25.

The parameter BMI was chosen so that this value would be independent of a person's height, thus expressing a single number or index indicative of whether a case subject is overweight, and by what relative amount.

Of course, one may also plot "height" as the abscissa (the horizontal x-axis) and "weight" as the ordinate (the vertical y-axis), as follows:

> plot(height, weight, pch=8) # *Outputting* Figure 3.14.

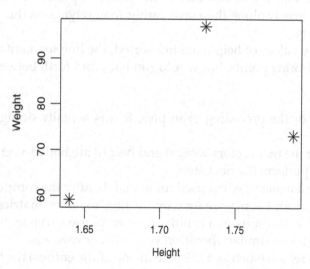

FIGURE 3.14   An x-y plot for > plot (height, weight, pch=8).

A normal BMI is between 18.5 and 25, averaging $(18.5 + 25)/2 = 21.75$. For this BMI value, then, the weight of a typical "normal" person would be $(21.75 \times height^2)$. Thus, one can superimpose a line of "expected" weights at BMI = 21.75 on Figure 3.14. This line may be accomplished in the R environment by the following code segments:

> ht <- c(1.79, 1.64, 1.73)
> lines(ht, 21.75*ht^2) # *Outputting* Figure 3.15.

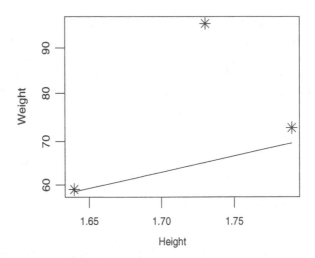

FIGURE 3.15 Superimposed reference curve using lines (ht, 21.75*ht^2).

In the last plot, a new variable for height (ht) was defined instead of the original (height) because:

- The relation between height and weight is quadratic, and hence nonlinear. Although it may not be obvious on the plot, it is preferable to use points that are spread evenly along the x-axis rather than relying on the distribution of the original data.
- Because the values of height are not sorted, the line segments would not connect neighboring points, but would run back and forth between distant points.

Remarks:

1. In the last of the preceding examples, R was actually doing the arithmetic of vectors.
2. Notice that the two vectors weight and height are both 3-vectors, making it reasonable to perform the next step.
3. The cbind statement, when used immediately after the computations have been completed, forms a new matrix by *bind*ing together matrices horizontally, or column-wise. It results in a multivariate response variable. Similarly, the rbind statement does a similar operation vertically, or *row*-wise.
4. If for some reason (such as a mistake in one of the entries) the two entries weight and height have *different* numbers of elements, R will output an error message. For example:

```
>
> weight <- c(73, 59, 97)          # a 3-vector
> height <- c(1.79, 1.64, 1.73, 1.48)  # a 4-vector
> bmi <- weight/height^2 # Outputting:
Warning message: # An error message!
In weight/height^2:
longer object length is not a multiple of shorter object length
>
```

x as Vectors and Matrices in Biostatistics

We have just seen that a variable, such as x or M, may be assigned as follows:

1. A number, such as $x = 7$
2. A vector or an array, such as $x = c(1, 2, 3, 4)$
3. A matrix, such as $x =$

	[,1]	[,2]	[,3]	[,4]	[,5]
[1,]	1	4	7	10	13
[2,]	2	5	8	11	14
[3,]	3	6	9	12	15

4. A character string, such as
    x = 'The rain in Spain falls mainly on the plain."
5. In fact, in R, a variable *x* may be assigned a complete dataset, which may consist of a multidimensional set of elements, each of which may in turn be any one of these kinds of variables. For example, besides being a numerical vector, as in number 2 in this list, *x* may be:

    (a) a *character vector*, which is a vector of text strings whose elements are expressed in quotation marks, using double, single, or mixed quotes:

    ```
    > c("one", "two", "three", "four", "five") # Double quotes
    [1] "one" "two" "three" "four" "five"
    >
    > c('one', 'two', 'three', 'four', 'five') # Single quotes
    [1] "one" "two" "three" "four" "five"
    >
    > c("one", 'two', "three", 'four', "five") # Mixed quotes
    [1] "one" "two" "three" "four" "five"
    ```

    However, a mixed pair of quotes, such as "xxxxx', will *not* be accepted. For example:

    ```
    > c("one", "two", "three", "four", "five')
    +
    ```

    (b) a *logical vector,* which takes the value TRUE or FALSE (or NA). For inputs, one may use the abbreviation T or F. These vectors are similarly specified using the c function:

    ```
    > c(T, F, T, F, T)
    [1] TRUE FALSE TRUE FALSE TRUE
    ```

    In most cases, there is no need to repeat specified logical vectors. It is acceptable to use a single logical value to provide the needed options, as vectors of more than one value will respond in terms of relational expressions. Observe:

    ```
    > weight <- c(73, 59, 97)
    > height <- c(1.79, 1.64, 1.73)
    > bmi <- weight/height^2
    ```

```
> bmi # Outputting:
[1]   22.78331   21.93635   32.41004
> bmi > 25 # A single logical value will suffice.
[1] FALSE FALSE TRUE
>
```

Some Special Functions That Create Vectors

Three functions that create vectors are c, seq, and rep.

c, for "concatenate"; the joining of objects end to end (this was introduced earlier). For example:

```
> x <- c(1, 2, 3, 4) # x is assigned to be a 4-vector.
> x
[1] 1 2 3 4
```

seq, for "sequence"; defining an equidistant sequence of numbers. For example:

```
> seq(1, 20, 2)   # To output a sequence from 1 to 20 in steps of 2.
[1]  1  3  5  7  9 11 13 15 17 19
> seq(1, 20)      # To output a sequence from 1 to 20 in steps of 1 (which may
>                 # be omitted).
[1]  1  2  3  4  5  6  7  8  9 10 11 12 13 14 15 16 17 18 19 20
> 1:20 # This is a simplified alternative to writing seq(1, 20).
[1]  1  2  3  4  5  6  7  8  9 10 11 12 13 14 15 16 17 18 19 20
> seq(1, 20, 2.5) # To output a sequence from 1 to 20 in steps of 2.5.
[1]  1.0  3.5  6.0  8.5 11.0 13.5 16.0 18.5
```

rep, for "replicate"; for generating repeated values. This function takes two forms, depending on whether the second argument is a single number or a vector. For example:

```
> rep(1:2, c(3,5))   # Replicating the first element (1) 3 times, and
>                    # then replicating the second element (2) 5 times
[1] 1 1 1 2 2 2 2 2 # This is the output.
> vector <- c(1, 2, 3, 4)
> vector # Outputting vector
[1] 1 2 3 4
> rep(vector, 5) # Replicating vector 5 times
[1] 1 2 3 4 1 2 3 4 1 2 3 4 1 2 3 4 1 2 3 4
```

Arrays and Matrices

In finite mathematics, a matrix M is a 2D array of elements (generally numbers), such as:

$$M = \begin{matrix} 1 & 4 & 7 & 10 & 13 \\ 2 & 5 & 8 & 11 & 14 \\ 3 & 6 & 9 & 12 & 15 \end{matrix}$$

The array is usually placed inside parentheses (), or some type of brackets {}, []. In R, the use of a matrix is extended to elements of many types, numbers as well as character strings. For example, in R, the preceding sample matrix M is expressed as follows:

```
      [,1]  [,2]  [,3]  [,4]  [,5]
[1,]    1     4     7    10    13
[2,]    2     5     8    11    14
[3,]    3     6     9    12    15
```

Use of the Dimension Function dim in R

In R, the preceding sample 3 × 5 matrix may be set up as vectors with dimension dim(x) using the following code segment:

```
> x <- 1:15
> x
[1] 1 2 3 4 5 6 7 8 9 10 11 12 13 14 15
> dim(x) <- c(3, 5) # A dimension of 3 rows by 5 columns
> x
      [,1]  [,2]  [,3]  [,4]  [,5]
[1,]    1     4     7    10    13
[2,]    2     5     8    11    14
[3,]    3     6     9    12    15
```

Remark: Here 15 total elements, 1 through 15, are set to be the elements of the matrix x. Then the dimension of x is set as c(3, 5), making x a 3 × 5 matrix. The assignment of the 15 elements follows a column-wise procedure, such that the elements of the first column are allocated first, followed by those of the second column, then the third column, and so on.

Use of the Matrix Function matrix in R

Another way to generate a matrix is to use the function matrix. The 3 × 5 matrix used in the previous subsection may be created by the following one-line code segment:

```
> matrix (1:15, nrow=3)
      [,1]  [,2]  [,3]  [,4]  [,5]
[1,]    1     4     7    10    13
[2,]    2     5     8    11    14
[3,]    3     6     9    12    15
```

However, if the 15 elements should be allocated by row, then the following code segment should be used:

```
> matrix (1:15, nrow=3, byrow=T)
      [,1]  [,2]  [,3]  [,4]  [,5]
[1,]    1     2     3     4     5
[2,]    6     7     8     9    10
[3,]   11    12    13    14    15
```

Some Useful Functions Operating on Matrices in R

■ colnames, rownames, and t (for *transpose*)

Using the same 3×5 matrix example, first the five columns of the 3×5 matrix x are assigned the names C1, C2, C3, C4, and C5, respectively. Then the transpose is obtained, and finally one takes the transpose of the transpose to obtain the original matrix x:

```
> matrix (1:15, nrow=3, byrow=T)
      [,1] [,2] [,3] [,4] [,5]
[1,]   1    2    3    4    5
[2,]   6    7    8    9   10
[3,]  11   12   13   14   15
> colnames(x) <- c("C1", "C2", "C3", "C4", "C5")
> x
     C1  C2  C3  C4  C5
[1,]  1   4   7  10  13
[2,]  2   5   8  11  14
[3,]  3   6   9  12  15
> t(x)
    [,1] [,2] [,3]
C1   1    2    3
C2   4    5    6
C3   7    8    9
C4  10   11   12
C5  13   14   15
> t(t(x)) # which is just x, as expected.
     C1  C2  C3  C4  C5
[1,]  1   4   7  10  13
[2,]  2   5   8  11  14
[3,]  3   6   9  12  15
```

Yet another way to do this is to use the function LETTERS, which is a built-in variable containing the capital letters A through Z. Other useful vectors include letters, month.name, and month.abb for lowercase letters, month names, and abbreviated names of months, respectively. Take a look:

```
> X <-LETTERS
> X
[1]  "A" "B" "C" "D" "E" "F" "G" "H" "I" "J" "K" "L" "M" "N" "O"
[16] "P" "Q" "R" "S" "T" "U" "V" "W" "X" "Y" "Z"
> x <-letters
> x
[1]  "a" "b" "c" "d" "e" "f" "g" "h" "i" "j" "k" "l" "m" "n" "o"
[16] "p" "q" "r" "s" "t" "u" "v" "w" "x" "y" "z"
> M <- month.name
> M
```

[6]   "June"   "July"   "August"   "September"   "October"
[11] "November" "December"
> m <- month.abb
> m
[1] "Jan" "Feb" "Mar" "Apr" "May" "Jun" "Jul" "Aug" "Sep" "Oct"
[11] "Nov" "Dec"

NA: "Not Available" for Missing Values in Datasets

NA is a logical constant of length 1, which contains a missing value indicator.

NA can be forced to any other vector type except raw. There are also constants NA_integer_, NA_real_, NA_complex_, and NA_character_ of the other atomic vector types that support missing values. All of these are reserved words in the R language.

■ The generic function .na indicates which elements are missing.
■ The generic function .na<- sets elements to NA.

The reserved words in R's parser are if, else, repeat, while, function, for, next, break, NA_complex_, NA_character_, ..., and ...1, ...2, and so on, which are used to refer to arguments passed down from an enclosing function.

Reserved words outside quotation marks are always parsed to be references to the objects linked to in the foregoing list, and are not allowed as syntactic names. They *are* allowed as nonsyntactic names.

Special Functions That Create Vectors

There are three useful R functions that are often used to create vectors:

1. c for "concatenate," which was introduced earlier in this section for joining items together end to end. For example:

    > c(2, 3, 5, 7, 11, 13, 17, 19, 23, 29) # *The first 10 prime numbers*
    [1] 2 3 5 7 11 13 17 19 23 29

2. seq for "sequence," which is used for listing equidistant sequences of numbers. For example:

    > seq(1, 20) # *Sequence from 1 to 20*
    [1] 1 2 3 4 5 6 7 8 9 10 11 12 13 14 15 16 17 18 19 20
    > seq(1, 20, 1) # *Sequence from 1 to 20 in steps of 1*
    [1] 1 2 3 4 5 6 7 8 9 10 11 12 13 14 15 16 17 18 19 20
    > 1:20 # *Sequence from 1 to 20 in steps of 1*
    [1] 1 2 3 4 5 6 7 8 9 10 11 12 13 14 15 16 17 18 19 20
    > seq(1, 20, 2) # *Sequence from 1 to 20 in steps of 2*
    [1] 1 3 5 7 9 11 13 15 17 19
    > seq(1, 20, 3) # *Sequence from 1 to 20 in steps of 3*

```
> seq(1, 20, 10) # Sequence from 1 to 20 in steps of 10
[1] 1 11
> seq(1, 20, 20) # Sequence from 1 to 20 in steps of 20
[1] 1
> seq(1, 20, 21) # Sequence from 1 to 20 in steps of 21
[1] 1
>
```

3. rep for "replicate," which is used to generate repeated values and may be expressed in two ways. For example:

```
> x <- c(3, 4, 5)
> rep(x, 4)            # Replicate the vector x 4 times.
[1] 3 4 5 3 4 5 3 4 5 3 4 5
> rep(x, 1:3)          # Replicate the elements of x: the first element once, the second
>                      # element twice, and the third element three times.
[1] 3 4 4 5 5 5
> rep(1:3, c(3,4,5))   # For the sequence (1, 2, 3), replicate its elements 3,
> # 4, and 5 times, respectively.
[1] 1 1 1 2 2 2 2 3 3 3 3 3
```

Review Questions for Section 3.3

1. Generate a "Tower of Powers" by computations using R. There is an interesting challenge in arithmetic which goes like this:

$$\sqrt{2}^{\sqrt{2}^{\cdots}}$$

What is the value of $\sqrt{2}^{\sqrt{2}^{\cdots}}$? This is an infinity of ascending "tower of powers" of the square root of 2.

Solution: Let x be the value of this "Tower of Powers." Then it is easily seen that $\sqrt{2}^{x} = x$ itself. Do you agree? Watch the lowest $\sqrt{2}$. Clearly, it follows that $x = 2$, because $\sqrt{2}^2 = 2$. This shows that the value of this infinite Tower of Powers of $\sqrt{2}$ is just 2.
   Now use the R environment to verify this interesting result:
   (a) Compute $\sqrt{2}$
       ```
       > sqrt(2)
       ```
   (b) Compute $\sqrt{2}^{\sqrt{2}}$
       ```
       > sqrt(2)^sqrt(2) [a 2-Towers of √2-s]
       ```
   (c) `> sqrt(2)^sqrt(2)^sqrt(2) [a 3-Towers of √2-s]`
   (d) `> sqrt(2)^sqrt(2)^sqrt(2)^sqrt(2) [a 4-Towers of √2-s]`
   (e) `> sqrt(2)^sqrt(2)^sqrt(2)^sqrt(2)^sqrt(2) [a 5-Towers of √2-s]`
   (f) Now try the following computations of 10-, 20-, 30-, and finally 40-Towers of Powers of $\sqrt{2}$, and finally reach the result of 2 (accurate to six decimal places).
       ```
       > sqrt(2)^sqrt(2)^sqrt(2)^sqrt(2)^sqrt(2)^sqrt(2)^sqrt(2)^sqrt(2)^
       sqrt(2)
       [1] 1.983668 [a 10-Tower of Powers of √2-s]
       ```

> sqrt(2)^sqrt(2)^sqrt(2)^sqrt(2)^sqrt(2)^sqrt(2)^sqrt(2)^sqrt(2)^sqrt(2)^s
qrt(2)^
+ sqrt(2)^sqrt(2)^sqrt(2)^sqrt(2)^sqrt(2)^sqrt(2)^sqrt(2)^sqrt(2)^sqrt(2)^s
qrt(2)
[1] 1.999586 [a 20-Tower of Powers of √2-s]
> sqrt(2)^sqrt(2)^sqrt(2)^sqrt(2)^sqrt(2)^sqrt(2)^sqrt(2)^sqrt(2)^sqrt(2)^s
qrt(2)^
+ sqrt(2)^sqrt(2)^sqrt(2)^sqrt(2)^sqrt(2)^sqrt(2)^sqrt(2)^sqrt(2)^sqrt(2)^s
qrt(2)^
+ sqrt(2)^sqrt(2)^sqrt(2)^sqrt(2)^sqrt(2)^sqrt(2)^sqrt(2)^sqrt(2)^sqrt(2)^s
qrt(2)
[1] 1.999989 [a 30-Tower of Powers of √2-s]
> sqrt(2)^sqrt(2)^sqrt(2)^sqrt(2)^sqrt(2)^sqrt(2)^sqrt(2)^sqrt(2)^sqrt(2)^s
qrt(2)^
+ sqrt(2)^sqrt(2)^sqrt(2)^sqrt(2)^sqrt(2)^sqrt(2)^sqrt(2)^sqrt(2)^sqrt(2)^s
qrt(2)^
+ sqrt(2)^sqrt(2)^sqrt(2)^sqrt(2)^sqrt(2)^sqrt(2)^sqrt(2)^sqrt(2)^sqrt(2)^s
qrt(2)^
+ sqrt(2)^sqrt(2)^sqrt(2)^sqrt(2)^sqrt(2)^sqrt(2)^sqrt(2)^sqrt(2)^sqrt(2)^s
qrt(2)
[1] 2 [a 40-Tower of Powers of √2-s]

Thus, this R computation verifies the solution.

2. (a) What are the equivalents in R for the basic mathematical operations: +, −, ×, / (division), √, and squaring of a number?
   (b) Describe the use of factors in R programming. Give an example.
3. If $x = (0, 1, 2, 3, 4, 5)$ and $y = (0, 1, 4, 9, 16, 25)$, use R to plot:
   (a) y versus x
   (b) x versus y
   (c) $\sqrt{y}$ versus x
   (d) y versus $\sqrt{x}$
   (e) $\sqrt{y}$ versus $\sqrt{x}$
   (f) $\sqrt{x}$ versus $\sqrt{y}$
4. Explain, giving an example, how the following functions may be used to combine matrices to form new ones: (a) cbind, (b) rbind.
5. (a) Describe the R function factor().
   (b) Give an example of using factor() to create new arrays.
6. Using examples, illustrate two procedures for creating:
   (a) a vector
   (b) a matrix
7. Describe, using examples, the following three functions for creating vectors:
   (a) c
   (b) seq
   (c) rep
8. (a) Use the function dim() to set up a matrix. Give an example.
   (b) Use the function matrix() to set up a matrix. Give an example.

9. Describe, using an example, the use of the following functions operating on a matrix in R: t(), colnames(), and rownames().
10. (a) What are reserved words in the R environment?
    (b) In R, how is the logical constant NA used? Give an example.

Exercises for Section 3.3 (Everitt & Hothorn, 2006; Virasakdi, 2011)

Enter the R environment and do the following exercises using R programming.

1. Perform the following elementary arithmetic exercises:
   (a) 7 + 31
   (b) 87 − 23
   (c) $3.1417 \times (7)^2$
   (d) 22/7
   (e) $e^{\sqrt{2}}$

2. BMI is calculated from your weight in kilograms and your height in meters:
$$BMI = kg/m^2$$
   Using 1 kg ≈ 2.2 lb and 1 m ≈ 3.3 ft ≈ 39.4 in.:
   (a) Calculate your BMI.
   (b) Is it in the "normal" range $18.5 \leq BMI \leq 25$?

3. In the MPH program, five graduate students taking the class called "Introductory Epidemiology" measured their weight (in kilograms) and height (in meters). The result is summarized in the following matrix:

	John	Chang	Michael	Bryan	Jose
WEIGHT	69.1	62.5	74.3	70.9	96.6
HEIGHT	1.81	1.46	1.69	1.82	1.74

   (a) Construct a matrix showing their BMIs as the last row.
   (b) Plot:
       (i) WEIGHT (on the y-axis) versus HEIGHT (on the x-axis)
       (ii) HEIGHT versus WEIGHT
       (iii) Assuming that the weight of a typical "normal" person is ($21.75 \times HEIGHT^2$), superimpose a line of "expected" weight at BMI = 21.75 on the plot from (i).

4. (a) To convert between temperatures in degrees Fahrenheit (F) and Celsius (C), the following conversion formulas are used:
$$F = (9/5)C + 32$$
$$C = (5/9) \times (F - 32)$$

   At standard temperature and pressure, the freezing and boiling points of water are 0 and 100 degrees Celsius, respectively. What are the freezing and boiling points of water in degrees Fahrenheit?
   (b) For C = 0, 5, 10, 15, 20, 25, ..., 80, 85, 90, 95, 100, compute a conversion table that shows the corresponding Fahrenheit temperatures.
   Note: To create the sequence of Celsius temperatures, use the R function seq(0, 100, 5).

5. Use the data in Table 3.1 (Aragon, 2011; CDC, 2005). Assume that a person is initially HIV-negative.

    If the probability of getting infected per act is p, then the probability of *not* getting infected per act is $(1 - p)$.

    The probability of *not* getting infected after two consecutive acts is $(1 - p)^2$, and the probability of *not* getting infected after three consecutive acts is $(1 - p)^3$.

    Therefore, the probability of not getting infected after n consecutive acts is $(1 - p)^n$, and the probability of getting *infected* after n consecutive acts is $1 - (1 - p)^n$.

    (a) For the non-blood-transfusion transmission probability (per-act risk) in Table 3.1, calculate the risk of being infected after 1 year (365 days) if one carries out needle-sharing injection-drug use (IDU) once daily for 1 year.

    (b) Do these cumulative risks seem reasonable? Why or why not?

TABLE 3.1   Estimated Per-Act Risk (Transmission Probability) for Acquisition of HIV by Exposure Route to an Infected Source

EXPOSURE ROUTE	RISK PER 10,000 EXPOSURES
Blood transfusion (BT)	9,000
Needle-sharing injection-drug use (IDU)	67

Source: CDC, 2005

SOLUTION:

```
> p <- 67/10000
> p
[1] 0.0067
> q <- (1 - p)
> q
[1] 0.9933
> q365 <- q^365
> q365
[1] 0.08597238
> p365 <- 1 - q365
> p365
[1] 0.9140276
```

=> Probability of being infected in a year = 91.40%. A high risk, indeed!

3.4   USING R IN DATA ANALYSIS IN BIOS

In epidemiologic investigations, after preparing the collected datasets to undertake biostatistical analysis (as discussed in Section 3.1), the first step is to enter the datasets into the R environment. Once the datasets are placed within the R environment, analysis will process the data to obtain results leading to creditable conclusions, and likely to recommendations for definitive courses of actions to improve public and personal health. Several methods for dataset entry are examined in this section.

Entering Data at the R Command Prompt

DATA FRAMES AND DATASETS (VIRASAKDI, 2011)

Many epidemiologic investigators use the terms *data frame* and *dataset* interchangeably. However, one can make distinctions.

In many applications, a complete **dataset** contains several data frames, including the real data that have been collected.

Rules for **data frames** are similar to those for arrays and matrixes, introduced earlier in Section 3.3. However, data frames are more complicated than arrays. In an array, if just one cell is a character, then all the columns will be characters. In contrast, a data frame can consist of:

- A column "IDnumber," in which the data are numeric
- A column "Name," in which the data are characters

In a data frame, each variable can have long variable descriptions, and a factor can have "levels" or value levels. These properties can be transferred from the original dataset in other software formats (such as SPS, Stata, etc.). They can also be created in R.

CREATING A DATA FRAME FOR R COMPUTATION USING AN EXCEL SPREADSHEET (WINDOWS PLATFORM)

As an example using a typical set of real **case–control** epidemiologic research data, consider the dataset in Table 3.2. These data were drawn from a clinical trial to evaluate the efficacy of maintenance chemotherapy for case subjects with acute myelogenous leukemia (AML), conducted at Stanford University, California, in 1977. After reaching a status of remission through treatment by chemotherapy, the patients who entered the study were assigned *randomly* to one of two groups:

(1)   Maintained: this group received maintenance chemotherapy.
(0)   Nonmaintained: this group did not receive chemotherapy; it is the control group.

The clinical trial was done to ascertain whether maintenance chemotherapy prolonged the time until relapse (="death").

We will use the following procedure (a) to *create* an AML data file, called AML. csv, in Windows; and (b) *to input* the new data file into R as a data file AML.

Creating a Data Frame for R Computation:

1.   Data input, using Microsoft Excel:
     (a)   Open the Excel spreadsheet.
     (b)   Type in data so that the variable names are in row 1 of the Excel spreadsheet.
     (c)   Consider each row of data to represent an individual case subject in the study.
     (d)   Start with column A

TABLE 3.2   Data for the AML Maintenance Clinical Study*

GROUP	DURATION FOR COMPLETE REMISSION (WEEKS)	A + INDICATES A CENSORED VALUE
1 = Maintained (11)	9,13,13+,18,23,28+,31,34,45+,48,161+ }	1 = Uncensored
0 = Nonmaintained (12)	5, 5, 8, 8, 12, 16+,23,27,30,33,43,45}	0 = Censored (+)

NB: The nonmaintained group may be considered as MBD.**

*Data points taken from *Survival Analysis Using S: Analysis of Time-to-Event Data*, by Mara Tableman and Jong Sung Kim (Boca Raton, FL: Chapman & Hall/CRC, 2004).

**The cancer epigenome is characterized by specific DNA methylation and chromatin modification patterns. The proteins that mediate these changes are encoded by the epigenetics genes defined here as:

- DNA methyltransferases (DNMT)
- methyl-CpG-binding domain (MBD) proteins
- histone acetyltransferases (HAT)
- histone deacetylases (HDAC)
- histone methyltransferases (HMT)
- histone demethylases

2. Save the spreadsheet as a .csv file:
   (a) *Click*: "File" → "Save as" → and then, in the file name box (the upper box at the bottom) type: AML.
   (b) In the "Save in:" box (at the top), *choose*: "Local Disc (C:)". The file AML then will be saved in the top level of the C drive; you may choose another level or location if you wish.
   (c) In the "Save as Type" box (the lower box at the bottom), *scroll down, select, and click* on: CSV (Comma delimited = Comma Separated Values).
   (d) To close Excel, *click* the big "X" at the top right-hand corner.
3. In Windows, check the C: drive for the AML.csv file.
4. Read AML into R:
   (a) Open R.
   (b) Use the read.csv() function:
   ```
   > aml <- read.csv("C:\\AML.csv", header = T,sep= ",").
   ```
   (c) This can be also be done by:
   ```
   > aml <- read.csv("C:\\AML.csv")
   > # Read in the AML.csv file from the C: drive of the computer, and call it
   > # aml.
   ```
5. Output the AML.csv file for inspection:
   ```
   > aml # Outputting:
       weeks   group   status
   1     9       1       1
   2    13       1       1
   3    13       1       0
   4    18       1       1
   5    23       1       1
   ```

6	28	1	0
7	31	1	1
8	34	1	1
9	45	1	0
10	48	1	1
11	161	1	0
12	5	0	1
13	5	0	1
14	8	0	1
15	8	0	1
16	12	0	1
17	16	0	0
18	23	0	1
19	27	0	1
20	30	0	1
21	33	0	1
22	43	0	1
23	45	0	1

```
>
```

Later in this book, in Section 7.3 of Chapter 7, this dataset will be revisited and further processed for survival analysis.

OBTAINING A DATA FRAME FROM A TEXT FILE

Data from various sources are often entered using many *different* software programs. They may be transferred from one format to another through the ASCII file format. For example, in Windows, a text file is the most common ASCII file, usually having a ".txt" extension. There are other files in ASCII format, including the "**.R**" command file.

Data from most software programs can be output or saved as an ASCII file. From Excel, a very popular spreadsheet program, the data can be saved in ".csv" (comma-separated values) format. This is an easy way to interface between Excel spreadsheet files and R. Open the Excel file and "save as" the .csv format.

Files with field separators: As an example, suppose that the file **csv1.xls** was originally an Excel spreadsheet. After it is saved in .csv format, the output file is called **csv1.csv**, the contents of which are:

```
"name","gender","age"
  "A",      "F",     20
  "B",      "M",     30
  "C",      "F",     40
```

The characters are enclosed in quotation marks and the *delimiters* (variable separators) are commas. Sometimes a file may not contain quotation marks, as in the file **csv2.csv**:

```
name,    gender,      age
  A,          F,       20
  B           M        30
```

For both files, the R command to read in the dataset is the same:

```
> a <- read.csv("csv1.csv", as.is=TRUE)
> a
  name gender age
1    A      F  20
2    B      M  30
3    C      F  40
```

The argument as.is=TRUE keeps all characters as they are; otherwise, the characters would have been coerced into factors. The variable "name" should not be factored, but "gender" should. The following command should therefore be entered as follows:

```
> a$gender <- factor(a$gender)
```

Note that the object a has a class data frame and that the names of the variables within the data frame "a" must be referenced using the dollar sign notation $. Otherwise, R will state that the object "gender" cannot be found.

For files with white space (spaces and tabs) as the separator, such as in the file **data1.txt**, the command to use is read.table():

```
> a <- read.table("data1.txt", header=TRUE, as.is=TRUE)
```

Files without field separators: Consider the file **data2.txt**, which is in a fixed field format *without* field separators.

```
  name gender age
1    A      F  20
2    B      M  30
3    C      F  40
```

To read in such a file, use the function read.fwf():

1. Skip the first line, which is the header.
2. The width of each variable and the column names must be specified:

```
> a <- read.fwf("data2.txt", skip=1, width=c(1,1,2), col.names
+               = c("name", "gender", "age"), as.is=TRUE)
```

DATA ENTRY AND ANALYSIS USING THE FUNCTION DATA.ENTRY()

The previous section dealt with creating data frames by reading in data created from programs outside R, such as Excel. It is also possible to enter data directly into R by using the function data.entry(). However, if the amount of data is large (say, more than 15 columns and/or more than 25 rows), the chance of human error is high with spreadsheet or text-mode data entry. A software program specially designed for data entry, such as *EpiData* (www.epidata.dk), is more appropriate.

DATA ENTRY USING SEVERAL AVAILABLE R FUNCTIONS

The dataset in Table 3.3 (Aragon, 2011), listing deaths among subjects who received a dose of tolbutamide or a placebo in the University Group Diabetes Program (1970),

TABLE 3.3 Deaths Among Subjects Who Received Tolbutamide or a Placebo in the University Group Diabetes Program (1970)*

	AGE < 55		AGE ≥ 55		COMBINED	
	TOLBUTAMIDE	PLACEBO	TOLBUTAMIDE	PLACEBO	TOLBUTAMIDE	PLACEBO
Deaths	8	5	22	16	30	21
Survivors	98	115	76	69	174	184

*Available at http://www.medepi.net/data/ugdp.txt

The R functions that can be used to import the data frame were introduced in Section 3.3, earlier in this chapter.

A convenient way to enter data at the command prompt is to use the R functions c(), matrix(), array(), apply(), list(), data.frame(), and odd.ratio(), as shown by the following examples, which use the data from Table 3.3:

```
> #Entering data for a vector
> vector1 <- c(8, 98, 5, 115) # Using data from Table 3.3.
> vector1
[1] 8 98 5 115
>
> vector2 <- c(22, 76, 16, 69); vector2 # Data from Table 3.3.
[1] 22 76 16 69
>
```

```
> # Entering data for a matrix
> matrix1 <- matrix(vector1, 2, 2)
> matrix1

     [,1]  [,2]
[1,]   8    5
[2,]  98  115

> matrix2 <- matrix(vector2, 2, 2); matrix2
     [,1]  [,2]
[1,]  22   16
[2,]  76   69
>
```

```
> # Entering data for an array
> udata <- array(c(vector1, vector2), c(2, 2, 2))
> udata

, , 1

     [,1]  [,2]
[1,]   8    5
```

```
, , 2

     [,1]  [,2]
[1,]  22    16
[2,]  76    69

> apply(udata, c(1, 2), sum); udata.tot
     [,1]  [,2]
[1,]  30    21
[2,] 174   184
>


> # Entering a list
> x <- list(crude.data = udata.tot, stratified.data = udata)
> x$crude.data

     [,1]  [,2]
[1,]  30    21
[2,] 174   184
> x$stratified

, , 1

     [,1]  [,2]
[1,]   8     5
[2,]  98   115

, , 2

     [,1]  [,2]
[1,]  22    16
[2,]  76    69
>


> # Entering a simple data frame
> subjectname <- c("Peter", "Paul", "Mary")
> subjectnumber <- 1:length(subjectname)
> age <- c(26, 27, 28) # These are the singers' true ages, respectively, in 1964.
> gender <- c("Male", "Male", "Female")
> data1 <- data.frame(subjectnumber, subjectname, age, gender)
> data1
    subjectnumber  subjectname  age    gender
1                1       Peter   26      Male
2                2        Paul   27      Male
3                3        Mary   28    Female
>
> # Entering a simple function
> odds.ratio <- function(aa, bb, cc, dd){ aa*dd / (bb*cc)}
> odds.ratio(30, 174, 21, 184) # Data from Table 3.3.
```

DATA ENTRY AND ANALYSIS USING THE FUNCTION SCAN() (TEETOR, 2011)

The R function scan() is taken from the CRAN package base. This function, which reads data into a vector or list from the console or file, takes the following usage form:

```
scan(file = "", what = double(), nmax = -1, n = -1, sep = "",
     quote = if(identical(sep, "\n")) "" else "'\"'", dec = ".",
     skip = 0, nlines = 0, na.strings = "NA",
     flush = FALSE, fill = FALSE, strip.white = FALSE,
     quiet = FALSE, blank.lines.skip = TRUE, multi.line = TRUE,
     comment.char = "", allowEscapes = FALSE,
     fileEncoding = "", encoding = "unknown", text)
```

Argument:

what	The type of what gives the type of data to be read. The supported types are logical, integer, numeric, complex, character, raw, and list. If what is a list, it is assumed that the lines of the data file are records, each containing length(what) items ("fields") and the list components should have elements that are one of the first six types listed or NULL.

The what argument describes the tokens that scan() should expect in the input file. For a detailed description of this function, execute:

```
> ?scan
```

The methodology of applying scan() is similar to that for c(), as described in the preceding subsection, except that it does not matter that the numbers are being entered on different lines. The result will still be a vector.

▪ Use scan() when accessing data from a file that has an irregular or a complex structure.

▪ Use scan() to read individual tokens and use the argument what to describe the stream of tokens in the file.

▪ scan() converts tokens into data and then assembles the data into records.
▪ Use scan() along with readLines(), especially when attempting to read an unorthodox file format. Together, these two functions will likely result in successful processing of the individual lines and tokens of the file.

The function readLines() reads lines from a file and returns them to a list of character strings:

```
> lines <- readLines("input.text")
```

One may limit the number of lines to be read, per pass, by using the n parameter, which gives the maximum number of lines to be read:

```
> lines <- readLines("input.text, n=5) # Read 5 lines and stop
```

The function scan() reads one token at a time and handles it as instructed. For example, assume that the file to be scanned and read contains triplets of data (like

15-Oct-1987	2439.78	2345.63	16-Oct-1987	2396.21	2207.73
19-Oct-1987	2164.16	1677.55	20-Oct-1987	2067.47	1616.23
21-Oct-1987	2087.07	1951.76			

Use a list to inform scan() that it should expect a repeating, 3-token sequence:

> triplets <- scan("triples.txt, what=list(character(0), numeric(0), numeric(0)))

Give names to the list elements, and scan() will assign those names to the data:

> triplets <- scan("triples.txt,
+   what=list(date=character(0), high=numeric(0), low=numeric(0)))

Here, it reads five records:

> triples # *Outputs:*
$date
[1] "15-Oct-1987" "15-Oct-1987" "19-Oct-1987" "20-Oct-1987" "21-Oct-1987"
$high
[1] 2439-78 2396.21 2164.16 2067.47 2081.07
$low
[1] 2345.63 2207.73 1677.55 1616.21 1951.76

DATA ENTRY AND ANALYSIS USING THE FUNCTION SOURCE() (ARAGON, 2011; TEETOR, 2011; VENABLES ET AL., 2004)

The R function source() is also taken from the CRAN package base. This function, which reads data into a vector or list from the console or file, takes the following usage form:

source() causes R to accept its input from the named file or URL or connection. Input is read and parsed from that file until the end of the file is reached; then the parsed expressions are evaluated sequentially in the chosen environment:

```
source(file, local = FALSE, echo = verbose, print.eval = echo,
      verbose = getOption("verbose"),
      prompt.echo = getOption("prompt"),
      max.deparse.length = 150, chdir = FALSE,
      encoding = getOption("encoding"),
      continue.echo = getOption("continue"),
      skip.echo = 0, keep.source = getOption("keep.source"))
```

Commands that are stored in an external file, such as **commands.R** in the working directory "work," can be executed in an R environment with the command:

> source("command.R")

The function source() instructs R to read the text and execute its contents. Thus, when you have a long or frequently used piece of R code, you may capture it inside a text file. This allows you to rerun the code without having to retype it, and use the function source() to read and execute the code.

For example: Suppose that the file **howdy.R** contains the familiar greeting:

By sourcing the file, you can execute the content of the file, as in the following R code segment:

```
> source("howdy.R")
[1] "Hi, My Friend!"
```

Setting echo-TRUE will echo the same script lines before they are executed, with the R prompt shown before each line:

```
> source("howdy.R", echo=TRUE)
> Print("Hi, My Friend!")
[1] "Hi, My Friend!"
```

DATA ENTRY AND ANALYSIS USING THE SPREADSHEET INTERFACE IN R (ARAGON, 2011)

Data entry with R's spreadsheet interface uses the following R functions in the package utils:

```
data.entry(..., Modes = NULL, Names = NULL)
dataentry(data, modes)
de(..., Modes = list(), Names = NULL)
```

The arguments of these R functions are as follows:

...	A list of variables; currently, these should be numeric or character vectors or a list containing such vectors.
Modes	The modes to be used for the variables.
Names	The names to be used for the variables.
Data	A list of numeric and/or character vectors.
Modes	A list of a length up to that of data giving the modes of (some of) the variables; list() is allowed.

The function data.entry() edits an existing object, saving the changes to the original object name. However, the function edit() edits an existing object but does *not* save the changes to the original object name; thus, one must assign it to an object name (even if it is the original name).

To enter a vector, one needs to initialize a vector and then use the function data.entry(). For example:

Start by entering the R environment, and set:

```
> x <- c(2, 4, 6, 8, 10) # X is initially defined as an array of five elements.
> x # Just checking to make sure.
[1] 2 4 6 8 10 # x is indeed set to be an array of five elements.
>
> data.entry(x) # Entering the Data Editor:
> # The Data Editor window opens. Looking at the first column:
> # it is now named "x", with the first five rows (all in the first column) filled
```

> # *respectively, by the numbers 2, 4, 6, 8, 10*
> # *One can now edit this dataset by, say, changing all the entries to 2, then*
> # *closing the Data Editor window and returning to the R console window.*
> x
[1] **2 2 2 2 2** # *x is indeed changed.*
> # *Thus, one can change the entries for x via the Data Editor, and save the changes.*

When using the functions data.entry(x) and edit() for data entry, there are a number of limitations (Aragon, 2011):

- Arrays and nontabular lists cannot be entered using a spreadsheet editor.
- When using the function edit() to create a new data frame, one must assign it an object name in order to save the data frame.
- This approach is not a preferred method for entering data because one often prefers to have the original data in a text editor or available to be read in from a data file.

EDITING A DATA FRAME IN R (ADLER, 2010)

To edit a data frame, one may use the function edit(). This calls up a spreadsheet editor with a column for each variable in the data frame. Within the editor spread-sheet, one may then direct the mouse/cursor and begin editing the existing cells by typing in the new data in place of the old data. One may also change the type of variable from real (numeric) to character (factor) by clicking on the column headers. The names of the variables may also be changed. When the Data Editor is closed, *the new edited data frame is assigned to the new name given, and the original data frame is left unchanged.*

For example, if the dataset cancer, in the package survival, is to be edited, one may use:

```
> data(cancer)
> cancer1 <- edit(cancer)
```

This is illustrated in the next example. Moreover, to enter data into a blank data frame, one may use:

```
> newdata <- data.frame()
> fix(newdata)
```

■ **Example:** In the data frame cancer, in the CRAN package survival, change the meal.cal value of the first row from 1175 to 1176.

Solution: The following R code segment is used to accomplish the required editing task:

```
> install.packages("survival") # Installing the package survival
> library(survival) # Bringing in the files of survival
> ls("package:survival")     # Listing all the files in survival, noting that
```

[1] "aareg"	"aml"	"attrassign"
[4] "basehaz"	"bladder"	"bladder1"
[7] "bladder2"	"cancer"	"cch"
[10] "cgd"	"clogit"	"cluster"
[13] "colon"	"cox.zph"	"coxph"
[16] "coxph.control"	"coxph.detail"	"coxph.fit"
[19] "dsurvreg"	"format.Surv"	"frailty"
[22] "frailty.gamma"	"frailty.gaussian"	"frailty.t"
[25] "heart"	"is.na.coxph.penalty"	"is.na.ratetable"
[28] "is.na.Surv"	"is.ratetable"	"is.Surv"
[31] "jasa"	"jasa1"	"kidney"
[34] "labels.survreg"	"leukemia"	"logan"
[37] "lung"	"match.ratetable"	"mgus"
[40] "mgus1"	"mgus2"	"nwtco"
[43] "ovarian"	"pbc"	"pbcseq"
[46] "pspline"	"psurvreg"	"pyears"
[49] "qsurvreg"	"ratetable"	"ratetableDate"
[52] "rats"	"ridge"	"stanford2"
[55] "strata"	"Surv"	"survConcordance"
[58] "survdiff"	"survexp"	"survexp.mn"
[61] "survexp.us"	"survexp.usr"	"survfit"
[64] "survfitcoxph.fit"	"survobrien"	"survreg"
[67] "survreg.control"	"survreg.distributions"	"survreg.fit"
[70] "survregDtest"	"survSplit"	"tcut"
[73] "tobin"	"tt"	"untangle.specials"
[76] "veteran"		

```
> data(cancer) # Calling in the data frame cancer
> cancer # Checking over the data frame (looking at the first 5 lines only)
```

	inst	time	status	age	sex	ph.ecog	ph.karno	pat.karno	meal.cal	wt.loss
1	3	306	2	74	1	1	90	100	1175	NA
2	3	455	2	68	1	0	90	90	1225	15
3	3	1010	1	56	1	0	90	90	NA	15
4	5	210	2	57	1	1	90	60	1150	11
5	1	883	2	60	1	0	100	90	NA	0

```
> cancer1 <- edit(cancer) # Editing cancer and renaming it cancer1
> # A spreadsheet with the dataset cancer opens. Within the spreadsheet,
> # manually change the first meal.cal entry from "1175" to "1176":
```

	inst	time	status	age	sex	ph.ecog	ph.karno	pat.karno	meal.cal	wt.loss
1	3	306	2	74	1	1	90	100	1176	NA
2	3	455	2	68	1	0	90	90	1225	15
3	3	1010	1	56	1	0	90	90	NA	15
4	5	210	2	57	1	1	90	60	1150	11
5	1	883	2	60	1	0	100	90	NA	0

> # *Close the spreadsheet. Return to the* R *environment and check the*
> # *newly edited data frame* cancer1:
> cancer1

	inst	time	status	age	sex	ph.ecog	ph.karno	pat.karno	meal.cal	wt.loss
1	3	306	2	74	1	1	90	100	1176	NA
2	3	455	2	68	1	0	90	90	1225	15
3	3	1010	1	56	1	0	90	90	NA	15
4	5	210	2	57	1	1	90	60	1150	11
5	1	883	2	60	1	0	100	90	NA	0

> # cancer1 *is the edited dataset, as required. The original data frame*
> # cancer *remains unchanged.*

The Function list() and the Making of data.frame() in R (Dalgaard, 2002; Teetor, 2011; Venables et al., 2004)

THE FUNCTION list()

A list in R consists of an ordered collection of objects—its **components**—which may be of any mode or type. For example, a list may consist of a matrix, a numeric vector, a complex vector, a logical value, a character array, a function, and so on. The following example shows a simple way to create a list.

■ **Example:** It's as easy as 1, 2, 3!

```
> x <- 1
> y <- 2
> z <- 3
> list1 <- list(x, y, z) # Forming a simple list
> list1 # Outputting:
[[1]]
[1] 1
[[2]]
[1] 2
[[3]]
[1] 3
```

The components are always numbered and may be referred to as such. Thus, if my.special.list is the name of a list with four components, they may be referred to individually as my.special.list[[1]], my.special.list[[2]], my.special.list[[3]], and my .special.list[[4]].

If one defines my.special.list as follows:

```
> my.special.list <- list(name="John", wife="Mary",
+    number.of.children=3, children.age=c(2, 4, 6))
```

then

```
> my.special.list[[1]] # Outputting:
```

```
> my.special.list[[2]]
[1] "Mary"
> my.special.list[[3]]
[1] 3
> my.special.list[[4]]
[1] 2 4 6
```

The Number of Components in a List: The number of (top-level) components in a list may be found by the function length(). Thus:

```
> length(my.special.list)
[1] 4
```

That is, the list my.special.list has four components.

To combine a set of objects into a larger composite collection for more efficient processing, the list function may be used to construct a list from its components. As an example, consider

```
> odds <- c(1, 3, 5, 7, 9, 11,13,15,17,19)
> evens <- c(2, 4, 6, 8, 10, 12, 14, 16, 18, 20)
> mylist <- list(before=odds, after=evens)
> mylist
$before
[1] 1 3 5 7 9 11 13 15 17 19
$after
[1] 2 4 6 8 10 12 14 16 18 20
> mylist$before
[1] 1 3 5 7 9 11 13 15 17 19
> mylist$after
[1] 2 4 6 8 10 12 14 16 18 20
```

Components of a List: Components of a list may be named. In such a case, the component may be referred to either:

1. By giving the component name as a character string in place of the number in double square brackets, or
2. By giving an expression of the form > name$component_name for the same object

■ **Example 2:** Concatenating Lists

Take any three, more or less, lists:

```
> list.A <- c("The", "quick", "brown")
> list.A
[1] "The" "quick" "brown"
> list.B <- c("fox", "jumps", "over")
> list.B
[1] "fox" "jumps" "over"
> list.C <- c("the", "lazy", "dog")
```

[1] "the" "lazy" "dog"
> list.ABC <- c(list.A, list.B, list.C) # *Concatenating the three lists*
> list.ABC # *Outputting:*
[1] "The" "quick" "brown" "fox" "jumps" "over" "the" "lazy" "dog"
>

THE CONSTRUCTION OF DATA FRAMES USING THE FUNCTION data.frame()

A *data frame* is a list with class "data.frame". Restrictions on lists that may be turned into data frames are as follows:

- The components in the list must be vectors (including numeric, logical, or character), numeric matrixes, lists, factors, or other data frames.
- Matrixes, lists, and data frames provide as many variables to the new data frame as that frame has columns, elements, and variables, respectively.
- Numeric and logical vectors and factors are included as is. Character vectors are restricted to being factors, whose levels are the unique values appearing in the vector.
- Vector structures appearing as variables of the data frame should all have the same row size.

For most purposes, a data frame may be considered a matrix with columns possibly of different modes and attributes. However, a data frame may be shown in matrix form, with its rows and columns extracted using matrix-indexing conventions.

The function data.frame(), from the R package base, creates data frames that are tightly coupled collections of variables sharing many of the properties of matrixes and of lists. This function is used as the fundamental data structure by most of R's modeling software. It is defined by

```
data.frame(..., row.names = NULL, check.rows = FALSE,
                check.names = TRUE,
                stringsAsFactors = default.stringsAsFactors())
```

Many rules used for arrays are also applicable to data frames. For example, the main structure of a data frame consists of columns (or variables) and rows (or records). The rules for subscripting, column or row binding, and selection of a subset in arrays apply to data frames.

However, data frames are more complicated than arrays:

- All columns in an array are forced to be character if just one cell is a character. In contrast, a data frame can have different classes of columns. For example, a data frame can consist of a column "Patient.ID"(which is numeric); and a column "name"(which is character).
- A data frame can also have extra attributes. For example, each variable can have lengthy variable descriptions.
- A factor in a data frame often has "levels" or value labels.

These attributes can be transferred from the original dataset in other formats, such as SAS, SPSS, or Stata. They can also be created in R during the analysis.

OBTAINING A DATA FRAME FROM A TEXT FILE

Obtaining a data frame from a text file was discussed earlier in this section, and examples were given. Those subsections dealt with creating data frames by reading in data created from programs outside R, such as Excel on the Windows platform. We also discussed, and gave examples of, obtaining a data frame by entering data directly into R using the function data.entry(). As noted there, the chance of human error is high when spreadsheet or text-mode data entry is undertaken. Hence, the software program *EpiData*, which is specially designed for data entry, is more appropriate.

EpiData has facilities for setting up useful constraints such as range checks, automatic jumps, and labeling of variables and values (codes) for each variable. One can do a direct transfer between *EpiData* and R (using "read.epiinfo"), but it is recommended to export data from *EpiData* (using the export procedure inside that software) to Stata format and use the function read.dta to read the dataset into R. Exporting data into Stata format maintains many of the attributes of the variables, such as the variable labels and descriptions (Virasakdi, 2011).

Review Questions for Section 3.4

1. To use R in data analysis in BIOS, the data to be processed must first be entered into the R environment. Discuss seven ways of entering data, giving examples.
2. How can the function list() be used to enter data into the R environment? Provide an example.
3. Use the function data.frame() to enter data into the R environment, giving an example.
4. Use the following functions to input data into the R environment, giving an example of each: c(), matrix(), and array().
5. Use the function source() to enter data into the R environment, giving an example.
6. What are the limitations when using the functions data.entry(x) and edit() for data entry?
7. Show that the function list() may be used to combine several components to form a new list, giving an example.
8. Write a code segment in R to extract the name of a component stored in another variable, giving an example.
9. Set up an example in which you use the concatenation function c() with given list arguments, and obtain a list whose components are those of the argument list joined together sequentially, in the following form:
   > list.ABC <- c(list.A, list.B, list.C)
10. Look up the *EpiData* software from its website (www.epidata.dk), and suggest an efficient method of data entry in R.

Exercises for Section 3.4 (Dalgaard, 2002; Everitt & Hothorn, 2006; Virasakdi, 2011)

1. Bladder cancer data in HSAUR2 (Everitt & Hothorn, 2006).
   The data were taken from 31 male patients who were treated for superficial bladder cancer. The data record the number of recurrent tumors during a particular

time after removal of the primary tumor, along with the size of the original tumor. Let us take an in-depth look at the dataset.

(a) Use the following code segments to enter the dataset to examine its contents:
```
> data("bladdercancer", package = "HSAUR2")
```
(b) Output the whole data frame using the code segment:
```
> bladdercancer
```
(c) Sort the data frame by components using the code segment:
```
> data1 <- c(~ number + tumorsize, data = bladdercancer)
> data1
```
(d) Using the following code segment, you can also reach the package HSAUR2, which contains the dataset bladdercancer.
```
> install.packages("HSAUR2")
```
You will be asked to select a CRAN site for support of your work:
Please select a CRAN mirror for use in this session ---

If you have no particular preference, select the site USA (CA1), which is the University of California at Berkeley:
```
> data ("bladdercancer")
```
2. Here is another data frame:

(a) Use the following code segments to enter the dataset to examine its contents:
```
> data("HELPrct", package = "mosaic")
> data
```
(b) Use the following code segment to extract the component from the dataset:
```
> data1 <- c(data = HELPrct)
> data1
```
3. Here is one more data frame of epidemiologic interest: the data frame USmelanoma, which may also be downloaded from the R package HSAUR2.

In this case, one can examine the annual mortality rate from a malignant melanoma by U.S. state, and also by the latitude of their geographical centers. These epidemiologic data were collected from the population of White males in the United States during 1950–1969. The study was of interest because it was thought that

◼ People with light skin color are more susceptible to the development of malignant melanoma.

◼ The geographic latitude of the location is related to the amount of sun exposure per unit time on average.

(a) Use the following code segments to download the dataset from HSAUR2:
```
> data("USmelanoma", package = "HSAUR2")
```
(b) Use the following code segment to extract the dataset USmelanoma:
```
> data
```
[1] "USmelanoma"
```
> USmelanoma
```
(c) Sort the data frame by components using the following code segment:
```
> data1 <- c(~ mortality + latitude, data = USmelanoma)
> data1
```

4. Here are some data frames from the study of genetics (genome size data from www.ornl.gov; Seefeld & Linder, 2005).

   (a) Use the following code segments to download the vectors that constitute the dataset and to create the data frame object:

   ```
   > organism<-c("Human","Mouse","Fruit Fly",
   +              "Roundworm","Yeast")
   > genomeSizeBP<-
   +    c(3000000000,3000000000,135600000,97000000,12100000)
   > estGeneCount<-c(30000,30000,13061,19099,6034)
   ```

   (b) If you have three vectors of equal length, you can join them in a data frame using the function data.frame() with the vectors as the arguments of this function. Note that the format is "column name"="vector to add" and the equals (not assignment <-) operator is used. Here, you are naming columns rather than creating new variables: the variable names are used as column names, but you could rename the columns with names other than the variable names:

   ```
   > comparativeGenomeSize<-
   + data.
   > comparativeGenomeSize<-
   + data.frame(organism=organism,genomeSizeBP=genomeSizeBP,
   + estGeneCount=estGeneCount)
   > comparativeGenomeSize
   ```

   (c) Sort the data frame by components using the following code segment:

   ```
   > data1 <- c(~ organism, data = comparativeGenomeSize)
   > data1
   ```

5. *Using the Data Editor:* From ISwR (*Introductory Statistics with R*; Dalgaard, 2002)

   (a) Bring the ISwR package onto the computer-desktop R environment using the following code segment:

   ```
   > install.packages("ISwR")
   > # For --- Please select a CRAN mirror for use in this session --- # select CA1
   ```

   (b) Edit the data frame airquality using the function edit() in the following code segment:

   ```
   > data(airquality)
   > aq <- edit(airquality)
   ```

   This brings up a spreadsheet-like editor with a column for each variable in the data frame.

   (c) Once inside the editor, move the cursor around with the mouse or the touch-pad, and edit the cells by typing in new data or changing the existing data. Then close the editor and enter:

   ```
   > aq
   ```

   The first two lines of the aq file will look like this:

	Ozone	Solar.R	Wind	Temp	Month	Day
1	41	190	7.4	67	5	10
2	36	118	8.0	72	5	2

   (d) Return to the Data Editor by entering:

   ```
   > aq <- edit(airquality)
   ```

   Once back inside the editor, change the data. For example, change the first row

```
> aq
```
The first two lines of the aq file will then look like this:

	Ozone	Solar.R	Wind	Temp	Month	Day
1	42	190	7.4	67	5	10
2	36	118	8.0	72	5	2

The value of the variable "Ozone" on the first row has been changed from 41 to 42. Has the data editing process been a success?

Remark: When the Data Editor is closed, the edited data frame is assigned to aq and the original file airquality is left unchanged.

3.5   UNIVARIATE, BIVARIATE, AND MULTIVARIATE DATA ANALYSIS

A **univariate** dataset has only one variable:$\{x\}$, such as {*patient name*}.

A **bivariate** dataset has two variables:$\{x_1, x_2\}$ or $\{x, y\}$, such as {*patient name, gender*}.

A **multivariate** dataset has more than two, or many, variables: $\{x_1, x_2, x_3, ..., x_n\}$, such as {*patient name, gender, age, diagnosis, treatment, ...*}.

Univariate Data Analysis

As an example, enter the following code segments:

```
> x <- rexp(100); x     # Outputting 100 exponentially distributed random
>                       # numbers:
```

[1] 0.39136880	0.66948212	1.48543076	0.34692128	0.71533079	0.12897216
[7] 1.08455419	0.07858231	1.01995665	0.81232737	0.78253619	4.27512555
[13] 2.11839466	0.47024886	0.62351482	1.02834522	2.17253419	0.37622879
[19] 0.16456926	1.81590741	0.16007371	0.95078524	1.26048607	5.92621325
[25] 0.21727112	0.07086311	0.83858727	1.01375231	1.49042968	0.53331210
[31] 0.21069467	0.37559212	0.10733795	2.84094906	0.17899040	1.34612473
[37] 0.00290699	1.77078060	1.79505318	0.09763821	1.96568170	0.15911043
[43] 4.36726420	0.33652419	0.01196883	0.35657882	0.72797670	0.91958975
[49] 0.68777857	0.29100399	0.22553560	1.56909742	0.20617517	0.37169621
[55] 0.53173534	0.26034316	0.21965356	2.94355695	1.88392667	1.13933083
[61] 0.31663107	0.23899975	0.01544856	1.30674088	0.53674598	1.72018758
[67] 0.31035278	0.81074737	0.09104104	1.52426229	1.35520172	0.27969075
[73] 1.36320488	0.56317216	0.85022837	0.49031656	0.17158651	0.31015165
[79] 2.07315953	1.29566872	1.28955269	0.33487343	0.20902716	2.84732652
[85] 0.58873236	1.54868210	2.93994181	0.46520037	0.73687959	0.50062507
[91] 0.20275282	0.49697531	0.58578119	0.49747575	1.53430435	4.56340237
[97] 0.90547787	0.72972219	2.60686316	0.33908320		

Note: The function rexp() is defined as follows:

```
rexp(n, rate = 1)
```

with arguments:

x	Vector
n	Number of observations. If length(n) > 1, the length is taken to be the number required.

The exponential distribution with rate λ has the following density: $f(x) = \lambda e^{-\lambda x}$, for $x \geq 0$. If the rate λ is not specified, it assumes the default value of 1.

Remark: The function rexp() is one of the functions in R under Exponential in the CRAN package stats.

To undertake a biostatistical analysis of this set of univariate data, call up the function univax(), in the package epibasix, using the following code segments:
```
> library(epibasix)
> univar(x) # Outputting:
Univariate Summary
Sample Size: 100
Sample Mean: 1.005
Sample Median: 0.646
Sample Standard Deviation: 1.067
>
```
Thus, for this sample, with a size of 100 elements, the mean, median, and standard deviation have been computed.

For data analysis of univariate datasets, the R package epibasix may be used. This CRAN (n.d.) package covers many elementary epidemiologic functions for biostatistics and epidemiology. It contains elementary tools for the analysis of common epidemiologic problems, ranging from sample-size estimation, through 2×2 contingency table analysis, and basic measures of agreement (kappa, sensitivity/specificity).

Appropriate print and summary statements have also been written to facilitate interpretation wherever possible. This work is appropriate for graduate biostatistics/epidemiology courses. This package is a work in progress.

To start, enter the R environment and use the following code segment:
```
> install.packages("epibasix")
Installing package(s) into 'C:/Users/bertchan/Documents/R/win-library/2.14'
    (as 'lib' is unspecified)
--- Please select a CRAN mirror for use in this session ---
> # Select CA1
trying URL
'http://cran.cnr.Berkeley.edu/bin/windows/contrib/2.14/epibasix_1.1.zip'
Content type 'application/zip' length 57888 bytes (56 Kb)
```

downloaded 56 Kb
package 'epibasix' successfully unpacked and MD5 sums checked
The downloaded packages are in
C:\Users\bertchan\AppData\Local\Temp\RtmpMFOrEn\downloaded_
packages

With epibasix loaded into the R environment, follow these steps to learn more about this package:

1. Go to the CRAN website (http://cran.r-project.org).
2. Select (single click) "Packages" in the left column.
3. On the "Packages" page, select E (for epibasix).

Available CRAN Packages by Name

A B C D E F G H I J K L M N O P Q R S T U V W X Y Z

4. Scroll down the list of packages whose names start with "E" or "e", and select:

epibasix	Elementary Epidemiological Functions for a Graduate Epidemiology\Biostatistics Course

5. When the epibasix page opens up, select: Reference manual: ***epibasix.pdf***
6. The information is now displayed as follows:

Package	**'epibasix'**
	January 2, 2012
Version	**1.1**
Date	**2009-05-13**
Title	**Elementary Epidemiological Functions for a Graduate Epidemiology\{}Biostatistics Course**
Author	**Michael A Rotondi <mrotondi@uwo.ca>**
Maintainer	**Michael A Rotondi mrotondi@uwo.ca**
Depends R	**(>= 2.01)**

For another example, consider the same analysis on the first 100 natural numbers, using the following R code segments:

```
> x <-1:100; x # Consider, and then output, the first 100 natural numbers:
 [1]   1   2   3   4   5   6   7   8   9  10  11  12  13  14  15  16  17  18
[19]  19  20  21  22  23  24  25  26  27  28  29  30  31  32  33  34  35  36
[37]  37  38  39  40  41  42  43  44  45  46  47  48  49  50  51  52  53  54
[55]  55  56  57  58  59  60  61  62  63  64  65  66  67  68  69  70  71  72
[73]  73  74  75  76  77  78  79  80  81  82  83  84  85  86  87  88  89  90
[91]  91  92  93  94  95  96  97  98  99 100
> # ANOVA Tables: Summarized in the following tables, ANOVA is used for
> # two different purposes:
> library(epibasix)
> univar(x) # Performing a univariate data analysis on the vector x, and
> # outputting:
```

Univariate Summary
Sample Size: 100

Sample Mean: 50.5
Sample Median: 50.5
Sample Standard Deviation: 29.011

Bivariate and Multivariate Data Analysis (Daniel, 2005)

When there are two variables, (X, Y), one needs to consider two cases:

Case I: In the classical regression model, only Y (called the *dependent variable*) is required to be random. X is defined as a fixed, nonrandom, variable, and is called the *independent variable*. Under this model, observations are obtained by preselecting values of X and determining the corresponding value of Y.

Case II: If both X and Y are random variables, the **correlation model** is used. Under this model, sample observations are obtained by selecting a random sample of the units of association, such as persons, characteristics (age, gender, locations, points of time, specific events/actions/...,), or elements on which the two measurements are based; and by recording a measurement of X and of Y. In this case, values of X are not preselected but rather occur at random, depending on the unit of association selected in the sample.

REGRESSION ANALYSIS

Case I—Correlation analysis cannot be meaningfully performed under this model.
Case II—Regression analysis can be performed under the correlation model.

Correlation for two variables implies a co-relationship between the variables and does not distinguish between them as to which is the dependent or independent variable. Thus, one may fit a straight line to the data either by minimizing $\sum(x_i - \underline{x})^2$ or by minimizing $\sum(y_i - \underline{y})^2$. The fitted regression line will generally be different in the two cases, so a logical question arises as to which line to fit.

Two situations do exist, and should be considered:

1. If the objective is to obtain a measure of strength of the relationship between the two variables, it does not matter which line is fitted; the measure calculated will be the same in either case.

2. If one needs to use the equation describing the relationship between the two variables to gauge the dependency of one upon the other, it *does* matter which line is to be fitted. The variable for which one wishes to estimate means or to make predictions should be treated as the dependent variable. That is, this variable should be regressed with respect to the other variable.

AVAILABLE R PACKAGES FOR BIVARIATE DATA ANALYSIS

Among the R packages for bivariate data analysis, a notable one available for sample-size calculations in the bivariate random intercept (RI) regression model is bivarRIpower.

■ **Example of Bivariate Data Analysis:** As an example, this package may be used to calculate the necessary sample size to achieve 80% power at 5% alpha level for null and alternative hypotheses so that the correlation between RIs is 0 and 0.2, respectively, across six time points. Other covariance parameters are set as follows:

■ Correlation between residuals = 0
■ Standard deviations: 1st RI = 1, 2nd RI = 2, 1st residual = 0.5, 2nd residual = 0.75

The following R code segment may be used:

```
> library(bivarRIpower)
> bivarcalcn(power=.80,powerfor='RI',timepts=6,d1=1,d2=2,
+ p=0,p1=.2,s1=.5,s2=.75,r=0,r1=.1) # Outputting:
```

Variance parameters

Clusters	=	209.2
Repeated measurements	=	6
Standard deviations		
1st random intercept	=	1
2nd random intercept	=	2
1st residual term	=	0.5
2nd residual term	=	0.75
Correlations		
RI under H_o	=	0
RI under H_a	=	0.2
Residual under H_o	=	0
Residual under H_a	=	0.1
Con obs under H_o	=	0
Con obs under H_a	=	0.1831984
Lag obs under H_o	=	0
Lag obs under H_a	=	0.1674957

Correlation variances under H_o

Random intercept	=	0.005096138
Residual	=	0.0009558759
Concurrent observations	=	0.00358999
Lagged observations	=	0.003574277

Power (%) for correlations

Random intercept	=	80%
Residual	=	89.9%
Concurrent observations	=	86.4%
Lagged observations	=	80%

```
>
```

BIVARIATE NORMAL DISTRIBUTION

Under the correlation model, the bivariates X and Y vary together in a *joint distribution*, which, if this joint distribution is normal, is called a **bivariate normal distribution**. From this distribution, inferences may be made based on the results of sampling properly from the population. If the joint distribution is known to be nonnormal, or if the form is unknown, inferential procedures are invalid. When sampling from a bivariate distribution, the following assumptions must hold if inferences about the population are to be valid:

- For each value of X, there is a normally distributed subpopulation of Y values.
- For each value of Y, there is a normally distributed subpopulation of X values.
- The joint distribution of X and Y is a normal distribution (the bivariate normal distribution).
- The subpopulation of Y values all have the same variance.
- The subpopulation of X values all have the same variance.

Two random variables X and Y are said to be **jointly normal** if they can be expressed in the form

$$X = aU + bV \tag{3.5-1}$$

$$Y = cU + dV \tag{3.5-2}$$

where U and V are independent normal random variables.

If X and Y are jointly normal, then any linear combination

$$Z = s_1 X + s_2 Y \tag{3.5-3}$$

has a normal distribution. The reason is that if one has $X = aU + bV$ and $Y = cU + dV$ for some independent normal random variables U and V, then

$$Z = s_1(aU + bV) + s_2(cU + dV) = (as_1 + cs_2)U + (bs_1 + ds_2) \tag{3.5-4}$$

Thus, Z is the sum of the independent normal random variables $(as_1 + cs_2)U$ and $(bs_1 + ds_2)V$, and is therefore normal.

A very important property of jointly normal random variables is that **zero correlation implies independence**. If two random variables X and Y are jointly normal and are uncorrelated, then they are independent. This property can be verified using multivariate transforms.

Multivariate Data Analysis (Daniel, 2005)

Two similar, but distinct, approaches are used for multivariate data analysis: multiple linear regression analysis and multiple correlation model analysis.

MULTIPLE LINEAR REGRESSION ANALYSIS

Multiple linear regression analysis assumes that a linear relationship exists between some variable Y (the dependent variable) and n independent variables X_1, X_2, X_3, ... , X_n, which are called *explanatory* or *predictor variables* because of the way they are used.

For multiple linear regression, the model equation is

$$y_j = \beta_0 + \beta_1 x_{1j} + \beta_2 x_{2j} + \beta_3 x_{3j} + \cdots + \beta_n x_{nj} + e_j \qquad (3.5\text{-}5)$$

where y_j is a typical value from one of the subpopulations of Y values and the β_i values are the regression coefficients.

$x_{1j}, x_{2j}, x_{3j}, \ldots, x_{nj}$ are particular values of the independent variables $X_1, X_2, X_3, \ldots, X_n$, respectively, and e_j is a random variable with mean 0 and variance β^2, the common variance of the subpopulation of Y values. Generally, e_j is assumed to be normal and independently distributed.

When Equation (3.5-1) consists of one dependent variable and two independent variables, the model becomes

$$y_j = \beta_0 + \beta_1 x_{1j} + \beta_2 x_{2j} + e_j \qquad (3.5\text{-}6)$$

A plane in three-dimensional (3D) space may be fitted to the data points. For models containing more than two variables, it is a **hyperplane.**

The parameter of interest in this model is the **coefficient of multiple determination,** $R^2_{y,12\ldots n}$, obtained by dividing the explained sum of squares by the total sum of squares:

$$R^2_{y,12\ldots n} = \sum (\underline{y}_i \, y)^2 / \sum (\underline{y}_i \, y)^2 = SSR/SSE \qquad (3.5\text{-}7)$$

where

$\sum (\underline{y}_i \, y)^2$ = the explained variation,
             = the original observed values from the calculated Y values,
             = the sum of squared deviation of the calculated values from the mean of the observed Y values, or
             = the sum of squares due to regression (SSR)

$\sum (\underline{y}_i \, y)^2$ = the unexplained variation,
             = the sum of squared deviations of the original observations from the calculated values,
             = the sum of squares about regression, or
             = the error sum of squares (SSE).

The total variation is the sum of squared deviations of each observation of Y from the mean of the observations:

$$\sum (y_j \, y)^2 = \sum (\underline{y}_i \, y)^2 + \sum (\underline{y}_i \, y)^2 \qquad (3.5\text{-}8A)$$

$$SST = SSR + SSE \qquad (3.5\text{-}8B)$$

or

Total sum of squares = Explained (regression) sum of squares

+ Unexplained (error) sum of squares $\qquad (3.5\text{-}8C)$

MULTIPLE CORRELATION MODEL ANALYSIS

The object of this approach is to gain insight into the strength of the relationship between variables.

The assumptions underlying **multiple regression model analysis** are:

1. The Xi items are nonrandom fixed variables, indicating that any inferences drawn from sample data apply only to the set of X values observed, but not to larger collections of X. Under this regression model, correlation analysis is not meaningful.
2. For each set of X_i values, there is a subpopulation of Y values. Usually, one assumes that these Y values are normally distributed.
3. The variances of Y are all equal.
4. The Y values are independent of the different selected sets of X values.

The multiple correlation model equation is

$$y_j = \beta_0 + \beta_1 x_{1j} + \beta_2 x_{2j} + \beta_3 x_{3j} + \dots + \beta_n x_{nj} + e_j \tag{3.5-9}$$

where y_j is a typical value from one of the subpopulations of Y values; the β_i values are the regression coefficients; $x_{1j}, x_{2j}, x_{3j}, \dots, x_{nj}$ are particularly known values of the random variables $X_1, X_2, X_3, \dots, X_n$, respectively; and e_j is a random variable with mean 0 and variance σ^2, the common variance of the subpopulation of Y values. Generally, e_j is assumed to be normal and independently distributed.

This model is similar to Equation (3.5-5), with one important distinction: In Equation (3.5-5), the X_i items are nonrandom variables, but in Equation (3.5-9), the X_i items are random variables. That is, in the correlation model Equation (3.5-9), there is a joint distribution of Y and X_i, which is called a **multivariate distribution**.

Under this model, the variables are no longer considered as being dependent or independent, because logically they are interchangeable, and any X_i may play the role of Y.

To analyze the relationships among the variables, consider the **multiple correlation coefficient**, which is the square root of the coefficient of multiple determination. Hence, the sample value may be computed by taking the square root of Equation (3.5-7):

$$R^2_{y,12\dots n} = \sqrt{R^2_{y,12\dots n}} = \sqrt{\{\sum (\hat{y}_i \, y)^2 / \sum (y_i \, y)^2\}} = \sqrt{(SSR/SSE)} \tag{3.5-10}$$

Analysis of Variance (ANOVA, n.d.)

In biostatistics, **AN**alysis **O**f **VA**riance (ANOVA) is a collection of biostatistical models in which the observed variance in a particular variable is partitioned into components from different sources of variation. ANOVA provides a biostatistical test of whether the means of several groups are all equal, and therefore generalizes the t-test to more than two groups. Doing multiple two-sample t-tests would result in an increased chance of committing a Type I error. For this reason, ANOVA is useful in comparing two, three, or multiple means.

As summarized in Tables 3.4 and 3.5, ANOVA is used for two different purposes:

1. To estimate and test hypotheses for simple linear regression about population variances
2. To estimate and test hypotheses about population means

TABLE 3.4 ANOVA Table for Testing Hypotheses About Simple Linear Regression

SOURCE	DF	SUM OF SQUARES	MEAN SQUARES	F VALUE	P-VALUE
Model	1	$\Sigma(\hat{y}_i - \bar{y})^2 = $ SSModel	SSM = MSM	MSG/MSE = $F_{1,\,n-2}$	$\Pr(F > F_{1,\,n-2}{}^*)$
Residual	$n-2$	$\Sigma e_i^2 = $ SSResidual	SSR/$(n-2)$ = MSE		
Total	$n-1$	$\Sigma(\hat{y}_i - \bar{y})^2 = $ SSTotal	SST/$(n-1)$ = MST		

Residuals are often called *errors* because they are the part of the variation that the line could not explain. In this case,

MSR = MSE = sum of squared residuals/df = $\hat{\sigma}$ = estimate for variance of the population regression line

$$\text{SSTot}/(n-1) = \text{MSTOT} = s_y^2 = \text{the total variance of the } ys$$

$$F = t^2 \text{ for simple linear regression}$$

The larger the F (the smaller the p-value), the more of y's variation the line explained, so the less likely it is that H_0 is true. We reject a hypothesis when the p-value $< \alpha$:

R^2 = proportion of the total variation of y explained by the regression line = SSM/SST = 1 – SSResidual/SST

The F test statistic has two different DFs: the numerator = $k-1$ and the denominator = $N-k \rightarrow F_{k-1,\,N-k}$.

Note: SSE/$(N-k)$ = MSE = s_p^2 = (pooled sample variance) = $\dfrac{(n_1 - 1)s_1^2 + ... + (n_k - 1)s_k^2}{(n_1 - 1) + ... + (n_k - 1)}$

= $\hat{\sigma}^2$ = estimate for assumed equal variance (this is the "average" variance for each group)
SSTot/$(N-1)$ = MSTOT = s^2 = the total variance of the data (assuming NO groups)
$F \approx$ variance of the (between) sample means divided by the approximate average variance of the data; the larger the F (the smaller the p-value), the more varied the means are, so the less likely it is that H_0 is true. It is rejected when the p-value $< \alpha$.

TABLE 3.5 ANOVA Table for Testing Hypotheses About Population Means

SOURCE	DF	SUM OF SQUARES	MEAN SQUARES	F VALUE	P-VALUE
Group (between)	$k-1$	$\Sigma n_i(\bar{x}_i\,\bar{x})^2 = $ SSG	SSG/$(k-1)$ = MSG	MSG/MSE = $F_{k-1,\,N-k}$	$\Pr(F > F_{k-1,\,N-k})$
Error (within)	$N-k$	$\Sigma(n_i - 1)s_i^2 = $ SSE	SSE/$(N-k)$ = MSE		
Total	$N-1$	$\Sigma(x_{ij} - \bar{x})^2 = $ SSTot	SSTot/$(N-1)$ = MST		

R^2 = proportion of the total variation explained by the difference in means =

$$\frac{SSG}{SSTot}$$

■ **Example 1 in Multivariate Data Analysis:** Cystic Fibrosis Epidemiologic Study (Dalgaard, 2002)

Consider an epidemiologic study of lung function in patients suffering from cystic fibrosis. The data frame may be obtained from CRAN using the following R code segments:

```
> install.packages("ISwR")
```
--- Please select a CRAN mirror for use in this session ---
```
> # Select CA1
> library(ISwR)
> data(cystfibr)
> cystfibr # Outputting a matrix with a heading of 10 items and 25 cases:
```

	age	sex	height	weight	bmp	fev1	rv	frc	tlc	pemax
1	7	0	109	13.1	68	32	258	183	137	95
2	7	1	112	12.9	65	19	449	245	134	85
3	8	0	124	14.1	64	22	441	268	147	100
4	8	1	125	16.2	67	41	234	146	124	85
5	8	0	127	21.5	93	52	202	131	104	95
6	9	0	130	17.5	68	44	308	155	118	80
7	11	1	139	30.7	89	28	305	179	119	65
8	12	1	150	28.4	69	18	369	198	103	110
9	12	0	146	25.1	67	24	312	194	128	70
10	13	1	155	31.5	68	23	413	225	136	95
11	13	0	156	39.9	89	39	206	142	95	110
12	14	1	153	42.1	90	26	253	191	121	90
13	14	0	160	45.6	93	45	174	139	108	100
14	15	1	158	51.2	93	45	158	124	90	80
15	16	1	160	35.9	66	31	302	133	101	134
16	17	1	153	34.8	70	29	204	118	120	134
17	17	0	174	44.7	70	49	187	104	103	165
18	17	1	176	60.1	92	29	188	129	130	120
19	17	0	171	42.6	69	38	172	130	103	130
20	19	1	156	37.2	72	21	216	119	81	85
21	19	0	174	54.6	86	37	184	118	101	85
22	20	0	178	64.0	86	34	225	148	135	160
23	23	0	180	73.8	97	57	171	108	98	165
24	23	0	175	51.1	71	33	224	131	113	95
25	23	0	179	71.5	95	52	225	127	101	195

```
> # To obtain pairwise scatter plots between all the variables
> par(mex=0.5)
> pairs(cystfibr, gap=0, cex.labels=0.9)
> # Outputting figure
```

Plotting the data frame: A simple plot of all 10 components of the data may be obtained by the following code segment:

> plot(cystfibr) # *Outputting* Figure 3.16.

The function plot() is generic, behaving differently depending on the class of its arguments.

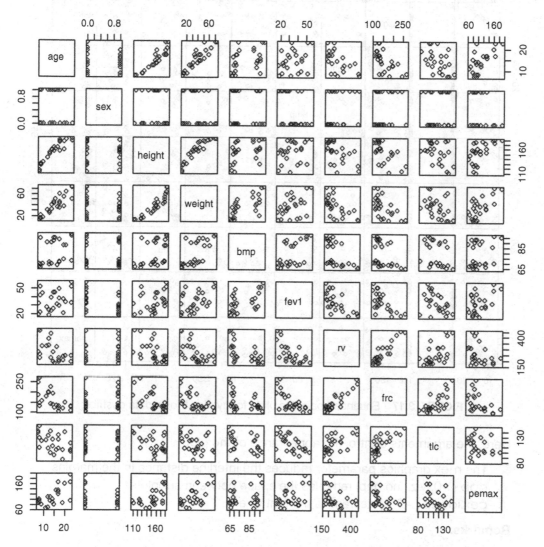

FIGURE 3.16 Plots for all 10 components of the cystic fibrosis data cystfibr.

Plotting multivariate data: To obtain pairwise scatter plots between all the variables in the data frame, the R function pairs() is used in the following code segment:

> par (mex=0.5)
> pairs(cystfibr, gap=0, cex.labels=0.9) # *Outputting* Figure 3.17.

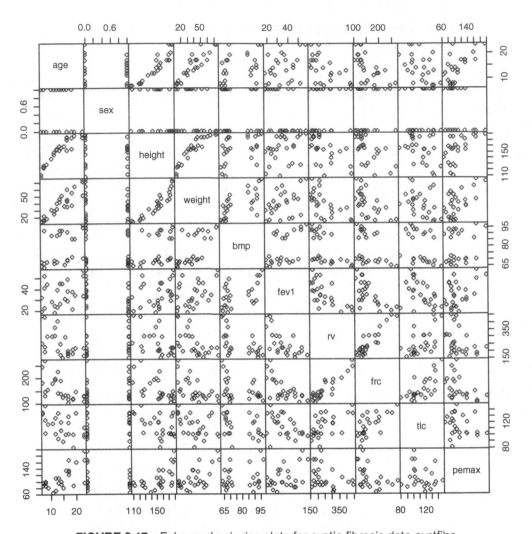

FIGURE 3.17 Enhanced pairwise plots for cystic fibrosis data cystfibr.

Here, the arguments control the appearance of the plot:

- The mex graphics parameter reduces the interline distance in the margins.
- gap (=0, viz., no gap) removes the space between subplots.
- cex.labels (=0.9) decreases the font size.

Remarks:

1. As the individual plots are small, the clarity may be compromised.
2. The 10 variables in the data frame are age, sex, height, weight, bmp, fev1, rv, frc, tlc, and pemax.
   They represent the following parameters:
   age: age, a numeric vector; age in years
   sex: sex, a numeric vector code; 0: male, 1: female
   height: height, a numeric vector; height (cm)
   weight: weight, a numeric vector; weight (kg)

fev1: fev1, a numeric vector; forced expiratory volume

rv: rv, a numeric vector; residual volume

frc: frc, a numeric vector; functional residual capacity

tlc: tlc, a numeric vector; total lung capacity

pemax: pemax, a numeric vector; maximum expiratory pressure

3. Nevertheless, some special characteristics and clear trends are apparent. For example:

(a) In the data frame cystfibr, there are 10 variables: age, sex, height, weight, bmp, fev1, rv, frc, tlc, and pemax. It appears that the tenth variable pemax may be considered the dependent variable, with the other nine considered as independent variables.

(b) In the age versus sex subplot (Row 1, Column 2), because there are only two sexes (M, F), all the data are stacked up on two piles: one column for M and another column for F.

(c) In the weight versus height subplot (Row 3, Column 4), there is a definite trend showing that, by a near-linear slope, weight is approximately directly proportional to height.

(d) This data frame contains common variable names such as age, height, weight, and so on. To eliminate possible confusion, it is prudent to ensure that these identically named objects are not involved elsewhere in the R environment at this workspace in the same work session.

Further Analysis Using Biostatistical Modeling

Additional information may be obtained by biostatistical modeling of the data frame cystfibr. For example, a linear R model lm() may be used to correlate the data. (Clearly, other biostatistical models may be used.)

The function lm() is used to fit linear models. It can be used to carry out regression, single-stratum ANOVA, and analysis of covariance.

The form for the use of lm() is

lm(formula, data, subset, weights, na.action,

```
method = "qr", model = TRUE, x = FALSE, y = FALSE,
qr = TRUE, singular.ok = TRUE, contrasts = NULL, offset, ...)
```

For a clinical diagnosis of cystic fibrosis using the collected data frame, one may consider the **maximum expiratory pressure (MEP)** parameter, pemax, which is a measure of the strength of the respiratory muscles and is obtained by having the patient exhale as strongly as possible into a mouthpiece. *The maximum value is near total lung capacity*. Hence, one may define the linear model correlation function to be

> lm(pemax ~ age + sex + height + weight + bmp + fev1 + rv + frc + tlc)

which means that pemax is being described using a linear model that is additive in the remaining nine variables. The output of this code segment is

Call:

lm(formula = pemax ~ age + sex + height + weight + bmp +

Coefficients:

(Intercept)	age	sex	height	weight
176.0582	−2.5420	−3.7368	−0.4463	2.9928
bmp	fev1	rv	frc	tlc
1.7449	1.0807	0.1970	−0.3084	0.1886

```
> # Using the summary command, more meaningful output was
> # obtained:
> summary(lm(pemax ~ age + sex + height + weight + bmp +
+                     fev1 + rv + frc + tlc))
> # Outputting the ANOVA table:
Call:
lm(formula = pemax ~ age + sex + height + weight + bmp + fev1 +
rv + frc + tlc)
```

Residuals:

Min	1Q	Median	3Q	Max
−37.338	−11.532	1.081	13.386	33.405

Coefficients:

	Estimate	Std. Error	t value	Pr(>|t|)
(Intercept)	176.0582	225.8912	0.779	0.448
age	−2.5420	4.8017	−0.529	0.604
sex	−3.7368	15.4598	−0.242	0.812
height	−0.4463	0.9034	−0.494	0.628
weight	2.9928	2.0080	1.490	0.157
bmp	−1.7449	1.1552	-1.510	0.152
fev1	1.0807	1.0809	1.000	0.333
rv	0.1970	0.1962	1.004	0.331
frc	−0.3084	0.4924	−0.626	0.540
tlc	0.1886	0.4997	0.377	0.711

Residual standard error: 25.47 on 15 degrees of freedom
Multiple R-squared: 0.6373, Adjusted R-squared: 0.4197
F-statistic: 2.929 on 9 and 15 DF, p-value: 0.03195

Remarks:

1. With the function lm(), there was not a great deal of output.
2. With the additional help of the function summary(), more output was obtained.
3. The t-values, in absolute terms, varied from 0.242 to 1.510; thus, there is not one single t-value that is biostatistically significant. However, in the joint F test, the p-value was 0.03195, which indicated that it is a significant result. The reason for this result is that the t-tests will say something about what happens only if one variable is removed while all the other variables are left in. The conclusion is, therefore, that not one particular variable should be included. It is not biostatistically clear whether any particular variable should be removed to form a reduced model.
4. The unadjusted R^2 of 0.6373 differs markedly from the adjusted R^2 of 0.4197. This is likely due to the large number of variables, 10, relative to the number of DF for variance, 15. This is consistent with the fact that the former is the change in residual sum of squares relative to an empty model, whereas the latter is a similar

The adjusted R^2 is computed as follows:

$$R1 = \text{Residual standard error} = 25.47$$

Returning to the R environment, the adjusted R-squared (denoted as R2 in the code) may be found by the following code segment:

```
>
> R1 <- 25.47 # This is the residual standard error
> R2 <- 1 - R1^2/var(pemax)
> R2 # Outputting the adjusted R-squared
[1] 0.4197626
>
```

Review Questions for Section 3.5

1. Define univariate, bivariate, and multivariate data analyses, giving an example of each.
2. (a) How are these analyses carried out in the R environment?
   (b) Give examples of the R code segments for these analyses.
3. (a) What is meant by *regression analysis*?
   (b) How is regression analysis used in data analysis?
4. (a) How is regression analysis carried out in the R environment?
   (b) Provide examples of the R functions used for regression analysis.
5. (a) Summarize the two uses of the ANOVA table in data analysis.
   (b) For data analysis, suggest an applicable R code segment.

Exercises for Section 3.5

1. Using the R code segment here:
   (a) Create a 50-vector x of 50 random numbers from the standard normal distribution.
   (b) Output x.
   (c) Perform a univariate data analysis on x:
   ```
   > x <- rnorm(1:50)
   > x
   > install.packages("epibasix")
   > library(epibasix)
   > univar(x)
   > x
   ```
2. Using the R code segment here:
   (a) Install the package ISwR.
   (a) Call up the files in this package.
   (b) Look into the "Blood Pressure Versus Obesity" dataset bp.obese.
   (c) Plot obesity versus blood pressure, distinguishing the data between men and women:
   ```
   > install.packages("ISwR")
   > library(ISwR)
   > bp.obese
   ```

3. *The Epidemiology of Heart Rates After Enalaprilat Treatment*

Enalaprilat is a modification of the drug enalapril, an angiotensin-converting enzyme (ACE) inhibitor used in the treatment of **hypertension** and some types of chronic **heart failure**. ACE raises blood pressure by constricting blood vessels; hence, **enalaprilat** is called a *pro-drug*.

The heart.rate dataset has 36 rows and 3 columns. It contains data for nine patients with congestive heart failure before and shortly after administration of enalaprilat, in a balanced two-way layout. This data frame contains the following columns:

hr a numeric vector; heart rate in beats per minute
subj a factor with levels 1 to 9
time a factor with levels 0 (before), 30, 60, and 120 (minutes after administration)

Using the R code segment here:

(a) Install the package ISwR.
(b) Call up the file heart.rate in this package.
(c) Inspect the dataset.
(d) For each of the nine patients, plot the mean heart rate versus time.

```
> install.packages("ISwR")
> library(ISwR)
> heart.rate
> evalq(interaction.plot(time,subj,hr), heart.rate)
```

4. *Nutritional Epidemiology: An Exercise in Multivariate Data Analysis and Analysis of Variance*

First, here are some more useful R functions for this application:

The function tapply(), in the CRAN R package base, applies a function to each cell of a ragged array; that is, to each nonempty group of values given by a unique combination of the levels of certain factors.

The function aov(), in the CRAN R package stats, fits an ANOVA model by a call to lm for each stratum.

The Investigation: Weight Gain in Laboratory Rats

Here is an interesting analysis in an investigation in nutritional epidemiology. The data arise from an experiment to study the gain in weight of laboratory rats fed on four different diets, distinguished by the amount of protein (low and high) and by the source of protein (beef and cereal).

Using the R code segment here:

(a) Install the package HSAUR.
```
> install.packages("HSAUR")
```

(b) Call up the file weightgain in this package:
```
> data("weightgain", package = "HSAUR")
```

(c) Inspect the dataset weightgain:
```
> weightgain
```

(d) Summarize the main features of this dataset by calculating the means and
standard deviation, using the function tapply():

```
> tapply(weightgain$weightgain, list(weightgain$source,
+                                    weightgain$type), mean)
```

(e) Plot the mean weight gain for the amount of protein factor, showing that the gain for the high-protein diet is far more than for the low-protein diet:
```
> plot.design(weightgain)
```

(f) Summarize the cell variances to show that they are relatively similar, and that there is no apparent relationship between cell mean and cell variance. This in turn shows that the homogeneity assumption of the ANOVA seems to be reasonable for this dataset:
```
> tapply(weightgain$weightgain, list(weightgain$source,
+                                    weightgain$type), sd)
```

(g) Use the R function aov() to perform an ANOVA for the dataset; then examine the result of the analysis. Finally, use the function summary() to produce an ANOVA table:
```
> wg_aov <- aov(weightgain ~ source * type, data = weightgain)
> wg_aov
> summary(wg_aov)
```

(h) The resulting ANOVA table shows that the main effect of type is highly significant, confirming what was seen in part (e) of this exercise. The main effect of the source is not significant, but interpretation of both these main effects is complicated by the type X source interaction, which approaches significance at the 5% level. To understand this interaction effect, plot the mean weight gain for low- and high-protein diets for each level of source protein: beef and cereal. Use the following R code segment:
```
> interaction.plot(weightgain$type, weightgain$source,
+                  weightgain$weightgain)
```

(i) From the resulting plot, it can be seen that for low-protein diets, the use of cereal as the source of protein resulted in a greater weight gain than the use of beef. For high-protein diets, the reverse is true, with the beef/high-protein diet leading to the highest weight gain. Obtain the estimates of the intercept and the main and interaction effects by extracting them from the model fit by using the following R code segment:
```
> coef(wg_aov)
```

(j) Note that the model was fitted with the following restrictions: $\gamma_1 = 0$ (corresponding to Beef) and $\beta_1 = 0$ (corresponding to High) because treatment contrasts were used as the default. This can be seen from the following R code segment:
```
> options("contrasts")
```

(k) Thus, the coefficient for a source of 14.1 (in the ANOVA table) may be considered an estimate of the differences $\gamma_2 - \gamma_1$. Also, one may use the following restriction:

$$\sum \gamma_i = 0$$

by the following R computations of the coefficients:

```
> coef(aov(weightgain ~ source + type + source:type, data =
+              weightgain, contrasts = list(source = contr.sum)))
```

5. ***Medicare Air Pollution Study* (MCAPS;** Peng & Domonici, 2008**)**

The MCAPS package contains maximum likelihood estimates and biostatistical variances of the county-specific log-relative risks of hospital admissions for each of the cardiovascular and respiratory diseases associated with lags 0, 1, and 2 exposure to $PM_{2.5}$. ($PM_{2.5}$ and PM_{10} are measures of particles in the **atmosphere** with a diameter of less than or equal to a nominal 2.5 and 10 micrometers, respectively.) The package also contains air pollution and weather data for the seven geographical regions used.

The following R code segments load the package, extract the datasets, and examine their contents critically.

(a) Run the code segment.

(b) Briefly explain the output at each stage:

```
> install.packages("MCAPS")
> library(MCAPS)
> initMCAPS("MCAPS")
> getData()
> estimates <-getData("estimates.subset")
> head(estimates[, c("CountyName", "outcome", "beta", "var")])
> sites <- getData("siteList")
> head(sites)
> apw <- getData("APWdata")
> chic <- apw[["17031"]]
> head(chic)
```

6. *Cystic Fibrosis: Polynomial Regression Analysis*

Returning to the cystic fibrosis dataset in Example 1 of Section 3.5, the plot of pemax versus height shows considerable nonlinearity. Under biostatistics theory, to test this observation, it may be instructive to add a nonlinear term in height, such as the square of the height: $(height)^2$.

(a) On this basis, provide an R code segment that adds the effect of $(height)^2$ to the correlation model.

(***Hint***: Use the R function predict() for the new model; and newdata, which allows the prediction of values for a chosen set of predictors. Choose a set of heights between 110 and 180 cm in steps of 2 cm.)

(b) Comment on the success or failure of this new nonlinear correlation model.

REFERENCES

Adler, J. (2010). *R in a nutshell: A desktop quick reference*. Sebastopol, CA: O'Reilly Media, Inc.

American Statistical Association. (n.d.). Biostatistician job search. Retrieved from http://jobs. amstat.org/jobs/4627784/biostatistician-1

ANOVA. (n.d.). Analysis of variance. Retrieved from http://en.wikipedia.org/wiki/

Aragon, T. J. (2011). *Applied epidemiology using R (epir)*. Berkeley, CA: UC Berkeley School of Public Health & San Francisco Department of Public Health.

BMI Notes. (2012). *Body mass index*. Retrieved from http://en.wikipedia.org/wiki/Body_mass_index

Centers for Disease Control and Prevention (CDC). (2005, January). Antiretroviral postexposure prophylaxis after sexual, injection-drug use, or other nonoccupational exposure to HIV in the United States: Recommendations from the U.S. Department of Health and Human Services. *MMWR Recommendations Reports, 54*(RR-2), 1–20. Retrieved from http://www.cdc .gov/mmwr/preview/mmwrhtml/rr5402a1.htm

CRAN. (n.d.). The Comprehensive R Archive Network. Retrieved from http://cran.r-project.org/

Dalgaard, P. (2002). *Introductory statistics with R* (Springer Statistics & Computing Series). New York, NY: Springer Science+Business Media.

Daniel, W. W. (2005). *Biostatistics: A foundation for analysis in the health sciences*. New York, NY: John Wiley & Sons.

Everitt, B. S., & Hothorn, T. (2006). *A handbook of statistical analysis using R*. Boca Raton, FL: Chapman & Hall/CRC.

Mittal, H. V. (2011). *R graphics cookbook*. Birmingham, UK: PACKT Publishing Ltd.

Murrell, P. (2006). *R graphics*. Computer Science and Data Analysis Series. Boca Raton, FL: Chapman & Hall/CRC.

Peng, R. D., & Domonici, F. (2008). *Statistical methods for environmental epidemiology with R: A case study in air pollution and health*. Springer Use R! Series. New York, NY: Springer Science+Business Media.

Seefeld, K., & Linder, L. (2005). *Statistics using R with biological examples*. Durham, NH: Department of Mathematics & Statistics, University of New Hampshire. (Also affiliated with the Department of Nephrology and the Biostatistics Research Center, Tufts-NEMC, Boston, MA.) Retrieved from http://cran.r-project.org/doc/contrib/Seefeld_StatsRBio.pdf

Statistics Canada. (2013, July 23). Data processing. Retrieved from http://www.statcan.gc.ca/edu/ power-pouvoir/ch3/5214785-eng.htm#a1

Teetor, P. (2011). *R cookbook: Proven recipes for data analysis, statistics, and graphics*. Sebastopol, CA: O'Reilly Media.

Venables, W. N., Smith, D. M., & the R Development Core Team. (2004). *An introduction to R*. Bristol, UK: Network Theory, Ltd.

Verzani, J. (2005). *Using R for introductory statistics*. Boca Raton, FL: Chapman & Hall/CRC.

Virasakdi, C. (2011). *Analysis of epidemiological data using R and Epicalc*. Songkhla, Thailand: Epidemiology Unit, Prince of Songkla University.

APPENDIX: DOCUMENTATION FOR THE plot FUNCTION

plot {graphics}   R Documentation

Generic X–Y Plotting

DESCRIPTION

Generic function for plotting of R objects. For more details about the graphical parameter arguments, see par.

For simple scatter plots, plot.default will be used. However, there are plot methods for many R objects, including functions, data.frames, density objects, and so on. Use methods(plot) and the documentation for these.

USAGE

plot(x, y, ...)

ARGUMENTS

x   The coordinates of points in the plot. Alternatively, a single plotting structure, function, or any R object with a plot method can be provided.

y   The y coordinates of points in the plot; optional, if x is an appropriate structure.

...   Arguments to be passed to methods, such as graphical parameters (see par). Many methods will accept the following arguments:
type
What type of plot should be drawn. Possible types are
- "p" for points
- "l" for lines
- "b" for both
- "c" for the lines part alone of "b"
- "o" for both "overplotted"
- "h" for "histogram" like (or "high-density") vertical lines
- "s" for stair steps
- "S" for other steps (see "Details" below)
- "n" for no plotting

All other types give a warning or an error; using, for example, type = "punkte" being equivalent to type = "p" for S compatibility. Note that some methods (e.g., plot.factor), do not accept this.
main
       An overall title for the plot; see title.
sub
       A subtitle for the plot; see title.
xlab
       A title for the x-axis; see title.
ylab
       A title for the y-axis; see title.
asp
       The y/x aspect ratio; see plot.window.

DETAILS

The two step types differ in their x–y preference. Going from $(x1,y1)$ to $(x2,y2)$ with $x1 < x2$, type = "s" moves first horizontally and then vertically, whereas type = "S" moves the other way around.
     See also **plot.defvault**, **plot.formula**, and other methods; **points, lines, par**.
     For X–Y–Z plotting, see **contour, persp**, and **image**.

Examples
require(stats)

```
lines(lowess(cars))
plot(sin, -pi, 2*pi) # see ?plot.function
## Discrete Distribution Plot:
plot(table(rpois(100,5)), type = "h", col = "red", lwd=10,
     main="rpois(100,lambda=5)")
## Simple quantiles/ECDF; see ecdf() {library(stats)} for a better one:
plot(x <- sort(rnorm(47)), type = "s", main = "plot(x, type = \"s\")")
points(x, cex = .5, col = "dark red")
```

FOUR

Graphics Using R

INTRODUCTION

Up to this point, you have been introduced to many graphical outputs in the R environment, all on a casual, ad hoc basis. Clearly, graphics are an important and versatile feature in the biostatistics of epidemiology and public health. This chapter investigates such graphics facilities in some detail.

R graphics functionality may be described in terms of two systems (Dalgaard, 2002; Mittal, 2011; Murrell, 2006; Venables, Smith, & R Development Core Team, 2005): base (or traditional) graphics and grid graphics.

The R graphics system may be considered as consisting of four levels:

1. **Graphics packages**: mostly listed on the CRAN website
2. **Graphics systems**: including the *graphics* and the *grid*, which will be discussed in some detail in this chapter
3. **Graphics engines:** known as *grDevices*; these allow users to deal with such aspects as font types and colors, output formats, and the like
4. **Graphics device packages:** including *add-on* graphics packages, which provide the details on graphical outputs

The base system, along with the graphics packages built on it, provides the majority of the high-level functions. The exception is the lattice package, which provides complete plots based on the grid system. Both the base and grid systems may be used in batch modes or interactively; however, the latter is more productive. For interactive use, at startup time, R initiates a *graphics device driver* that opens a graphics window for the display of interactive graphics. In Microsoft Windows, the command is simply windows().

As soon as the device driver is started, R plotting commands may be used to produce graphs and create various displays. The available plotting commands are classified into three groups:

Group I: High-level functions that create a new, complete plot on the graphics device (with the axes, lines, points, labels, titles, etc.)

Group II: Low-level functions that add information to an existing plot (such as lines, extra points, labels, etc.)

Group III: Interactive functions that interactively add information to, or remove information from, an existing plot using a pointing device such as a touchpad or mouse

The foregoing R facilities are known as *base graphics*. A subsystem, coexisting with the base, is a package called grid graphics; this contains the package lattice, which provides codes to produce multilevel plots similar to the Trellis system in S.

Choice of System

Because R can produce complete plots with a single function call, the choice of which graphics systems to use depends only on what type of plot is needed. If it is necessary to add further outputs to an initial plot, it is important to know the specific system that was used to produce the original plot: in general, the same graphics systems should be used to add output to existing plots (though there are exceptions). The grid system usually gives more flexibility.

Packages

Functions in R are organized in terms of *packages*, which allows:

- Loading of only the packages that contain the required functions; this requires less memory and thus enables R to run faster.
- Use of functions that others have written and loaded into the package; there are now hundreds of these contributed packages.

To download and install packages from within an R session, use:

> install.packages("PACKAGE NAME")

and

> update.packages("PACKAGE NAME")

Upon installation, to load the functions in that package, use:

> library("PACKAGE NAME")

Notes:

1. The base graphics system is provided by the graphics package, which is installed and loaded, by default, in a standard installation of R.
2. The Grid Graphics System is provided by the grid package, which, together with the lattice package, is also installed by default when the Grid Graphics System is loaded.
3. To automate the loading of packages, use:
   > help(Startup)
4. To get help on any function FUNCTION, use:
   > help(FUNCTION)
   For more help, try one or all of the following:
   > help(help) # *For additional help*
   > example() # *For some examples to run the function under study*

> help.start() # *Takes you to further available help*
> help.search() # *To locate a function for a special purpose*
> vignette() # *Vignettes have more extensive help*

Finally, the R home page has a guide for the R-help forum, to which one submits questions for online assistance.

4.1   BASE (OR TRADITIONAL) GRAPHICS

High-Level Functions

R's high-level plotting functions generate a complete plot of the data that have been passed as arguments of the function. Unless otherwise requested, axes, labels, and titles are generated. A high-level command starts a new plot, erasing the current plot if needed.

THE FUNCTION plot()

This is the most commonly used plotting command; it is a *generic* function. That is, the type of plot produced depends on the *class* or type of the first argument of the function. The following are some typical examples.

■ **Example 4.1**

> plot(x)

If *x* is a time series, plot(x) will produce a time-series plot. If *x* is numeric vector, this function will produce a plot of the values in the vector against their respective indexes in the vector. If *x* is a vector of imaginary numbers, this function will produce a plot of the imaginary versus real parts of the vector components.

As an illustration of the function in the R environment, consider:

> x <- 1:25 # *Let x be the vector of the first 25 natural numbers*
> x # *Outputting x:*

[1] 1 2 3 4 5 6 7 8 9 10 11 12 13 14 15 16 17 18 19 20 21 22 23 24 25

> plot(x) # *Outputting* Figure 4.1.

PLOTTING MULTIVARIATE DATASETS

For plotting multivariate data in R, there are several special functions: pairs(), coplot(), stars(), and mosaicplot(). Some are described here, with examples.

pairs(X), where X is a numeric matrix or data frame, outputs a pairwise scatter plot of the variables defined by the columns of X. In this plot, every column of X is plotted against every other column of X, and the $n(n - 1)$ plots, where n is the number of variables, are arranged in a matrix with plot scales constant over its rows and columns.

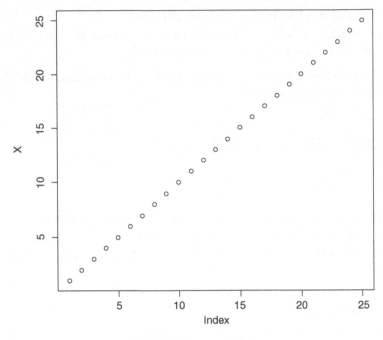

FIGURE 4.1 > plot(x).

■ **Example 4.2:** A simple numerical example of the function pairs(X)

```
> x <- c(1, 2, 3, 4, 5)
> y <- c(1, 4, 9, 16, 25) # Note: yi = xi2, i = 1,2,3,4,5
> X <- data.frame(x, y)
> X
```

	x	y
1	1	1
2	2	4
3	3	9
4	4	16
5	5	25

```
> pairs(X)
> # Outputs: Figure 4.2.
```

■ **Example 4.3:** Output of a simple coplot()

```
> ## Tonga Trench Earthquakes
> coplot(lat ~ long | depth, data = quakes) # Outputting: Figure 4.3.
```

If c is a factor, a is then plotted against b for values of c within the interval. The number and position of intervals may be controlled with the given.values= argument in coplot(). Also, one may use two given variables with the command coplot(a ~ b | c + d), which

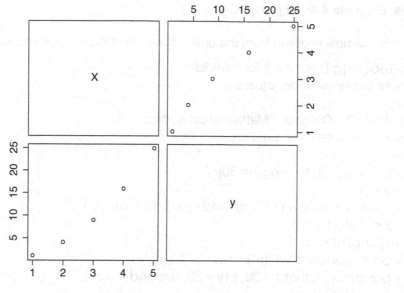

FIGURE 4.2 pairs(x).

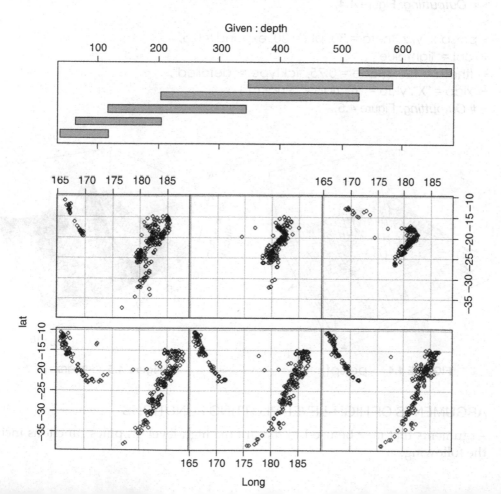

■ **Example 4.4:** for persp(x, y, z, …)

This example is drawn from the online "Documentation" page of the function persp().[1]

```
> require(grDevices) # for trans3d
> ## Examples in demo(persp)
>
> # (1)  The Obligatory Mathematical surface.
> #      Rotated sinc function.
>
> x <- seq(-10, 10, length= 30)
> y <- x
> f <- function(x,y) { r <- sqrt(x^2+y^2); 10 * sin(r)/r }
> z <- outer(x, y, f)
> z[is.na(z)] <- 1
> op <- par(bg = "white")
> persp(x, y, z, theta = 30, phi = 30, expand = 0.5,
+ col = "lightblue")
> # Outputting: Figure 4.4.
>
> persp(x, y, z, theta = 30, phi = 30, expand = 0.5,
+   col = "lightblue",
+   ltheta = 120, shade = 0.75, ticktype = "detailed",
+   xlab = "X", ylab = "Y", zlab = "Sinc( r )")
> # Outputting: Figure 4.5.
```

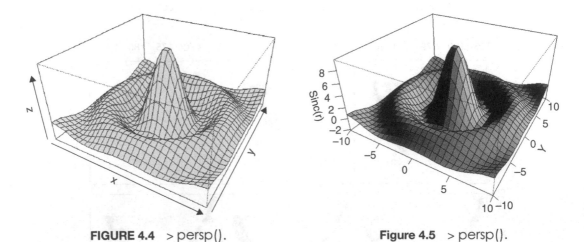

FIGURE 4.4 > persp().   **Figure 4.5** > persp().

ARGUMENTS OF HIGH-LEVEL PLOTTING FUNCTIONS

Arguments that may be used to modify the high-level graphics functions include the following:

add=TRUE   This additional argument will cause the function to act as a low-level function, superimposing the plot on the current plot.

add=FALSE   This argument suppresses the generation of axes and may be used when adding custom axes with the function axis().

log ="x", log="y", log"xy"   These arguments cause the respective axes to be logarithmic.

type=   This argument controls the types of plots produced, as follows:

"p"	plots individual points
"l"	plots lines
"b"	plots points connected by lines
"o"	plots points overlaid by lines
"h"	plots vertical lines from the points to the zero axis
"s", "S"	plots step functions, with the top/bottom, respectively, of the vertical defining the point
"n"	no plotting

xlab/ylab=(string)	Inserts axis labels for the x- and y-axes, respectively.
main/sub=(string)	Inserts figure title/subtitle, respectively, placing the text at the top of the plot/just below the x-axis.

Low-Level Plotting Functions

Low-level plotting may be used to add extra information, such as points, lines, text, and so on, to an existing display. Some useful low-level plotting functions are:

points (x, y)   Draws a sequence of points at the specified coordinates. The specified character(s) are plotted, centered at the coordinates.

lines (x, y)   Adds points or connecting lines to the existing plot.

A type=argument may be used with these functions, defaulting to "p" for points() and "l" for lines().

text(x, y, labels, ...)   Adds text to a plot at points x, y. labels is usually an integer or character vector; labels[i] is plotted at the points (x[i], y[i]). The default is 1:length(x). Thus, to plot a set of labeled points, the following sequence may be used:
> plot(x, y, type="n"; text(x, y, names)

Here, type="n" suppresses the points but sets up the axes, while the function text() supplies special characters, specified by the character vector names for the points.

abline()   adds one or more straight lines through the current plot.

abline(a, b)   adds a straight line with intercept a and slope b to the existing plot.

abline(v=x)   specifies x-coordinates for the widths of vertical lines to go across a plot.

abline(h=y)   specifies y-coordinates for the heights of horizontal lines to go across a plot.

abline(lm.obj)   specifies a list, lm/obj, with a coefficient component of length 2, which are taken as an intercept and slope, respectively.

axis(side, ...)   adds an axis to the existing plot on the side specified by the first

Other arguments control the positions of the axes within or next to the plot, and tick positions and labels. It is useful for adding axes after first calling plot() with the axes=FALSE argument.

title(main, sub)   adds a title main to the top of the current plot in a large font, and optionally a subtitle sub at the bottom (in a smaller font).

legend(x, y, legend, …)   adds a legend to the existing plot as the position labels in the character vector legend. At least one additional argument v (a vector with the same length as legend), with the corresponding values of the plotting unit, should also be specified, as follows:

legend(, fill=v)   specifies colors for filled boxes.
legend(, col=v)   specifies colors in which lines or points will be drawn.
legend(, lty=v)   specifies line styles.
legend(, lwd=v)   specifies line widths.
legend(, pch=v)   specifies plotting characteristics (a character vector).

■ **Example 4.5:** legend(x, y, legend, …)

This function can be used to add legends to plots. Its documentary form is:

```
legend(x, y = NULL, legend, fill = NULL, col = par("col"),
        border="black", lty, lwd, pch,
        angle = 45, density = NULL, bty = "o", bg = par("bg"),
        box.lwd = par("lwd"), box.lty = par("lty"),
        box.col = par("fg"),
        pt.bg = NA, cex = 1, pt.cex = cex, pt.lwd = lwd,
        xjust = 0, yjust = 1, x.intersp = 1, y.intersp = 1,
        adj = c(0, 0.5), text.width = NULL, text.col = par("col"),
        merge = do.lines && has.pch, trace = FALSE,
        plot = TRUE, ncol = 1, horiz = FALSE, title = NULL,
        inset = 0, xpd, title.col = text.col, title.adj = 0.5,
        seg.len = 2)
```

To illustrate its use, for a given existing plot, legends will be added to each of the nine major positions on the plot:

```
> x <- 0:1
> y <- sin(x)
> plot(x, y, type='n')
> # Outputting: Figure 4.6.
> legend("bottomright", "(x,y)", pch=1, title="bottomright")
> legend("bottom", "(x,y)", pch=1, title="bottom")
> legend("bottomleft", "(x,y)", pch=1, title="bottomleft")
> legend("left", "(x,y)", pch=1, title="left")
> legend("topleft","(x,y)", pch = 1, title = "topleft, inset = 0.05",
+  inset = .05)
> legend("top", "(x,y)", pch=1, title="top")
> legend("topright", "(x,y)", pch=1, title="topright, inset = 0.02",
```

> legend("right", "(x,y)", pch=1, title="right")
> legend("center", "(x,y)", pch=1, title="center")
> # *Outputting:* Figure 4.7.

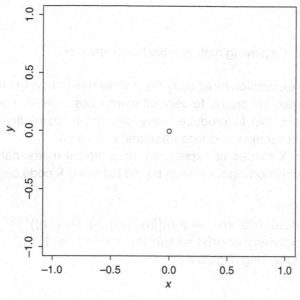

FIGURE 4.6 > plot().

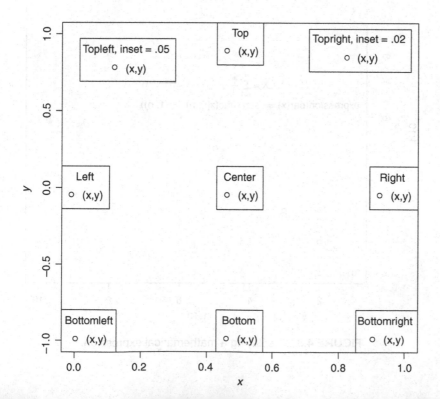

MATHEMATICAL ANNOTATION

In the R environment, to output a given mathematical expression as a graphic, one may use the function plotmath(), in the package grDevices. Features of this function may be found in demo(plotmath) or help(plotmath), among others. Some examples follow.

■ **Example 4.6:** Displaying mathematical expressions[2]

A mathematical expression must obey the normal rules of syntax for any R expression, but it is interpreted according to very different rules than for normal R expressions. However, it is possible to produce many different mathematical symbols, generate superscripts or subscripts, produce fractions, and so on.

   Observe the R modes of expression for a typical mathematical expression that includes the summation sign, as given by the following R code segment:

```
> plot(1:10, 1:10)
> text(4, 7, expression(bar(x) == sum(frac(x[i], n), i==1, n)))
> text(4, 6.4, "expression(bar(x) == sum(frac(x[i],n), i==1, n))",
+   cex = .8) # Outputting: Figure 4.8.
```

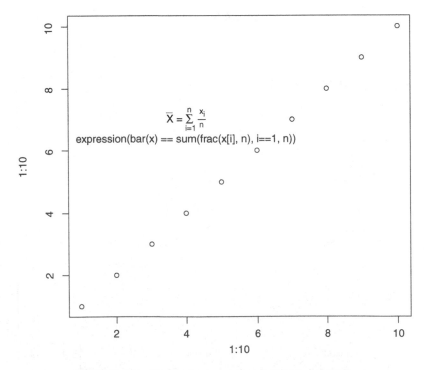

FIGURE 4.8   Displaying a mathematical expression.

Interacting With Graphics

R functions that permit users to add to, or remove from, information on a plot (using a mouse) include locator(n = 512, type = "n", ...):

locator(n = 512, type = "n", ...).   This function waits for the user to select certain locations on the existing plot using the left mouse button. This process continues until *n* points have been selected or another mouse button is pressed. The type argument permits plotting at the selected points and has the same effect for high-level graphics. The default is no plotting. This function returns the locations of the selected points. When called without an argument, this function has a large (512) default value.

identify(x, y, labels)   This function allows the highlighting of any points by x and y, using the left mouse button by plotting the corresponding component of labels nearby. It returns the indexes of the selected points.

Using Graphics Parameters

One may change many aspects of a graphical display using graphics parameters that control features such as line types and widths, colors, figure arrangements, text manipulations, and so forth. Each graphics parameter has a name; for example, col controls colors and a value (e.g., a color number).

Graphics parameters may be set either permanently (affecting all graphics functions that access the existing device), or temporarily (affecting only a single graphics call).

PERMANENT CHANGES: THE FUNCTION par()

par(), in the package graphics, may be used to query or set graphical parameters. Parameters may be set by specifying them as arguments to par in tag = value form, or by passing them as a list of tagged values. Some typical examples are:

par()   Without arguments, this function returns a list of all graphics parameters and their values for the existing graphics device.

par(c("lty", "lwd", "col"))   With a character vector argument, this function returns only the named graphics parameter, which in this case are the line type, line width, and line color, respectively.

par(col=3, lty=1)   With named arguments setting the values of the named graphics parameters, this function returns only the original values of the parameter as a list.

By saving the result of par() when making changes, one may restore the original values when the plotting is complete.

■ **Example 4.7:** The function par()

```
> par1 <- par(mfrow = c(3, 3),    # 3 x 3 pictures on one plot
+              col=3, pty = "s")    # with color square plotting region
```

```
> # At end of plotting, reset to previous settings:
> par(par1)
```

TEMPORARY CHANGES BY ADDING ARGUMENTS TO GRAPHIC FUNCTIONS

By adding graphics parameters to a graphic function such as plot(), the result has the same effect as passing the arguments to effect changes expressed in a par() function, except that the indicated changes will last only for the duration of the graphic function call. Thus, for example,

```
> plot(x, y, pch=20)
```

will produce a scatter plot using "bullets" (small solid circles) as the plotting character, without making changes in the default character for any future plots.

Parameters List for Graphics

Many useful graphical parameters are outlined in the following subsections.

GRAPHICAL ELEMENTS

A complete list of parameters for graphics may readily be found in the following two R function documentation sites, which may be called up as follows:

```
> ?par
> ?points or ?pch
```

1. par() {graphics} may be used to set or query graphical parameters. Parameters may be set by specifying them as arguments to par().
2. points() {graphics} is a generic function for drawing a sequence of points at specified coordinates. The specified characters are plotted and centered at the coordinates. The documentation includes that of pch().

TICK MARKS AND AXES

For high-level plots that call for axes, one may construct axes with the low-level graphics function axis(). The three components of a set of axes are:

1. The **axis line**, with the line style controlled by the graphics parameter lty (line type)
2. The **tick marks** that mark off unit divisions along the axis line
3. The **tick labels** that mark the units

Examples of these features are:

```
xaxs="r", yaxs="i"
```

The above is the style of axis interval calculation to be used for the x- and y-axes. Possible values are "r" and "i". The styles are generally controlled by the range of data or xlim, if given. Style "r" (regular) first extends the data range by 4% at each end and then finds an axis with pretty or visually attractive labels that fits within the extended range. Style "i" (internal) just finds an axis with pretty labels that fits within the original data range.

tck=0.5

The above is the length of tick marks as a fraction of the smaller of the width or height of the plotting region. If tck ≥ 0.5, it is interpreted as a fraction of the relevant side, so if tck = 1, grid lines are drawn. The default setting is tck = NA.

lab=c(3, 6, 12)

A numerical vector of the form c(x, y, len) that modifies the default way of annotating axes. The values of x and y give the (approximate) number of tick marks on the x- and y-axes, and len specifies the label length. The default is c(5, 5, 7).

FIGURE MARGINS

In R, a single plot, known as a *figure*, comprises a **plot region** surrounded by margins that may contain titles, subtitles, axis labels, and so on. This region is usually bounded by the axes. The parameters controlling figure layout include:

mai=c(1.5, 1.0, 1.5, 1.0)   These four parameters are the width at the bottom, left, top, and right margins, respectively, measured in inches (Figure 4.9).
mar=c(4, 3, 4, 3) Similar to mai, with the measurement unit in text lines.

These two sets of parameters are equivalent because specifying one set changes the value of the other. For further details or other sets of parameters for figure margins, refer to the documentation par {graphics} in CRAN.

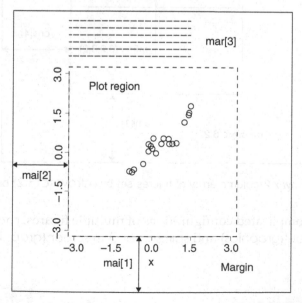

FIGURE 4.9 mar = c(a, b, c, d): A numerical vector of the form c(bottom, left, top, right),

MULTIPLE FIGURE OUTPUTS

In R, one may create an $n \times m$ array of figures in a page, with each figure having its own margins and with the array of figures optionally surrounded by an outer margin or border. In the documentation of par {graphics}, this configuration may be specified as follows:

mfcol, mfrow   A vector of the form c(nr, nc). Subsequent figures will be drawn in an nr-by-nc array on the device by *columns* (mfcol), or *rows* (mfrow), respectively.

oma, omi A vector of the form c(bottom, left, top, right) giving the size of the outer margins in lines of text, or inches, respectively.

A 3-row × 2-column array is shown in Figure 4.10.

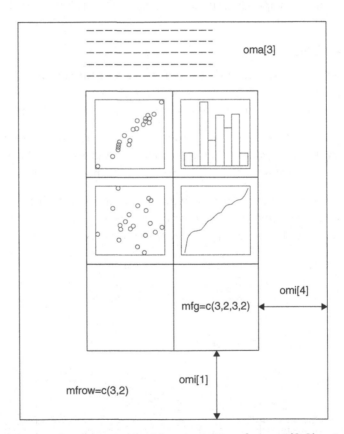

FIGURE 4.10   A 3-row x 2-column array of figures set by mfrow=c(3,2) or by mfcol=c(2,3).

For more complicated configurations of multiple figures, consider the functions layout() in layout{graphics} and split.screen() in screen{graphics}.

Device Drivers

In R computing, the device driver converts graphical instructions (e.g., plot(x, y))

windows()	For use on Windows
quartz()	For use on MacOS X
X11()	For use with an X11 window system on Unix-like systems
postscript()	For printing on PostScript printers or creating PostScript graphics
pdf()	For producing a portable document format (PDF) file
png()	For producing a bitmap portable network graphics (PNG) file
jpeg()	For producing a bitmap joint photographic experts group (JPEG; good for image plots)

When the run is finished, terminate the device driver as follows:

> dev.off()

POSTSCRIPT DIAGRAMS

The graphic function postscript(), also in the grDevices package, starts the graphics device driver for producing PostScript graphics. The function has the general form:

```
postscript(file = ifelse(onefile, "Rplots.ps", "Rplot%03d.ps"),
           onefile, family, title, fonts, encoding, bg, fg,
           width, height, horizontal, pointsize,
           paper, pagecentre, print.it, command,
           colormodel, useKerning, fillOddEven)
```

Passing the file argument by the postscript() device driver function, one stores the plot in PostScript format in a designated file. That plot will be in landscape orientation unless the horizontal=FALSE argument is passed. The size of the graphic may be controlled using the width and height arguments.

For example, the code

> postscript("file.ps", horizontal=FALSE, height=3, pointsize=8)

produces a file containing PostScript code for a figure 3 inches high. Refer to the documentation of postscript {grDevices} for further details.

MULTIPLE GRAPHICS DEVICES

When it is necessary to have several graphics devices open simultaneously, even when only one device can accept graphics commands at any given instance (that being the **current device**), the multiple devices form a numbered sequence with names giving the kind of device at any position. Each new call to a device extends the device list by one. That new device becomes the current device to which graphics output will then be directed.

This R function, dev(), also within the package grDevices, is defined in one of the following forms:

dev.cur()
dev.list()

= return the numbers and names of all active devices.

dev.next(which = dev.cur())

= return the numbers and names of the following, or prior, active devices.

dev.off(which = dev.cur())

= terminates the graphics device.

dev.set(which = dev.next())

= changes the current device to the next, as specified.

dev.new(...)

= returns the return value of the device opened, usually invisible NULL.

graphics.off()
= terminates all graphics devices on the list, except the null device.

These functions may be used with the following arguments:

which = an integer specifying a device number
...   = arguments to be passed to the device selected

Review Questions for Section 4.1

1. (a) What are the two systems of R graphics functionality?
   (b) What are the four levels that constitute the R graphics system?
2. (a) What are the three groups of plotting commands in R? Briefly describe each.
   (b) Suggest an R command for installing a package called PACKAGENAME.
3. (a) When the package PACKAGENAME has been installed, suggest a command to load all the functions in that package.
   (b) We want to obtain helpful information regarding a function called FUNCTION. Suggest a command to obtain the appropriate documentation for that function.
4. (a) Suggest a function to plot the values of an arbitrary vector x.
   (b) Use this function to plot the vector x = (1, 3, 5, 7, 9, 11, 13, 15, 17, 19).
5. x and y are vectors given by x = (1, 3, 5, 7, 9) and y = (2, 4, 6, 8, 10). Construct a matrix of two columns, in which the elements of x and y are the elements of Column 1 and Column 2, respectively.
6. Suggest a command to plot the elements of x and y (from question 5) to obtain a pairwise scatter plot of x and y; then obtain the scatter plot.
7. For plotting multivariate datasets, describe the graphics obtained by coplot().
8. What do the following low-level functions add to the graphic display of an already completed plot?
   (a) text()
   (b) abline()
   (c) axis()
   (d) legend()
9. (a) In the package graphics, what graphical parameters may be set by the following parameters in the function par(): "lty", "lwd", and "col"?
   (b) When preparing for multiple figure outputs, describe the configurations of the plot

Exercises for Section 4.1

1. Using R as a calculator, compute the answers to the following:
   (a) $1 + 2$
   (b) $13 - 5$
   (c) 17×29
   (d) $851/37$
   (e) $(3.1416)^2$
   (f) π^2
   (g) e^{-3}
   (h) $\sqrt{(11^2 - 4 \times 3 \times 7)}$
   (i) $\log_{10}(1234567)$
   (j) $\sin^2(30°)$

2. **Blood pressure** is the pressure of the circulating blood against the walls of the blood vessels. It is measured as part of an evaluation of a person's health. Adult blood pressure is considered normal at 120/80; the first number is the *systolic pressure* and the second is the *diastolic pressure*.

   The systolic pressure is measured *during* the contraction of the left ventricle of the heart, and the diastolic pressure is measured *after* the contraction of the heart while the chambers of the heart refill with blood.

   The following is the measured systolic pressure of Patient A taken daily for 10 consecutive days:

   145, 150, 135, 140, 160, 170, 138, 168, 155, 165

   (a) Enter these 10 readings into the variable bpsystolic.
   (b) Use the function diff() on this variable. What do the results mean?
   (c) Use the command mean(bpsystolic). What do the results mean?
   (d) Use the command mean(diff(bpsystolic)). What do the results mean?

3. Using the function boxplot(), enter the 10 blood pressure readings and obtain a plot of these 10 readings (see Figure 4.11).

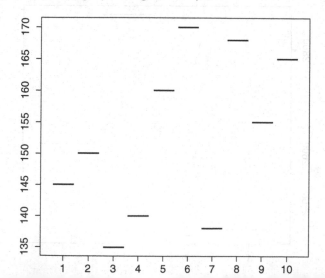

4. Four successive national health surveys, for the population of male subjects in their 20s, showed that the average amount of daily calories was:

2450, 2439, 2866, 2618.

The percentage of calories from fat was 37.0%, 36.2%, 34.0%, 32.1%.
The percentage of calories from carbohydrates was 43.1%, 42.2%, 50.0%, 48.1%.

(a) Is the average number of fat calories increasing or decreasing?
(b) Is this result consistent with the information that over the same time period, the prevalence of obesity in the country increased from 14.5% to 30.9%?

5. For the data in Exercise 4, use the function boxplot() to write down the three commands to obtain plots of the relative levels of:
(a) calories
(b) percentage of calories from fat
(c) percentage of calories from carbohydrates

```
> boxplot(2450, 2439, 2866, 2618)
> boxplot(37.0, 36.2, 34.0, 32.1)
> boxplot(43.1, 42.2, 50.0, 48.1)
```

The results are shown in Figures 4.12, 4.13, and 4.14.

6. The following are some data on accident rates by age group (Dalgaard, 2002). The age groups are 0–4, 5–9, 10–15, 16, 17, 18–19, 20–24, 25–59, and 60–79 years old. The recorded data are summarized as follows:

```
> group.midage<-c(2.5, 7.5, 13, 16.5, 17.5, 19, 22.5, 44.5, 70-5)
> accidents <- c(28, 46, 58, 20, 31, 64,149, 316, 103)
```

Combine these two parameters as follows:

```
> age.acc <- rep(group.midage, accidents)
```

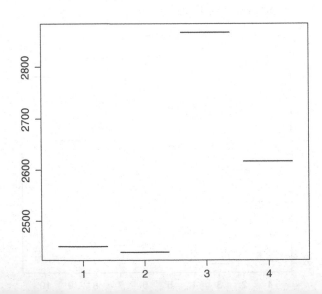

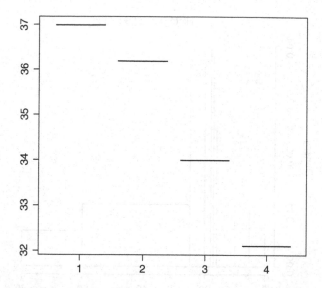

FIGURE 4.13 Percentage of calories from fat for four tests.

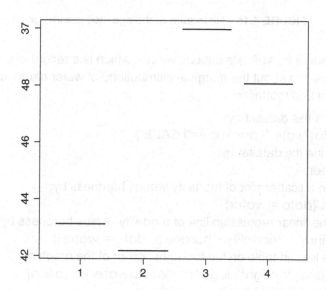

FIGURE 4.14 Percentage of calories from carbohydrates for four tests.

Note: The function rep(x) replicates the values in *x*.
  Now, define the break points as follows:

```
> breakpoint <- c(0, 5, 10, 16, 17, 18, 20, 25, age.acc
60, 80)
```

Plot a histogram of the parameter age.acc, to display the distribution by age groups, as follows:

```
> hist(age.acc, breaks=breakpoint)
```

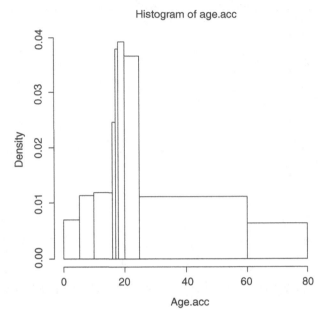

FIGURE 4.15 Histogram of the age–acc parameter.

7. In the package HSAUR is a dataset water, which is a record of 61 towns in Britain with information about the marginal distributions of water hardness (concentration of calcium) and mortality.

   (a) Access this dataset by:
       > data("water", package="HSAUR")
   (b) Examine the dataset by:
       > water
   (c) Obtain a scatter plot of mortality versus hardness by:
       > plot (data = water)
   (d) Plot the linear regression line of mortality versus hardness by:
       > abline(lm(mortality ~ hardness, data = water))
   (e) Add a legend table on the top-right corner of the graph by:
       > legend("topright", legend = levels(water$location),
       +   pch=c(1, 2), bty= "n")
   (f) Display a histogram of water versus hardness by:
       > hist(water$hardness)
   (g) Show a boxplot of water versus mortality by:
       > boxplot(water$mortality)

   The results are shown in Figures 4.16–4.20.

8. Displaying multivariate data.
   In a Danish study on the effect of screening for breast cancer (Dalgaard, 2002; Olsen et al., 2005), four groups or cohorts were collected:
   (i) The study group, consisting of the population of women in the appropriate age range in Copenhagen and Frederiksberg after the introduction of routine mammography screening

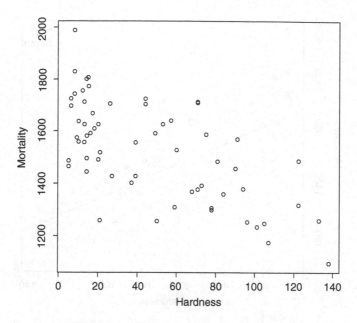

FIGURE 4.16 Mortality vs. water hardness.

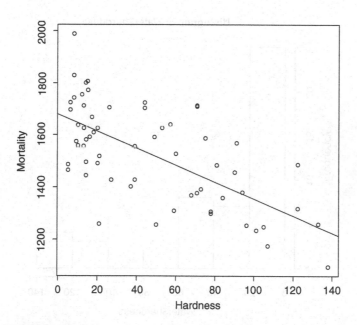

FIGURE 4.17 Mortality vs. water hardness with regression line.

(ii) The national control group, consisting of the population in the parts of Denmark in which routine mammography screening was *not* available

These two groups were collected in 1991–2001.

(iii) The historical control group

(iv) The historical national control group

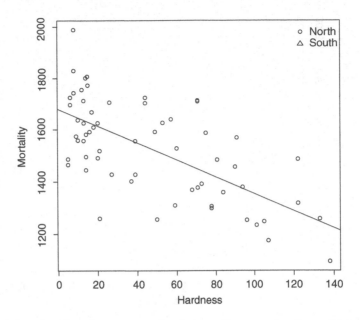

FIGURE 4.18 Mortality vs. water hardness with regression line, with legend.

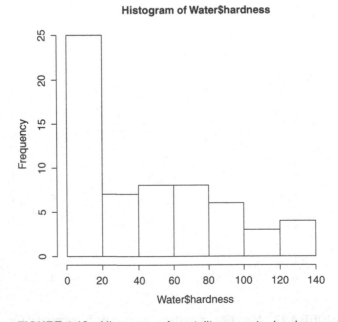

FIGURE 4.19 Histogram of mortality vs. water hardness.

These latter two are similar cohorts from 10 years earlier, before the introduction of screening in Copenhagen and Frederiksberg. The study group comprises the entire population, not just those accepting the invitation to be screened.

(a) Examine the dataset, using the following R code segment:
```
> install.packages("ISwR")
> library("ISwR")
```

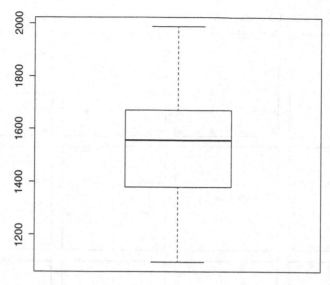

FIGURE 4.20 Boxplot of data.

> data(bcmort)
> bcmort

(b) Display the dataset by:
> plot(bcmort)

(c) Remove the gaps using the function pair():
> par(mex=1)
> pairs(bcmort, gap=0, cex.labels=2.0)

The results are shown in Figures 4.21 and 4.22.

9. Displaying more multivariate data.

A public health study investigated the effect of body weight on the resting metabolic rate (rmr) for women (Dalgaard, 2002; Altman, 1991).

The rmr data frame has 44 rows and 2 columns, containing the rmr and body weight data for 44 women. The two columns are:

body.weight   A numeric vector, body weight (kg)
metabolic.rate   A numeric vector, metabolic rate (kcal/24 hr)

(a) Examine the dataset, using the following R code segment:
> install.packages("ISwR")
> library("ISwR")
> data(rmr)
> rmr

(b) Display the dataset by:
> plot(rmr)

The result is shown in Figure 4.22.

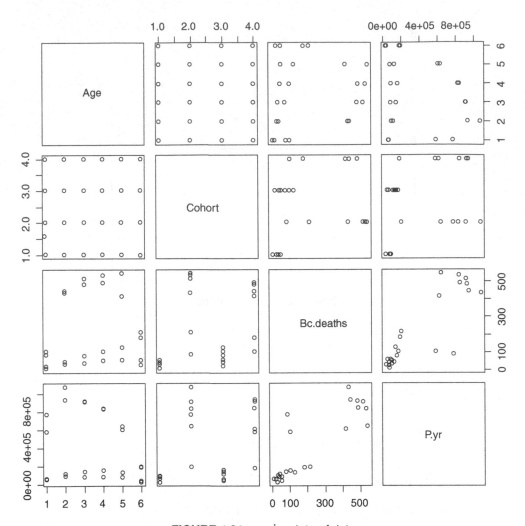

FIGURE 4.21 pairs plots of data.

(c) Execute the following plot:

> plot(metabolic.rate~body.weight,data=rmr)

The result is shown in Figure 4.24.

(d) Notice any difference between this plot and the last plot?

(e) Add a linear regression line on the display using:

> abline(lm(metabolic.rate ~ body.weight, data = rmr))

The result is shown in Figure 4.25.

10. A step-by-step procedure to display a plot with labeling (Murrell, 2006).

(a) Get ready by using:

> plot.new()

(b) Set up a window by using:

> plot.window(range(pressure$temperature),

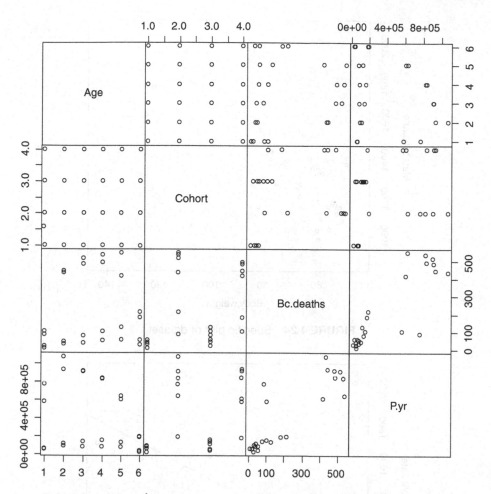

FIGURE 4.22 pairs plots of data, removing gaps between individual plots.

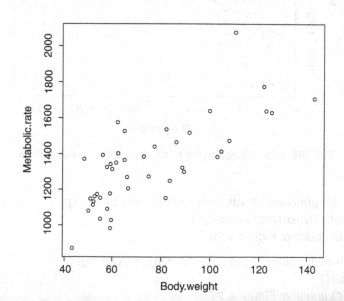

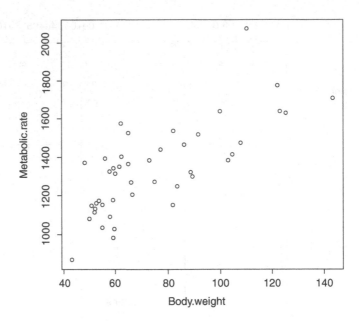

FIGURE 4.24   Specific plot of dataset.

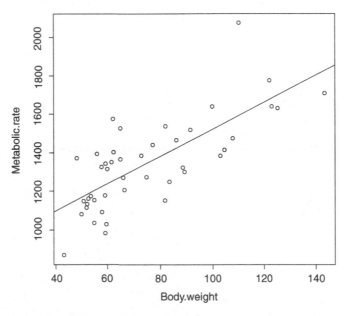

FIGURE 4.25   Specific plot of dataset, with regression line.

(c) Plot the pressure versus temperature data by using:
> plot.xy(pressure, type="p")
> # *Outputting:* Figure 4.26.

(d) Put a rectangular frame over the display by using:
> box()
> # *Outputting:* Figure 4.27

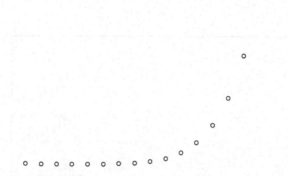

FIGURE 4.26   > plot.xy(pressure, type="p").

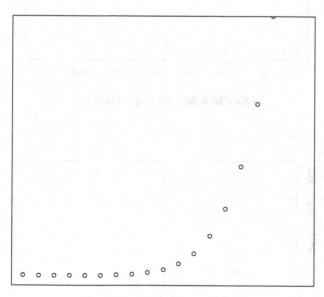

FIGURE 4.27   Adding > box().

(e) Add the horizontal (temperature) axis by using:
> axis(1)
> # *Outputting:* Figure 4.28.

(f) Add the other axis, the vertical (pressure) axis, by using:
> axis(2)
> # *Outputting:* Figure 4.29.

(g) Finally, label the plot centered at the position (100 units horizontal, 250 units vertical) by using:

> text(100, 250, "Pressure (mm Hg)\nversus\nTemperature
+ (Centigrade)")
> # *Outputting:* Figure 4.30.

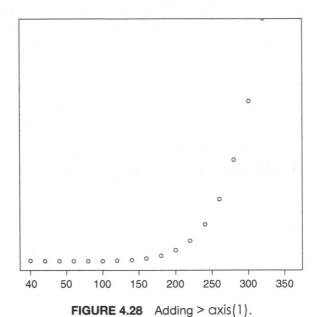

FIGURE 4.28 Adding > axis(1).

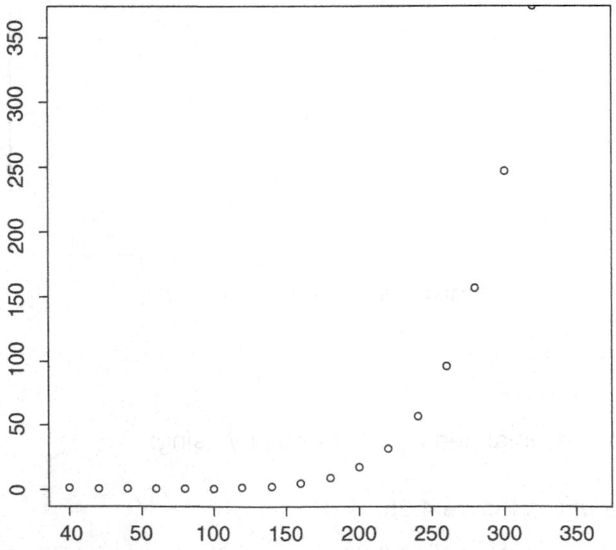

FIGURE 4.29 Adding > axis(2).

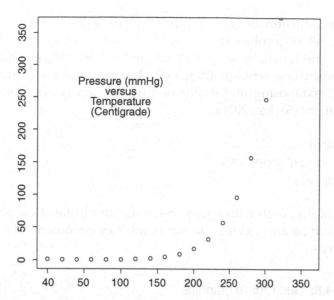

FIGURE 4.30   Adding > text(100, 250, "Pressure (mm Hg)\nversus\nTemperature (Centigrade)").

4.2   GRID GRAPHICS

Within the R environment for statistical computing and graphics, the **Grid Graphics System** is an add-on package. It provides a set of graphical functions, with substantial flexibility, that support graphics display. Several other R packages also use grid graphics (Murrell, 2006), including:

- Deepayan Sarkar's lattice package, distributed with R
- Frank Harrell's Hmisc and Design
- M. Kondrin's RGrace
- Paul Murrell's gridBase (available from CRAN) and gridSVG (available from Murrell's home page)

The grid graphics system is now part of the base R distribution.

This section introduces grid graphics in terms of the seminal CRAN package lattice (Sarkar, 2011b) package and the definitive treatise of Murrell (2006).

The lattice Package: Trellis Graphics

The lattice package (http://r-forge.r-project.org/projects/lattice) is a powerful, elegant, high-level data visualization system, with an emphasis on multivariate data, which is sufficient for typical graphics needs. It is also flexible enough to handle most nonstandard requirements. (Strictly speaking, lattice graphics produce an object of class "trellis," containing a description of the plot, and the function print() draws the plot.)

As an introduction to grid graphics, in this section, we consider one of the best-known lattice graphics functions, xyplot(), as a time-series plotting method. Other useful grid functions are also shown in the following examples. The xyplot() function handles time-series plotting, including cut-and-stack plots, and allows the superposing, juxtaposing, and styling of different time series. Consider the following code segment (Sarkar, 2011a):

```
> library(lattice)
> install.packages("graphics")
> library("graphics")
```

Two examples, each with special reference to biostatistical applications, from the package lattice are selected and run in the R environment. The resulting graphics are displayed.

■ **Example 4.8:** Grid lattice graphics

xyplot.ts   Time-series plotting methods (Sarkar, 2011a)
```
> ### Example with simpler data, few data points
> set.seed(1)
> z <- ts(cbind(a = 1:5, b = 11:15, c = 21:25) + rnorm(5))
> xyplot(z, screens = 1)
> # Outputting: > xyplot(z, screens = list(a = "primary (a)", "other (b & c)"),
+ type = list(a = c("p", "h"), b = c("p", "s"), "o"),
+ pch = list(a = 2, c = 3), auto.key = list(type = "o"))
> # Outputting: Figures 4.31 and 4.32.
```

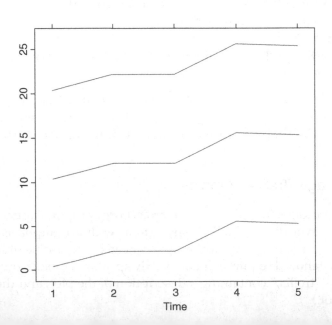

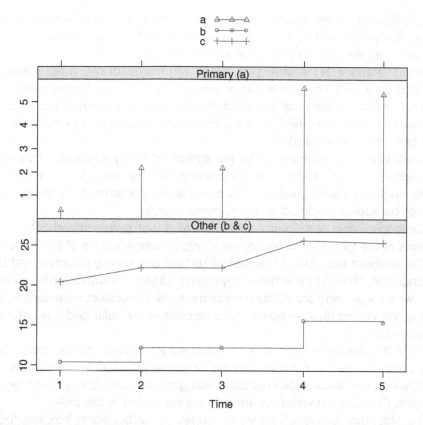

FIGURE 4.32   Grid lattice graphics: xyplot(), separating a dataset into two groups.

■ **Example 4.9:** Lattice grid graphics plot cloud(x, data, ...)

> ?cloud # *The following documentation is presented*[3]:
B_07_cloud {lattice}

3D Scatter Plot and Wireframe Surface Plot

Description:
Generic functions to draw three-dimensional (3D) scatter plots and surfaces. The formula methods do most of the actual work.

Use:
cloud(x, data, ...)
wireframe(x, data, ...)

Details:
These functions produce 3D plots in each panel (so long as the default panel functions are used). The orientation is obtained as follows: The data are scaled to fall within a bounding box that is contained in the [0.5, 0.5] cube (and even smaller for nondefault values of aspect). The viewing direction is given by a sequence of rotations specified

by the screen argument, starting from the positive z-axis. The viewing point (camera) is located at a distance of 1/distance from the origin. If perspective=FALSE, distance is set to 0 (i.e., the viewing point is at an infinite distance).

cloud draws a 3D scatter plot, while wireframe draws a 3D surface (usually evaluated on a grid). Multiple surfaces can be drawn by wireframe using the groups argument (although this is of limited utility because the display is incorrect when the surfaces intersect). Specifying groups with cloud results in a panel.superpose-like effect (via panel.3dscatter).

wireframe can optionally render the surface as being illuminated by a light source (no shadows, though). Details can be found in the help page for panel.3dwire. Note that although arguments controlling these are actually arguments for the panel function, they can be applied to cloud and wireframe directly.

For single-panel plots, wireframe can also plot parametrized 3D surfaces [i.e., functions of the form f(u,v) = (x(u,v), y(u,v), z(u,v)], where values of (u,v) lie on a rectangle. The simplest example of this sort of surface is a sphere parametrized by latitude and longitude. This can be achieved by calling wireframe with a formula x of the form z~x*y, where x, y, and z are all matrixes of the same dimension, representing the values of x(u,v), y(u,v), and z(u,v) evaluated on a discrete rectangular grid [the actual values of (u,v) are irrelevant].

When this feature is used, the heights used to calculate drape colors or shading colors are no longer the z-values, but the distances of (x,y,z) from the origin.

Note that this feature does not work with groups, subscripts, subset, or other such functions. Conditioning variables are also not supported in this case.

The algorithm for identifying which edges of the bounding box are "behind" the points does not work in some extreme situations. Also, panel.cloud automatically tries to figure out the optimal location of the arrows and axis labels, but it can fail on occasion (especially when the view is from "below" the data). This can be manually controlled by the scpos argument in panel.cloud.

These and all other high-level Trellis functions have several other arguments in common. These are extensively documented only in the help page for xyplot, which should be consulted to learn more detail on use.

```
> cloud(Sepal.Length ~ Petal.Length * Petal.Width | Species,
+ data=iris, screen=list(x=-90, y=70), distance =0.4, zoom =0.6)
> # Outputting: Figure 4.33.
```

CONTROLLING LATTICE PLOTS

To control the color, text font size, line types/widths of the graphic display, and so on in a lattice plot, graphical parameters may be used. Large lists of parameter groups are in the documentation files of each lattice function, and each parameter group consists of a list of parameter settings. For each function, reference information is readily available online, in conjunction with the help(function) route within the R environment.

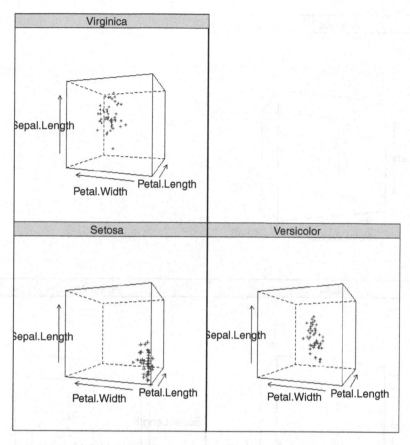

FIGURE 4.33 Lattice grid graphics plot cloud(x, data, ...).

- *Controlling text font size:*

■ **Example 4.10:** To control the text font size of the lattice plot in Example 4.9

Here, one may use the following code segment to control the font size:

```
> fontsize <- trellis.par.get("fontsize")
> fontsize$text <- 10
> trellis.par.set("fontsize", fontsize)
>
> cloud(Sepal.Length ~ Petal.Length * Petal.Width | Species,
+ data=iris, screen=list(x=-90, y=70),distance =0.4, zoom =0.6)
> # Outputting: Figure 4.34.
```

- *Controlling line color/type/width:* Refer to plot.lone.
- *Controlling data symbols, size, shape, and color:* Refer to plot.symbol and the pch settings, as well as the fontsize and strip.background settings.
- The current value of graphical parameter setting may be obtained using the functions trellis.par.get().
- Font size settings may be specified using the function trellis.par.set(), or using the par settings argument within a plotting command.

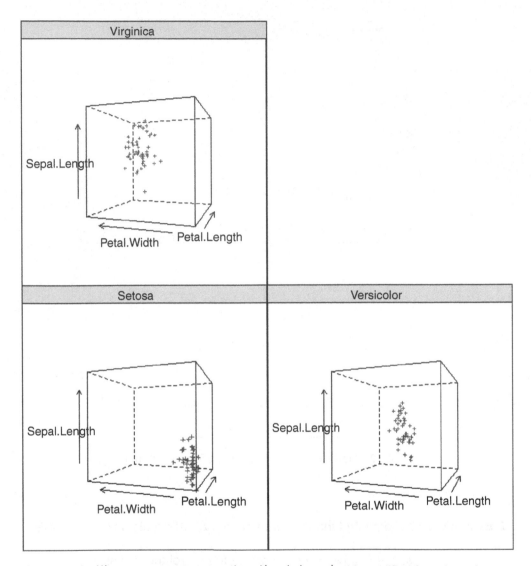

FIGURE 4.34 Lattice grid graphics plot cloud(x, data, ...) with modified font size using
> fontsize$text.

ARRANGING LATTICE PLOTS

Two types of arrangements must be considered when doing lattice plots:

Type I: Within a single plot, the arrangement of strips and panels
Type II: On a given page, the arrangement of several complete plots together

For Type I, two arguments may be specified: the layout argument and the aspect
argument.

1. The layout argument consists of up to three values; the first two indicate the
   number of rows and columns of panels on each page, and the third indicates the
   number of pages.

2. The aspect argument specifies the aspect ratio (the height divided by the width) of the panel. The default value is fill, which makes panels expand to fill as much space as possible. aspect=1 forces all panels to be square, because a square has an aspect ratio of 1.0.

The Grid Model for R Graphics (Murrell, 2006)[3]

As noted earlier, the Grid Graphics System is an add-on package within the R environment. The grid system consists of basic features such as functions for drawing geometric objects (point, lines, triangles, rectangles, etc.); texts; and concepts such as layouts, viewports, and units, which permit outputs to be sized and located as required. The grid system may be loaded into R as follows:

```
> library(grid)
```

with additional online documentation accessible via the functions help() and vignette().

```
> ?grid # To examine the function grid in the graphics package
    grid adds an nx by ny rectangular grid to an existing plot.
```

Use:
```
> grid(nx = NULL, ny = nx, col = "lightgray", lty = "dotted",
+       lwd = par("lwd"), equilogs = TRUE)
```

Arguments:

nx,ny	Number of cells of the grid in the x- and y-directions. When NULL, as per default, the grid aligns with the tick marks on the corresponding *default* axis (i.e., tick marks as computed by axTicks). When NA, no grid lines are drawn in the corresponding direction.
Col	Character or (integer) numeric; color of the grid lines.
Lty	Character or (integer) numeric; line type of the grid lines.
Lwd	Nonnegative numeric giving line width of the grid lines.
equilogs	Logical; only used when *log* coordinates and alignment with the axis tick marks are active. Setting equilogs = FALSE in that case gives *nonequidistant* tick-aligned grid lines.

■ **Example 4.11:** A demonstration of the Grid Graphics System

```
> plot(1:3)
> grid(NA, 5, lwd = 2) # grid only in y-direction
> # Outputting: Figure 4.35.
> ## maybe change the desired number of tick marks:
> ## par(lab=c(mx,my,7))
> op <- par(mfcol = 1:2)
```

```
> with(iris,
+     {
+       plot(Sepal.Length, Sepal.Width, col = as.integer(Species),
+            xlim = c(4, 8), ylim = c(2, 4.5), panel.first = grid(),
+            main = "with(iris, plot(...., panel.first = grid(), ..) )")
+       plot(Sepal.Length, Sepal.Width, col = as.integer(Species),
+            panel.first = grid(3, lty=1,lwd=2),
+            main = "... panel.first = grid(3, lty=1,lwd=2), ..")
+     }
+     ) # Outputting: Figure 4.36.
># At end of plotting, reset to previous settings:

> par(op)
```

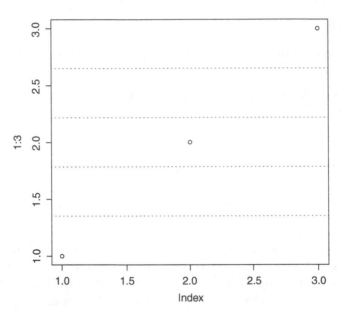

FIGURE 4.35   Grid Graphics System plot(1:3) with grid only in the y-direction.

◼ Controlling the output:

A set of grid functions exists for producing basic graphical output such as points, lines, rectangles, circles, and text. These functions are of the form grid.*(). For each one, there is a corresponding Grob() function that creates an object containing a description of primitive graphical output, but does not draw anything.

The full set of these functions is listed in Table 4.1.[3]

Notes:

1. In most cases, the first argument of each of these functions is a set of locations and dimensions for the graphical object to be drawn. For example, grid.rect() has arguments x, y, width, and height, specifying the locations and dimensions of the rectangles to be drawn. An exception is the function grid.text(), which requires the text to be drawn as its first argument.

2. Multiple primitives can be produced when multiple locations and dimensions are

with(iris, plot(...., panel.first = grid() ... panel.first = grid(3, lty = 1, lwd = 2)))

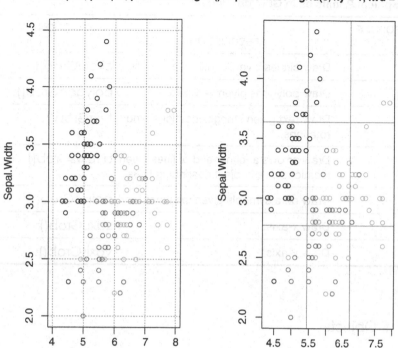

FIGURE 4.36   Grid Graphics System plot() with specified grid lines, titles, labels, and data points in different colors.

TABLE 4.1   Graphical Primitives in Grid

This is the complete set of low-level functions that produce graphical output. For each function that produces graphical output (leftmost column), there is a corresponding function that returns a graphical object containing a description of graphical output instead of producing graphical output itself (rightmost column). The latter set of functions is described later in this chapter.

FUNCTION TO PRODUCE OUTPUT	DESCRIPTION	FUNCTION TO PRODUCE OBJECT
grid.move.to()	Set the current location.	moveToGrob()
grid.line.to()	Draw a line from the current location to a new location and reset the current location.	lineToGrob()
grid.lines()	Draw a single line through multiple locations in sequence.	linesGrob()
grid.segments()	Draw multiple lines between pairs of locations.	segmentsGrob()
grid.rect()	Draw rectangles given locations and sizes.	rectGrob()

TABLE 4.1 Graphical Primitives in Grid (*continued*)

FUNCTION TO PRODUCE OUTPUT	DESCRIPTION	FUNCTION TO PRODUCE OBJECT
grid.circle()	Draw circles given locations and radii.	circleGrob()
grid.polygon()	Draw polygons given vertexes.	polygonGrob()
grid.text()	Draw text given strings, locations, and rotations.	textGrob()
grid.arrows()	Draw arrows at either end of lines given locations or an object describing lines.	arrowsGrob()
grid.points()	Draw data symbols given locations.	pointsGrob()
grid.xaxis()	Draw *x*-axis.	xaxisGrob()
grid.yaxis()	Draw *y*-axis.	yaxisGrob().

Grid Graphics Objects

In grid graphics, a **grob** is a *graphic ob*ject. A grob may be used to interactively edit a scenario produced by grid. Because lattice is built on grid, this approach allows one to interactively edit a lattice plot.

In the following code segment, which has 10 graphical outputs, notice the grob function barbedGrob(), described in the CRAN package gridExtra (Baptiste, 2012).

```
> set.seed(1234)
> grid.barbed(name="test") # Outputting: Figure 4.37.
> grid.edit("test", gp=gpar(fill="blue", lwd=3))
> # Outputting: Figure 4.38.
> grid.edit("test::points", pch=22) # Outputting: Figure 4.39.
> grid.newpage()
> g <-
+ barbedGrob(size=unit(1:5, "char"), only=FALSE,
+ gp=gpar(col="red", lex=3, fill="blue", alpha=0.5, pch=3))
>
> pushViewport(vp=viewport(width=1, height=1))
> grid.rect(gp=gpar(fill="thistle2")) # Outputting: Figure 4.40.
> grid.grill(gp=gpar(col="lavenderblush1",lwd=3,lty=3))
> # Outputting: Figure 4.41.
> grid.draw(g) # Outputting: Figure 4.42.
> x <- c(0.2, 0.7)
> y <- x
> dev.new(width=3, height=7) # Outputting: Figure 4.43.
> grid.newpage()# Outputting: Figure 4.44.
> grid.draw(g) # Outputting: Figure 4.45.
```

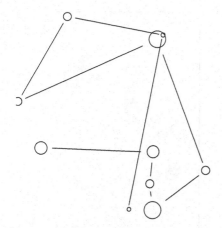

FIGURE 4.37 grid.barbed() Output.

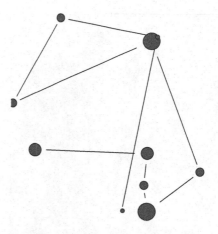

FIGURE 4.38 grid.edit() Output.

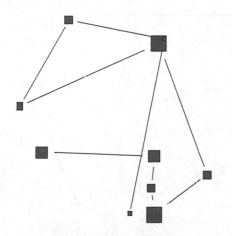

FIGURE 4.39 grid.edit() Output.

FIGURE 4.40 grid.rect() Output.

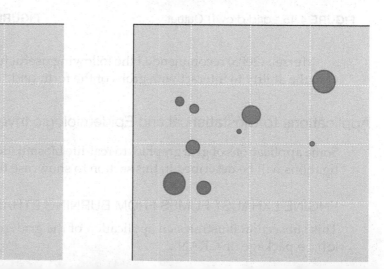

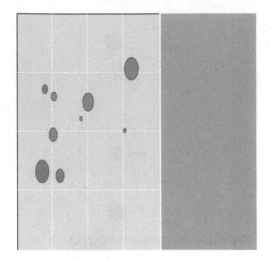

FIGURE 4.43   dev.new() Output.

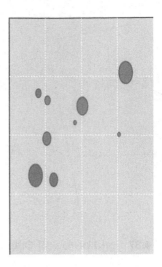

FIGURE 4.44   grid.newpage() Output.

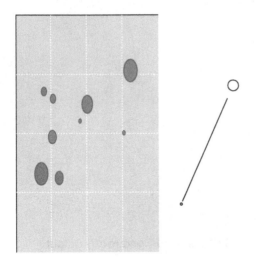

FIGURE 4.45   grid.draw() Output.

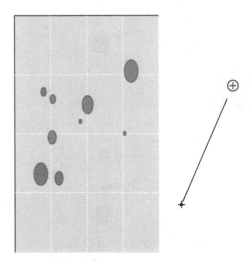

FIGURE 4.46   grid.points() Output.

Murrell (2006) recommended the following useful functions (Table 4.2) that provide the ability to interact with grobs of the form grid.*().

Applications to Biostatistical and Epidemiologic Investigations

Some applications of grid graphics to real-life biostatistical and epidemiologic investigations will be described in this section to showcase the grid graphics techniques.

ENGINE EXHAUST FUMES FROM BURNING ETHANOL

This subsection illustrates an application of the grid graphics–Trellis plot from the lattice package (in CRAN).[4]

TABLE 4.2   Some Useful Functions for Working With Grobs

FUNCTION TO WORK WITH OUTPUT	DESCRIPTION	FUNCTION TO WORK WITH GROBS
grid.get()	Returns a copy of one or more grobs	getGrob()
grid.edit()	Modifies one or more grobs	editGrob()
grid.add()	Adds a grob to one or more grobs	addGrob()
grid.remove()	Removes one or more grobs	removeGrod()
grid.set()	Replaces one or more grobs	setGrob()

Description of the Investigation:
Ethanol fuel was burned in a single-cylinder engine. For various settings of the engine compression and equivalence ratio, the emissions of nitrogen oxides were recorded. A data frame was constructed with 88 observations on the following three variables:

NOx   Concentration of nitrogen oxides (NO and NO_2) in micrograms/J
C   Compression ratio of the engine
E   Equivalence ratio (a measure of the richness of the air and ethanol fuel mixture)

Authors:
Documentation: Wright, K.
Source: Brinkman (1981).
Reference: Cleveland, William S. (1993). *Visualizing data.* Summit, NJ: Hobart Press.

```
>
> # H_ethanol
> install.packages("lattice")
> library("lattice")
>
> # The 88 sets of data in the dataframe ethanol may be inspected by
> # outputting the data using: > ethanol
>
> ## Constructing panel functions on the fly
> EE <- equal.count(ethanol$E, number=9, overlap=1/4)
> xyplot(NOx ~ C | EE, data = ethanol,
+ prepanel = function(x, y) prepanel.loess(x, y, span = 1),
+ xlab = "Compression ratio", ylab = "NOx (micrograms/J)",
+ panel = function(x, y) {
+ panel.grid(h=-1, v= 2)
+ panel.xyplot(x, y)
+ panel.loess(x,y, span=1)
+ },
```

```
> # Outputting: Figure 4.47 ethanol-1
>
>
> # Wireframe loess surface fit (see Figure 4.48).
> require(stats)
> with(ethanol, {
+ eth.lo <- loess(NOx ~ C * E, span = 1/3, parametric = "C",
+ drop.square = "C", family="symmetric")
+ eth.marginal <- list(C = seq(min(C), max(C), length.out = 25),
+ E = seq(min(E), max(E), length.out = 25))
+ eth.grid <- expand.grid(eth.marginal)
+ eth.fit <- predict(eth.lo, eth.grid)
+ wireframe(eth.fit ~ eth.grid$C * eth.grid$E,
+ shade=TRUE,
+ screen = list(z = 40, x = -60, y=0),
+ distance = .1,
+ xlab = "C", ylab = "E", zlab = "NOx")
+ })
> # Outputting: Figure 4.48 ethanol-2
>
```

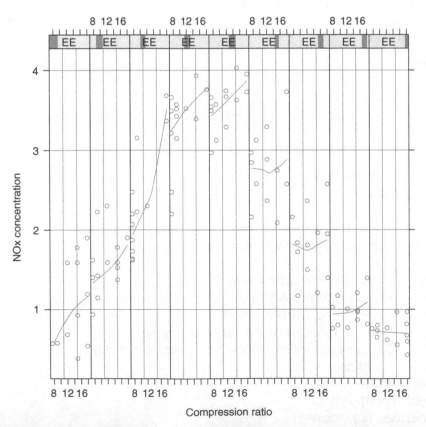

FIGURE 4.47 ethanol-1: Grid lattice panel.xyplot() of NOx concentration vs. compression

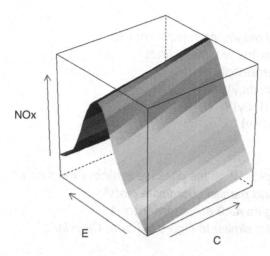

FIGURE 4.48 ethanol-2: Wireframe loess surface fit of NOx concentration vs. compression ratio C, for varying fuel mixture equivalence ratios E.

ENVIRONMENTAL EPIDEMIOLOGY: ATMOSPHERIC CONDITIONS IN NEW YORK CITY

Description of the Investigation:

Daily measurements of ozone concentration, wind speed, temperature, and solar radiation in New York City from May to September of 1973.

A data frame with 111 observations on the following four variables:

ozone—Average ozone concentration (hourly measurements) in parts per billion
radiation—Solar radiation (from 08:00 a.m. to 12:00 p.m.) in langleys
temperature—Maximum daily temperature in degrees Fahrenheit
wind—Average wind speed (at 07:00 a.m. and 10:00 a.m.) in miles per hour

Authors:

Documentation: Wright, K.

Source: Bruntz, S. M., Cleveland, W. S., Kleiner, B., & Warner, J. L. (1974). The dependence of ambient ozone on solar radiation, wind, temperature, and mixing height. In *Symposium on atmospheric diffusion and air pollution* (pp. 125–128). Boston, MA: American Meteorological Society.

Reference: Cleveland, W. S. (1993). *Visualizing data*. Summit, NJ: Hobart Press.

This environmental epidemiology example shows three different graphical ways for presenting four environmental factors (ozone, radiation, temperature, and wind conditions) using grid graphics–Trellis plot from the lattice package (in CRAN).[4]

■ **Example:** environmental {lattice} (Murrell, 2006)

```
> install.packages("lattice")
> library("lattice")
>
> # The 111 sets of data in the dataframe environmental may be inspected by
```

```
>
> # splom() plot of dataframe environmental
> # Scatter plot matrix with loess lines
> splom(~environmental,
+   panel=function(x,y){
+     panel.xyplot(x,y)
+     panel.loess(x,y)
+   }
+ )
```
> # *The function* splom(), *in the package* lattice, *draws conditional scatter*
> # *plot matrixes and parallel coordinate plots*[5]
> # *Outputting:* Figure 4.49 environmental-**1**
> # *Conditioned plot similar to Figure 5.3 from Cleveland*

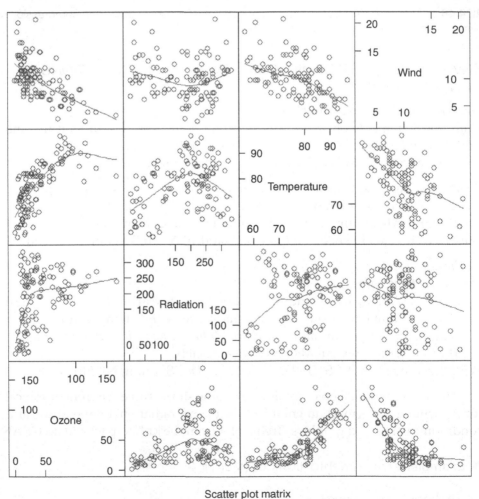

Scatter plot matrix

FIGURE 4.49 environmental-1: Grid lattice splom() plot of ozone, radiation, temperature, and wind conditions.

```
> attach(environmental)
> Temperature <- equal.count(temperature, 4, 1/2)
> Wind <- equal.count(wind, 4, 1/2)
> xyplot((ozone^(1/3)) ~ radiation | Temperature * Wind,
+    aspect=1,
+ prepanel = function(x, y)
+ prepanel.loess(x, y, span = 1),
+ panel = function(x, y){
+ panel.grid(h = 2, v = 2)
+ panel.xyplot(x, y, cex = .5)
+ panel.loess(x, y, span = 1)
+ },
+ xlab = "Solar radiation (langleys)",
+ ylab = "Ozone (cube root ppb)")
> # Outputting: Figure 4.50 environmental-2
> detach()
>
```

■ **Example:** environmental-**2** {lattice}

```
> install.packages("lattice")
> library("lattice")
>
> # Conditioned plot similar to Figure 5.3 from Cleveland
> attach(environmental)
> Temperature <- equal.count(temperature, 4, 1/2)
> Wind <- equal.count(wind, 4, 1/2)
> xyplot((ozone^(1/3)) ~ radiation | Temperature * Wind,
+    aspect=1,
+ prepanel = function(x, y)
+ prepanel.loess(x, y, span = 1),
+ panel = function(x, y){
+ panel.grid(h = 2, v = 2)
+ panel.xyplot(x, y, cex = .5)
+ panel.loess(x, y, span = 1)
+ },
+ xlab = "Solar radiation (langleys)",
+ ylab = "Ozone (cube root ppb)")
> # Outputting: Figure 4.50 environmental-2
> detach()
>
```

■ **Example:** environmental-**3** {lattice}

```
> install.packages("lattice")
> library("lattice")
>
```

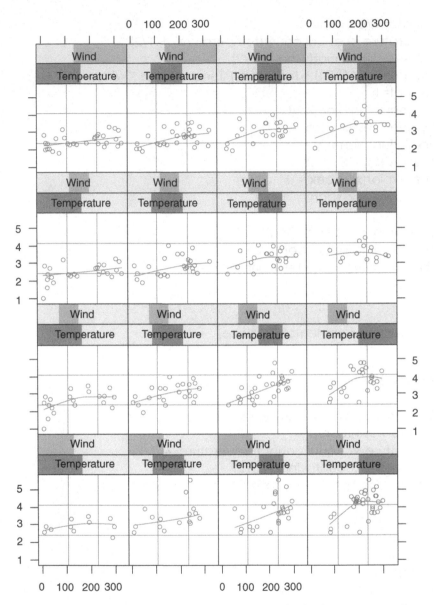

FIGURE 4.50 environmental-2: Grid lattice panel.xyplot() of ozone, radiation, temperature, and wind conditions.

```
> with(environmental,{
+   coplot((ozone^.33) ~ radiation | temperature * wind,
+   number=c(4,4),
+   panel = function(x, y, ...) panel.smooth(x, y, span = .8, ...),
+   xlab="Solar radiation (langleys)",
+   ylab="Ozone (cube root ppb)")
+ })
> # Outputting: Figure 4.51 environmental--3
```

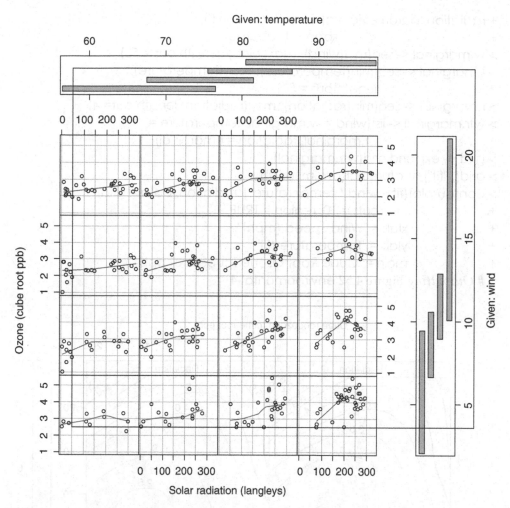

FIGURE 4.51 environmental-3: Grid lattice coplot() of ozone, radiation, temperature, and wind conditions.

ENVIRONMENTAL EPIDEMIOLOGY II

This subsection uses "Lattice-p.44: B_06_levelplot—Level plots and contour plots" to produce the desired graphics.

Description of the Investigation:
This is the same investigation as the examples in the preceding subsection.

Analytical Approach:
To display the variations within the multivariate dataset environmental by drawing color level plots and contour plots, using the following function in the lattice package: contourplot(x, data, ...)

```
>
> require(stats)
> attach(environmental)
```

```
+ radiation, parametric = c("radiation", "wind"),
+                          span = 1, degree = 2)
> w.marginal <- seq(min(wind), max(wind), length.out = 50)
> t.marginal <- seq(min(temperature), max(temperature),
+                   length.out = 50)
> r.marginal <- seq(min(radiation), max(radiation),length.out= 4)
> wtr.marginal <- list(wind = w.marginal, temperature =
+                      t.marginal, radiation = r.marginal)
> grid <- expand.grid(wtr.marginal)
> grid[, "fit"] <- c(predict(ozo.m, grid))
> contourplot(fit ~ wind * temperature | radiation, data = grid,
+             cuts = 10, region = TRUE,
+             xlab = "Wind Speed (mph)",
+             ylab = "Temperature (F)",
+             main = "Cube Root Ozone (cube root ppb)")
> # Outputting Figure 4.52 environmental-4
```

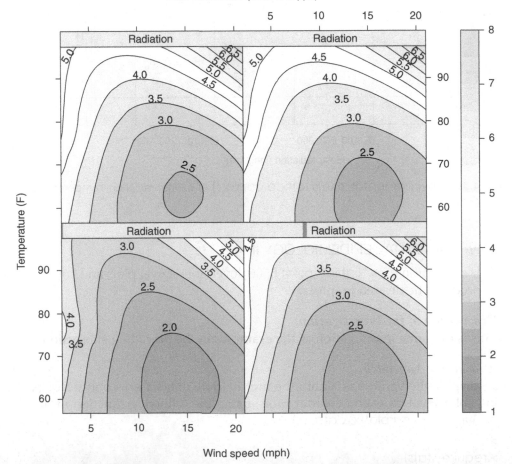

FIGURE 4.52 environmental-4: Grid lattice contourplot() of ozone, radiation, temperature

CANCER EPIDEMIOLOGY: MELANOMA SKIN CANCER INCIDENCE

This subsection uses grid graphics–Trellis plot from the lattice package (in CRAN)[4] to produce a time-series plot (Sarkar, 2011a).

Description of the Investigation:

The data from the Connecticut Tumor Registry present age-adjusted numbers of melanoma skin cancer incidences per 100,000 people in the U.S. state of Connecticut for the years from 1936 to 1972. It consists of a data frame with 37 observations on the following two variables:

year—Years 1936 to 1972
incidence—Rate of melanoma cancer per 100,000 population

Author(s):

Documentation: Wright, K.
Source: Houghton, A., Munster, E. W., & Viola, M. V. (1978). Increased incidence of malignant melanoma after peaks of sunspot activity. *Lancet, 8,* 759–760.
Reference: Cleveland, W. S. (1993). *Visualizing data.* Summit, NJ: Hobart Press.

```
> # Time-series plot (Figure 3.64 from Cleveland).
> xyplot(incidence ~ year,
+ data = melanoma,
+ aspect = "xy",
+ panel = function(x, y)
+ panel.xyplot(x, y, type="o", pch = 16),
+ ylim = c(0, 6),
+ xlab = "Year",
+ ylab = "Incidence"
+ )
> # Outputting: Figure 4.53 melanoma
```

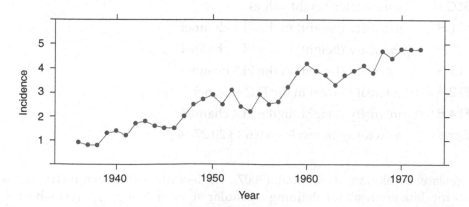

FIGURE 4.53 melanoma grid lattice panel.xyplot(x, y) time-series plot.

EXAMPLES FROM THE CRAN PACKAGE {latticeExtra}

In 2011, Sarkar (2011b) published the CRAN package latticeExtra, which contains a number of grid graphics functions that may support graphic displays for biostatistical datasets reported in research and investigational activities in epidemiology and public health. Some examples of applications of these functions to reported datasets are shown here.

■ **Example 4.12:** Grid graphics in R: gvhd10 in latticeExtra

Dataset: gvhd10—Flow cytometry (FCM) data from five samples from a patient

Note: FCM is a technique for examining and *counting* microscopic particles, such as *chromosomes* and cells, by suspending them in a stream of fluid and passing them by an electronic detection apparatus. It allows simultaneous multiparametric analysis of the physical and chemical characteristics of up to thousands of particles per second. FCM is used in the diagnosis of health disorders, especially blood cancers, but it has many other applications in both research and clinical practice.

Description of the Investigation:
FCM data are recorded from blood samples taken from a leukemia patient before and after allogenic bone marrow transplant (a transplant procedure in which the patient receives stem cells from a genetically compatible, but not identical, donor). The data cover five visits.

Use: data(gvhd10)

Format of Data: A data frame with 113,896 observations on the following eight variables:

FSC.H	forward scatter height values
SSC.H	side scatter height values
FL1.H	intensity (height) in the FL1 channel
FL2.H	intensity (height) in the FL2 channel
FL3.H	intensity (height) in the FL3 channel
FL2.A	intensity (area) in the FL2 channel
FL4.H	intensity (height) in the FL4 channel
Days	a factor with levels −6 0 6 13 20 27 34

Reference: Brinkman, R. R., et al. (2007). High-content flow cytometry and temporal data analysis for defining a cellular signature of graft-versus-host disease. *Biology of Blood and Marrow Transplantation, 13*(6), 691–700.

The R code segment for the analysis is as follows:

```
> install.packages("latticeExtra")
> library("latticeExtra")
Loading required package: RColorBrewer
Loading required package: lattice
> data(gvhd10)
>
> # The many thousands of datasets in the dataframe gvhd10 may be
> # inspected by outputting the data using: > gvhd10
>

> histogram(~log2(FSC.H) | Days, gvhd10, xlab = "log Forward
+ Scatter", type = "density", nint = 50, layout = c(2, 4))
> # Outputting: Figure 4.54.
```

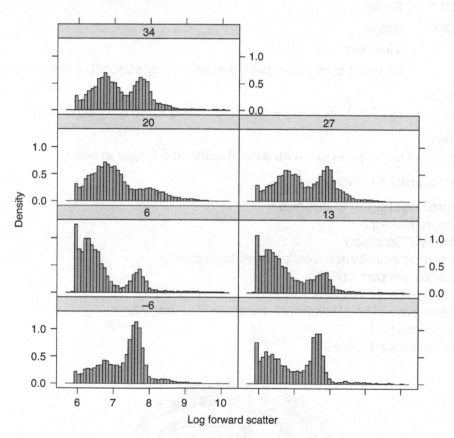

FIGURE 4.54 R grid graphics: Histogram for ghvd10 in latticeExtra with the Days factor labeled above each panel.

pixmapGrob(x): A SPECIAL GRID PLOT FOR ALL R USERS

To display the R insignia, the grid function pixmapGrob() may be used to create a grob from a pixmap object.

Description of the grid function: Using the R grid function pixmapGrob(), in the package RGraphics, one may create a grob from a pixmap object and produce the familiar insignia of the R program itself.

Use:
pixmapGrob(pic, x = 0.5, y = 0.5, scale = 1,

raster = FALSE, angle = 0, vp = NULL, ...)

Arguments:

Pic	Pixmap object
X	x-unit
Y	y-unit
Scale	Scale
Raster	Raster
Angle	Angle
Vp	Viewport
...	Optional grob parameters, passed to imageGrob() or rasterGrob()

Details:
Very primitive function, using R Graphics' imageGrob or rasterGrob (R > = 2.11)

Value:
A gTree of class "pixmap," with natural width and height in points

The requisite R code segment is:

```
> install.packages("RGraphics")
> library(pixmap)
> library(RGraphics)
> x <- read.pnm(system.file("pictures/logo.ppm",
+ package="pixmap")[1])
> g1 <- pixmapGrob(x)
> dev.new(width=g1$width/72, height=g1$height/72)
> grid.draw(g1)
> # Outputting: Figure 4.55.
```

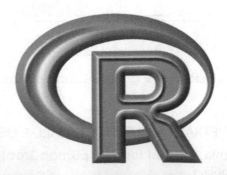

Review Questions for Section 4.2

1. (a) What is the Grid Graphics System?
   (b) Name some packages within this system.
2. (a) Contrast the plotting functions in the grid {lattice} graphics with base (traditional) graphics.
   (b) Give an example of dotplot().
3. (a) What two types of arrangements are available for multiple plots on a single page using lattice plots?
   (b) Give an example of each type.
4. When annotating a lattice plot of several panels, which function is available for
   (a) controlling the scaling and size of the panels?
   (b) controlling the contents in the strips of a lattice plot?
   Give an example of each.
5. (a) In grid graphics, what is a grob?
   (b) Write an R code segment that defines a grob.
6. In grid graphics, to draw circles at given locations and radii, which function is available
   (a) to create an object?
   (b) to produce an output of the object created?
   Give an example of each.
7. In grid graphics, describe the functions:
   (a) viewport()
   (b) pushViewport()
   Give an example of each.
8. In working with grobs in grid graphics, describe the functions:
   (a) getGrob()
   (b) grid.get()
   Provide an example of each.
9. (a) Describe the CRAN package latticeExtra.
   (b) Contrast the two functions map() and mapplot() from this package.
10. (a) Describe the CRAN package RGraphics.
    (b) Use the grid function pixmapGrob() from this package to create a pixmap object of your choice.

Exercises for Section 4.2

1. This is a practice session in using the grid graphics package lattice to produce Trellis graphics. In the R environment, execute the following code segment, command by command. For *each* command:
   (a) Explain the action expected of the command.
   (b) After executing the command, describe the results and outputs.
2. Compare the final output display obtained in Exercise 1 with the lattice plot type: the name of the R function for producing each plot type is shown on the strip above each plot. To obtain the same output, rewrite the code segment to obtain a more

```
> library(lattice)
> trellis.device()
> library(grid)
> x <- 1:5
> x
> y <- 1:5
> y
> g <- factor(1:5)
> g
> types <- c("barchart", "bwplot", "densityplot", "dotplot",
+         "histogram", "qqmath", "stripplot", "qq",
+         "xyplot", "levelplot", "contourplot",
+         "cloud", "wireframe", "splom", "parallel")
> types
> angle <- seq(0, 2*pi, length=21)[-21]
> angle
> xx <- cos(angle)
> xx
> yy <- sin(angle)
> yy
> gg <- factor(rep(1:2, each=10))
> gg
> aaa <- seq(0, pi, length=10)
> aaa
> xxx <- rep(aaa, 10)
> xxx
> yyy <- rep(aaa, each=10)
> yyy
> zzz <- sin(xxx) + sin(yyy)
> zzz
> doplot <- function(name, ...) {
+   do.call(name,
+     list(..., scales=list(draw=FALSE), xlab=NULL, ylab=NULL,
+          strip=function(which.panel, ...) {
+          grid.rect(gp=gpar(fill="grey90")); grid.text(name)
+                                          }))}
> plot <- vector("list", 15)
> plot
> plot[[1]] <- doplot("barchart", y ~ g | 1)
> plot[[1]]
> plot[[2]] <- doplot("bwplot", yy ~ gg | 1,
+              par.settings=list(box.umbrella=list(lwd=0.5)))
> plot[[2]]
> plot[[3]] <- doplot("densityplot", ~ yy | 1)
> plot[[3]]
```

```
> plot[[4]] <- doplot("dotplot", y ~ g | 1)
> plot[[4]]
> plot[[5]] <- doplot("histogram", ~ yy | 1)
> plot[[5]]
> plot[[6]] <- doplot("qqmath", ~ yy | 1)
> plot[[6]]
> plot[[7]] <- doplot("stripplot", yy ~ gg | 1)
> plot[[7]]
> plot[[8]] <- doplot("qq", gg ~ yy | 1)
> plot[[8]]
> plot[[9]] <- doplot("xyplot", xx ~ yy | 1)
> plot[[9]]
> plot[[10]] <- doplot("levelplot", zzz ~ xxx + yyy | 1,
+ colorkey=FALSE)
> plot[[10]]
> plot[[11]] <- doplot("contourplot", zzz ~ xxx + yyy | 1,
+                      labels=FALSE, cuts=8)
> plot[[11]]
> plot[[12]] <- doplot("cloud", zzz ~ xxx + yyy | 1, zlab=NULL,
+           zoom=0.9, par.settings=list(box.3d=list(lwd=0.01)))
> plot[[12]]
> plot[[13]] <- doplot("wireframe", zzz ~ xxx + yyy | 1,
+             zlab=NULL, zoom=0.9, drape=TRUE,
+        par.settings=list(box.3d=list(lwd=0.01)), colorkey=FALSE)
> plot[[13]]
> plot[[13]]
> plot[[14]] <- doplot("splom", ~ data.frame(x=xx[1:10],
+                      y=yy[1:10]) | 1, pscales=0)
> plot[[14]]
> plot[[15]] <- doplot("parallel", ~ data.frame(x=xx[1:10],
+                      y=yy[1:10]) | 1)
> plot[[15]]
>
> grid.newpage()
> pushViewport(viewport(layout=grid.layout(4, 4)))
> for (i in 1:15) {
+   pushViewport(viewport(layout.pos.col=((i - 1) %% 4) + 1,
+                 layout.pos.row=((i - 1) %/% 4) + 1))
+   print(plot[[i]], newpage=FALSE,
+                 panel.width=list(1.025, "inches"),
+                 panel.height=list(1.025, "inches"))
+   popViewport()}
>
> popViewport()
```

REFERENCES

Altman, D. G. (1991). Exercise 11.2. In *Practical statistics for medical research*. Boca Raton, FL: Chapman & Hall.

Baptiste, A. (2012, February 14). CRAN package "gridExtra." Retrieved from http://cran.cnr .berkeley.edu/

Brinkman, N. D. (1981). Ethanol fuel—A single-cylinder engine study of efficiency and exhaust emissions. *SAE Transactions, 90*, 1410–1424.

Dalgaard, P. (2002). *Introductory statistics with R* (Statistics and Computing Series). New York, NY: Springer.

Mittal, H. V. (2011). *R graphs cookbook*. Birmingham, UK: PACKT Publishing.

Murrell, P. (2006). *R graphics* (Computer Science and Data Analysis Series). Boca Raton, FL: Chapman & Hall/CRC. Retrieved from http://www.stat.auckland.ac.nz/~paul/grid/grid.html

Olsen, A. H., Njor, S. H., Vejborg, I., Schwartx, W., Dalgaard, P., Jensen, M. B., . . . Lynge, E. (2005). Breast cancer mortality in Copenhagen after introduction of mammography screening. *British Medical Journal, 330*, 220–222.

Sarkar, D. (2011a). Lattice Graphics—Package "lattice," Version 0.20-0. Retrieved from http://r-forge.r-project.org/projects/lattice/

Sarkar, D. (2011b). CRAN package "latticeExtra." Retrieved from http://cran.cnr.berkeley.edu/; http://latticeextra.r-forge.r-project.org/

Venables, W. N., Smith, D. M., & the R Development Core Team. (2005). *An introduction to R* (Rev. ed.). Bristol, UK: Network Theory Limited.

## FIVE

Probability and Statistics in Biostatistics

INTRODUCTION

Why study probability? As discussed in Chapter 2, different schools of biostatistical inference have become established. These schools, or paradigms, are not mutually exclusive; methods that work satisfactorily under one paradigm often yield attractive interpretations under other paradigms as well. The two main paradigms in use are Bayesian biostatistics and frequentist biostatistics.

The foundation for biostatistical inference, under any approach, is the **theory of probability**. Although this theory, often considered a branch of mathematics, is not the main focus of this book, it is beneficial to examine its fundamental concepts as they apply to biostatistical analysis within the disciplines of epidemiology and public health.

The concept of probability is familiar to epidemiologic investigators and workers in public health and preventive medicine. For example, one may learn from a health worker that someone has a "90% chance" of contracting malaria under certain environmental conditions, or hear an oncologist say that a patient has a "50–50 chance" of surviving a particular cancer diagnosis.

As shown by these informal examples, probabilities are often expressed in terms of percentages or fractions. The probability of occurrence of an event is a number between 0 (for no chance at all) and 1 (for absolute certainty). The more likely it is that the event will occur, the closer the probability gets to 1; the more unlikely it is that the event will occur, the closer the probability is to 0.

In epidemiology and public health/preventive medicine, investigators often must ask if the initially observed results of their work could have occurred by pure chance or if some other definitive factors have been operating to produce the observed efforts. For instance, if 5 out of 10 patients are cured of a certain illness upon receiving a particular treatment, the question may be posed as follows:

> Would that cure rate likely have occurred if the patients had not received the treatment, or can the result be considered evidence of a true healing effect from the treatment?

Applications of the theory of probability (Dalgaard, 2002; Daniel, 2005; Kolmogorov, 1964; Triola & Triola, 2006) are helpful in addressing such questions.

5.1   THEORIES OF PROBABILITY

What Is Probability?

Probability has been considered in at least two ways: subjective and objective.

Subjective probability considers probability as a measure of the confidence that one has in the truth of a particular proposition. It does not depend on any process or on repeatability. This concept allows one to determine the probability of a single event that can happen only once: for example, the probability that a complete cure for cancer will be found in 25 years.

Biostatisticians generally subscribe to the other concept of probability, **objective probability**, which is itself divided into two categories: classical and relative frequency.

Classical probability was developed in the 17th century to solve problems in games of chance, such as card games or the rolling of a six-sided die:

- If a card is drawn at random from a deck of 52 (well-shuffled) playing cards, the probability of drawing the ace of spades is 1/52, the probability of drawing a diamond is 13/52, and so on.
- If a fair die is rolled, then the probability of getting the six-spot face is 1/6, the probability of getting the four-spot face is 1/6, and so on.

Using this concept, one considers only the *equally likely* events—and the physical presence of a deck of cards, or a die, is not necessary.

The following is a good definition of classical probability:

When an event can occur in N equally likely (and mutually exclusive) ways, and if m of these events always occur with a property E, then the probability of the occurrence of E is m/N.

The common notation for this definition is

$$P(E) = m/N \tag{5.1-1}$$

which is read as "the probability of E is m divided by N."

The **relative frequency probability** approach depends on the repeatability of a process, as well as the ability to enumerate the repetitions and the number of times that some event of interest occurs. Thus, to state the probability of observing the occurrence of some characteristic E of an event, one uses the following definition of relative frequency probability:

If a process is repeated n (a large number of) times, and if some event with the characteristic E occurs m times, then the relative frequency of the occurrence of E, being m/n, will be *approximately* equal to the probability of E.

This definition may be expressed as

$$P(E) = m/n \tag{5.1-2}$$

with the caveat that m/n is only an *estimate* of $P(E)$.

Basic Properties of Probability

The whole system of probability theory rests on the following three properties:

Property 1: In an experiment or process with n **mutually exclusive** outcomes or events: $E_1, E_2, E_3, ..., E_n$, the probability of a particular event E_i is given a nonnegative number:

$$P(E_i) \geq 0 \qquad (5.1\text{-}3)$$

Thus, all events must have a nonnegative probability. According to this definition, two events are mutually exclusive if and only if they cannot occur simultaneously.

Property 2: The sum of the probabilities of the outcomes is equal to 1:

$$P(E_1) + P(E_2) + P(E_3) + ... + P(E_i) + ... + P(E_n) = 1 \qquad (5.1\text{-}4)$$

This is called the **property of exhaustiveness.** It requires the observer of a probabilistic process to allow all possible events, while the mutually exclusive property guarantees that the n events do not overlap (i.e., no two of them can occur simultaneously).

Property 3: For any two mutually exclusive events E_j and E_k, the probability of the occurrence of either event is equal to the sum of their individual probabilities:

$$P(E_j \text{ or } E_k) = P(E_j) + P(E_k) \qquad (5.1\text{-}5)$$

■ **Example 5.1:** Calculating the probability of having girls and boys in a family

Assume that, within a family, having girls and having boys is equally likely, and that the gender of any child is not influenced by the gender of the other children in the family. If a married couple, John and Mary Smith, plans to have four children, find the probability that they will have

- 4 girls (and no boys)
- 3 girls and 1 boy
- 2 girls and 2 boys
- 1 girl and 3 boys
- 4 boys (and no girls)

Solution:
To solve this problem, use Equation (5.1-1): $P(E) = m/N$.

To find m and N for each of the five cases, one should first enumerate all equally likely scenarios for the case of having four children. One may begin by examining the **sample space**—all possible combinations of the ways that four children can occur—which is as shown in Table 5.1.

This sample space shows that there are 16 equally likely possible outcomes for Mr. and Mrs. Smith. They represent the 16 *different possible* outcomes: $N = 16$.

(i) Characteristic $E_1 = 4$ girls (and no boys):
Only 1 possible outcome corresponds to exactly 4 girls and no boys:
Case #1, so $m = 1$.
Hence, by Equation (5.1-1): $P(E_1) = m/N = 1/16$, or 0.0625, or 6.25%.

TABLE 5.1   Sample Space: All Possible Combinations of Having Four Children

							G = GIRL, B = BOY									
Case #:	1	2	3	4	5	6	7	8	9	10	11	12	13	14	15	16
1st child	G	G	G	G	B	G	G	G	B	B	B	G	B	B	B	B
2nd child	G	G	G	B	G	G	B	B	B	G	G	B	G	B	B	B
3rd child	G	G	B	G	G	B	G	B	G	B	G	B	B	G	B	B
4th child	G	B	G	G	G	B	B	G	G	G	B	B	B	B	G	B

(ii) Characteristic E_2 = 3 girls and 1 boy:
Only 4 possible outcomes correspond to exactly 3 girls and 1 boy:
Cases #2, #3, #4, and #5, so m = 4.
Hence, by Equation (5.1-1): $P(E_2)$ = m/N = 4/16, or 1/4, or 0.25, or 25%.

(iii) Characteristic E_3 = 2 girls and 2 boys:
Only 6 possible outcomes correspond to exactly 2 girls and 2 boys:
Cases #6, #7, #8, #9, #10, and #11, so m = 6.
Hence, by Equation (5.1-1): $P(E_3)$ = m/N = 6/16, or 3/8, or 0.375, or 37.5%.

(iv) Characteristic E_4 = 1 girl and 3 boys:
Only 4 possible outcomes correspond to exactly 1 girl and 3 boys:
Cases #12, #13, #14, and #15, so m = 4.
Hence, by Equation (5.1-1): $P(E_4)$ = m/N = 4/16, or 1/4, or 0.25, or 25%.

(v) Characteristic E_5 = 4 boys (and no girls):
Only 1 possible outcome corresponds to exactly 4 boys and no girls:
Case #16, so m = 1.
Hence, by Equation (5.1-1): $P(E_5)$ = m/N = 1/16, or 0.0625, or 6.25%.

Remarks:
Note the two steps in determining the probability of any characteristic:
Step 1: *List* the sample space of all possible outcomes.
Step 2: For a specific characteristic, search the entire sample space and *enumerate* the number of possible outcomes that carry the specific characteristic.

Now we can check the results with respect to the three basic properties of probability:

Property I: Because each of the probabilities $P(E_i)$ is positive, clearly

$$P(E_i) \geq 0, \text{ as required.}$$

Property 2: $P(E_1) + P(E_2) + P(E_3) + P(E_4) + P(E_5)$

$$= 1/16 + 4/16 + 6/16 + 4/16 + 1/16$$

$$= (1 + 4 + 6 + 4 + 1)/16$$

$$= 16/16$$

$$= 1, \text{ or } 100\%, \text{ as required.}$$

Property 3: The condition $P(E_j \text{ or } E_k) = P(E_j) + P(E_k)$ is clearly satisfied, as may be seen by inspection of Table 5.1, and the values of the five calculated probabilities $P(E_i) \mid i = 1, 2, 3, 4, 5$.

The concept of probability may be discussed in terms of the following special properties (each defined in a following subsection):

- The probability for complement events
- Conditional probability
- Joint probability
- The multiplication rule for probabilities
- The addition rule for probabilities
- Independence and dependence of occurrences
- Marginal probability

THE PROBABILITY FOR COMPLEMENT EVENTS

If one wants to find the probability that a certain event E does *not* occur, then it is said that one is looking for the **complement** of event E, denoted by $\underline{E}$.

Because it must be true that either event E occurs or event E does not occur, one may write:

$$P(E) + P(\underline{E}) = P(\text{all possible occurrences}) = 1$$

so that

$$P(\underline{E}) = 1\ P(E) \tag{5.1-6}$$

which may be considered the definition of the **complement** of event E.

■ **Example 5.2:** Using the complement to calculate the probability of having girls and boys in a family

Again using the case of Mr. and Mrs. Smith, suppose that they would still like to have four children, but only with the condition of:

- No girls (i.e., only boys)
- 2 girls and 2 boys
- All except 2 girls and 2 boys
- No boys (i.e., only girls)

What are the probabilities for each of these conditions?

Solution:
Here we can use Equation (5.1-6): $P(\underline{E}) = 1\ P(E)$.

(i) $P(\text{an event for "no girls"})$

$= P(\underline{E_g})$ where E_g = the "no girls" event

$= 1\ P(E_g)$ by Equation (5.1-6), where E_g = the "any girls"

$= 1\ \{P(E_1) + P(E_2) + P(E_3) + P(E_4)\}$ from Example 5.1

$= 1\ \{1/16 + 4/16 + 6/16 + 4/16\}$ from Example 5.1(i), (ii), (iii), (iv)

$= 1\ 15/16$

(ii) P(an event for "only 2 girls and 2 boys")
  = 6/16, or 3/8, or 0.375, or 37.5%   from Example A1(iii)
(iii) Pan event for "all except 2 girls and 2 boys")
  = 1 $P(E)$ where E = "just 2 girls and 2 boys"
  = 1 – 6/16   from Example A1(iii), and part (ii) of this example
  = 10/16
  = 5/8, or 0.625, or 62.5%
(iv) P(an event for "no boys") = $P(E_1)$ where E_1 = the "1-boy" event, and E_1 = an
                                       event *without* a boy
  = 1 – 15/16, by counting the events in Table 5.1
  = 1/16, or 0.0625, or 6.25%

Remarks:
1. Both Cases (i) and (iv) have the same probability, 0.0625%. This implies that it is very unlikely—about a 6% chance—that there will be no girls at all or no boys at all.
2. Cases (ii) and (iii) are interesting results. One might be inclined to believe that, for a family with 4 children, the probability for a 2-girls-and-2-boys outcome would be 50%—but that is not the case for 62.5% of the possible outcomes.
3. Note that if the family has only 2 children, the probability for a 1-girl-and-1-boy outcome would indeed be 50%. (Show that this is indeed the case!)

CONDITIONAL PROBABILITY

Given any two events A and B, if it is first assumed that event A **has already occurred**, then the probability of event B occurring is the **conditional probability** $P(B \mid A)$, which is read as the probability of B occurring given A, or as the probability of event B occurring after event A has already occurred.

■ **Example 5.3:** Using the conditional probability concept to calculate the probability of a daughter, in a family of four children, having a sister or a brother

Again we use the case of the four-child family of Mr. and Mrs. Smith. If this family already has a daughter, what are the probabilities that this daughter would have a sister or would have a brother?

(i)   The probability of a daughter having a sister:
  If A is a daughter in this family, for A to have a sister, there must be at least 2 girls among the set of 4 children in the Smith family. Hence, the probability for A to have a sister is the conditional probability of having at least 2 girls in the set of 4 children.
  From Table 5.1, we find that there are 16 possible outcomes ($N = 16$). By enumeration, we see that there are 11 possible outcomes with at least 2 girls each: they are Cases #1 through #11 ($G = 11$). Hence, the conditional probability, written as $P(G|N)$, is

$$P(G|N) = 11/16, \text{ or } 0.6875, \text{ or } 68.75\%$$

(ii) The probability of a daughter having a brother:

If A is a daughter in this family, for A to have a brother, there must be at least 1 girl and 1 boy among the set of 4 children in the Smith family. Hence, the probability for A to have a brother is the conditional probability of having at least 1 girl and 1 boy in the set of 4 children.

From Table 5.1, we find that there are 16 possible outcomes ($N = 16$). By enumeration, we find that there are 14 possible outcomes with at least 1 girl and 1 boy: they are Cases #2 through #15 ($B = 14$). Hence, the conditional probability, written as $P(B|N)$, is

$$P(B|N) = 14/16, \text{ or } 7/8, \text{ or } 0.875, \text{ or } 87.5\%$$

Thus, A has an almost 90% chance of having a brother.

JOINT PROBABILITY

Given two random variables A and B, the **joint distribution** for A and B defines the probability of events defined in terms of both A and B. For two random variables, this yields a **bivariate distribution**; for any number of random variables, this yields a **multivariate distribution**.

■ **Example 5.4:** Using the concept of joint probability to calculate the probabilities of a first-born daughter, in a family of 4 children, having 2 sisters and 1 brother or 1 sister and 2 brothers

Yet again we use the case of the four-child family of Mr. and Mrs. Smith. If the first-born child of this family is a girl, G1, the question is: What are the probabilities that G1 will have (i) 2 sisters and 1 brother? (ii) 1 sister and 2 brothers?

In this example, it is assumed that a family's having a girl or a boy is an independent event from the probability viewpoint. (In some families, genetic factors, as well as other factors, may skew the odds in favor of having one sex or the other; girls or boys may just "run in the family." For purposes of these examples, though, we ignore these factors.)

From Table 5.1, we see that out of the 16 possible outcomes, there are 8 in which the first-born is a girl: Cases #1, #2, #3, #4, #6, #7, #8, and #12.

(Likewise, there are 8 in which the first-born is a boy.) Hence, $N_g = 8$.

Of these 8 cases, only 3 have 2 other girls and 1 boy: Cases #2, #3, and #4. Hence, $G_{21} = 3$, and

$$P(G_{21}/N_g) = G_{21}/N_g = 3/8$$

Also, of these 8 cases, only 3 have 1 other girl and 2 boys: Cases #6, #7, and #9. Hence, $G_{12} = 3$, and

$$P(G_{12}/N_g) = G_{12}/N_g = 3/8$$

The required probability is the joint probability of these two events. Because these are independent events, their joint probability is the sum of their individual probabilities. Let this joint probability be $P[(G_{21}, G_{12})/N_g]$. Then

$$P[(G_{21}, G_{12})/N_g] = P(G_{21}/N_g) + P(G_{12}/N_g) = 3/8 + 3/8 = 6/8, \text{ or } 3/4, \text{ or } 75\%$$

Hence, a first-born girl has a 75% chance of having either 2 sisters and 1 brother or 1

THE MULTIPLICATION RULE FOR PROBABILITIES

In symbolic notation, the multiplication rule for probabilities may be written as:
For any two events A and B,

$$P(A \cap B) = P(A)\,P(B \mid A), \text{ if } P(A) \neq 0 \qquad (5.1\text{-}7A)$$

or

$$P(A \cap B) = P(B)\,P(A \mid B), \text{ if } P(B) \neq 0 \qquad (5.1\text{-}7B)$$

in which the symbol $\cap$ is read either as "and" or "intersection" (as used in set theory). The statement $A \cap B$ indicates the joint occurrence of conditions A and B.

■ **Example 5.5:** Using the multiplication rule for probabilities to calculate the probability of having a first-born son, in a family of 4 children, who will have 2 brothers and 1 sister after him

Using the case of the four-child family of Mr. and Mrs. Smith, we posit that the first-born child of this family is a son, B1. The question is: What are the probabilities that B1 will have 2 brothers and 1 sister?

Table 5.1 shows that out of the 16 possible outcomes, $N = 16$, there are 8 in which the first-born is a boy: Cases #5, #9, #10, #11, #13, #14, #15, and #16. Hence, $N_b = 8$.

Thus, the probability of having a son as the first-born is

$$P(B) = N_b/N = 8/16$$

Now, of these 8 cases, 3 have 2 boys and a girl: Cases #13, #14, and #15. Hence, $N_{bbg} = 3$, and the probability of being the first-born with 2 brothers and 1 sister is

$$P(A|B) = N_{bbg}/N_b = 3/8$$

Using the multiplication rule for probabilities,

$$P(A \cap B) = P(B)\,P(A|B), \text{ if } P(B) \neq 0 \qquad (5.1\text{-}7B)$$

$$= (8/16) \times (3/8)$$

$$= 3/16, \text{ or } 0.1875, \text{ or } 18.75\%$$

Hence, the Smith family can expect a somewhat less than 20% chance of having a first-born son to be followed by 2 boys and 1 girl.

THE ADDITION RULE FOR PROBABILITIES

The addition rule for probabilities states that, given two events A and B, the probability that event A or B, or both, will occur is equal to the probability that event A occurs, **plus** the probability that event B occurs, **less** the probability that these two events occur jointly.

In symbolic form, this rule may be expressed as

$$P(A \cup B) = P(A) + P(B)\,P(A \cap B) \qquad (5.1\text{-}8)$$

in which the symbol ∪ is read either as "or" or "union" (as used in set theory).

■ **Example 5.6:** Using the addition rule for probabilities to calculate the probability of having either a first-born son, in a family of 4 children, who will have at least 1 brother after him; or a first-born son, in a family of 4 children, who will also have at least 1 sister after him

Table 5.1 shows that out of the 16 possible outcomes, $N = 16$, there are 8 in which the first-born is a boy: Cases #5, #9, #10, #11, #13, #14, #15, and #16. Hence, $N_b = 8$, and the probability of having a son as the first-born is

$$P(N_b) = N_b/N = 8/16$$

Now, of these 8 cases, 7 have at least 1 boy to follow: Cases #9, #10, #11, #13, #14, #15, and #16. Hence, $N_{bb} = 7$, and the probability of being the first-born with 1 younger brother is

$$P(N_{bb}/N_b) = N_{bb}/N_b = 7/8$$

Using the multiplication rule for probabilities:

$$P(N_{bb}\cap N_b) = P(N_b)\, P(N_{bb}|N_b),\ \text{if}\ P(N_b) \neq 0\ \text{from Equation (5.1-7B)}$$

$$= (8/16) \times (7/8)$$

$$= 7/16,\ \text{or}\ 0.4375,\ \text{or}\ 43.75\%$$

Designate this probability as $P(A)$.

From Table 5.1, out of the 16 possible outcomes, $N = 16$, there are 8 in which the first-born is a boy: Cases #5, #9, #10, #11, #13, #14, #15, and #16. Hence, $N_b = 8$, and the probability of having a son as the first-born is

$$P(N_b) = N_b/N = 8/16$$

Now, of these 8 cases, 7 have 1 girl to follow: Cases #9, #10, #11, #13, #14, #15, and #16. These are the same seven cases as those in the first part of this example.

Hence, $N_{bg} = 7$, and the probability of being a first-born son with 1 younger sister will be

$$P(N_{bg}\backslash N_b) = N_{bg}/N_b = 7/8.$$

Using the multiplication rule for probabilities,

$$P(N_{bg}\cap N_b) = P(N_b)\, P(N_{bg}N_b),\ \text{if}\ P(N_b) \neq 0\ \text{from Equation (5.1-7B)}$$

$$= (8/16) \times (7/8)$$

$$= 7/16,\ \text{or}\ 0.4375,\ \text{or}\ 43.75\%$$

Designate this probability as $P(B)$.

The probability that these two events will occur simultaneously is those 7 cases indicated earlier, out of a total of 16 possible cases. Hence,

$$P(A\cap B) = 7/16$$

Now we apply the **addition rule for probabilities**. For both events to occur simultaneously, the probability is given by

$$P(A\cup B) = P(A) + P(B)\, P(A\cap B) \tag{5.1-8}$$

$$= 7/16 + 7/16\ 7/16$$

Hence, if the Smith family has its four children, they may expect to have a greater than 40% chance of having a boy as the first-born, with either a brother or a sister to follow after him.

INDEPENDENCE AND DEPENDENCE OF OCCURRENCES

Given two events A and B, if event B has occurred, but it has no effect on the probability of A (i.e., the probability of event A is unchanged whether or not event B occurs), then

$$P(A \mid B) = P(A) \qquad\qquad (5.1\text{-}9)$$

In such a case, one says that A and B are **independent** events (in the probability sense).

Thus, for two independent events, the multiplication rule [Equation (5.1-7B)] may be written as

$$P(A \cap B) = P(B) \, P(A \mid B), \text{ if } P(B) \neq 0 \qquad\qquad (5.1\text{-}7B)$$

$$= P(B) \, P(A) \qquad\qquad (5.1\text{-}10)$$

according to Equation (5.1-9). That is:

$$P(A \cap B) = P(B) \, P(A), \text{ if } P(A) \neq 0, \text{ if } P(B) \neq 0 \qquad\qquad (5.1\text{-}11)$$

When two events, A and B, with nonzero probabilities are independent, each of the following statements is true:

$$P(A \mid B) = P(A); \; P(B \mid A) = P(B); \; P(A \cap B) = P(A) \, P(B)$$

Remarks:

1. In the theory of probability, the terms *independent* and *mutually exclusive* do **not** necessarily mean the same thing.
2. If events A and B are not independent, they are said to be *dependent*.

■ **Example 5.7:** Using the independence and dependence of occurrences to calculate the probabilities of having a first-born daughter, in a family of 4 children, who then also has sisters

We return to the case of the four-child family of Mr. and Mrs. Smith. If the first-born child of this family is a daughter, G1, the question is: What are the probabilities that G1 will have (i) no sister, (ii) only 1 sister, (iii) only 2 sisters, or (iv) 3 sisters?

In this example, it is again assumed that a family's having a girl or a boy is an independent event from the probability viewpoint. (As noted earlier, genetic factors that "run in the family" may skew these odds.)

(i) Table 5.1 shows that out of the 16 possible outcomes, $N = 16$, there are 8 in which the first-born is a girl: Cases #1, #2, #3, #4, #6, #7, #8, and #12. Hence, $N_g = 8$, and

$$P(A) = P(N_g) = N_g/N = 8/16$$

Of these 8 cases, only 1 has no more girls: Case #12. Hence, $N_{g=0} = 1$, and

Because these two events are independent,

$$P(A \cap B) = P(B) \, P(A)$$

$$= (1/8) \times (8/16)$$

$$= 1/16, \text{ or } 0.0625, \text{ or } 6.25\%$$

(ii) Table 5.1 shows that out of the 16 possible outcomes, $N = 16$, there are 8 in which the first-born is a girl: Cases #1, #2, #3, #4, #6, #7, #8, and #12. Hence, $N_g = 8$, and

$$P(A) = P(N_g) = N_g/N = 8/16$$

Of these 8 cases, only 3 have one more girl: Cases #6, #7, and #8. Hence, $N_{g=1} = 3$, and

$$P(B) = P(N_{g=1}) = N_{g=1}/N_g = 3/8$$

Because these two events are independent,

$$P(A \cap B) = P(B) \, P(A)$$

$$= (3/8) \times (8/16)$$

$$= 3/16, \text{ or } 0.1875, \text{ or } 18.75\%$$

(iii) Table 5.1 shows that out of the 16 possible outcomes, $N = 16$, there are 8 in which the first-born is a girl: Cases #1, #2, #3, #4, #6, #7, #8, and #12. Hence, $N_g = 8$, and

$$P(A) = P(N_g) = N_g/N = 8/16$$

Of these 8 cases, only 3 have two more girls: Cases #2, #3, and #4. Hence, $N_{g=2} = 3$, and

$$P(B) = P(N_{g=2}) = N_{g=2}/N_g = 3/8$$

Because these two events are independent,

$$P(A \cap B) = P(B) \, P(A)$$

$$= (3/8) \times (8/16)$$

$$= 3/16, \text{ or } 0.1875, \text{ or } 18.75\%$$

(iv) Table 5.1 shows that out of the 16 possible outcomes, $N = 16$, there are 8 in which the first-born is a girl: Cases #1, #2, #3, #4, #6, #7, #8, and #12. Hence, $N_g = 8$, and

$$P(A) = P(N_g) = N_g/N = 8/16$$

Of these 8 cases, only 1 has three more girls: Case #1. Hence, $N_{g=3} = 1$, and

$$P(B) = P(N_{g=3}) = N_{g=2}/N_g = 1/8$$

Because these two events are independent,

$$P(A \cap B) = P(B) \, P(A)$$

$$= (1/8) \times (8/16)$$

Thus, in this family of 4 children, if the first-born is a girl, the chance that she will have

- no more sisters is 6.25%
- only 1 more sister is 18.87%
- only 2 more sisters is 18.75%
- 3 more sisters is 6.25%

MARGINAL PROBABILITY

If a variable can be divided into n categories $A_1, A_2, A_3, \ldots, A_i, \ldots, A_n$, and another jointly occurring variable can be divided into m categories $B_1, B_2, B_3, \ldots, B_j, \ldots, B_m$, then the **marginal probability** of A_i, $P(A_i)$, is equal to the sum of the joint probabilities of A_i with all the categories of B; that is:

$$P(A_i) = \sum_j P(A_i \cap B_j), \text{ for all values of } j \qquad (5.1\text{-}12)$$

The following example (Table 5.2) further illustrates the special properties of marginal probability.

■ **Example 5.8:** Using Equation (5.1-12) and the data on the frequency of illegal drug use by adult males (M) and females (F), calculate the marginal probability for males, P(M)

Solution:
The variable GENDER is separated into two categories: M and F.

The variable lifetime frequency of illegal drug use is separated into three categories: 1–19 times (A), 20–99 times (B), and ≥ 100 times (C).

The category M occurs jointly with all three categories of the variable frequency of illegal drug use. Thus, the three joint probabilities that may be compared are

$$P(M \cap A) = 32/111; \qquad P(M \cap B) = 18/111; \qquad P(M \cap C) = 25/111$$

To obtain the marginal probability for males, $P(M)$, apply Equation (5.1-12):

$$P(A_i) = \sum_j P(A_i \cap B_j), \text{ for all values of } j \qquad (5.1\text{-}12)$$

TABLE 5.2 Frequency of Illegal Drug Use by Gender

LIFETIME FREQUENCY OF ILLEGAL DRUG USE	MALE (M)	FEMALE (F)	TOTAL
1–19 times (A)	32	7	39
20–99 times (B)	18	20	38
≥ 100 times (C)	25	9	34
Total	75	36	111

Source: Daniel (2005).

or

$$P(M) = P(M \cap A) + P(M \cap B) + P(M \cap C)$$

$$= 32/111 + 18/111 + 25/111$$

$$= (32 + 18 + 25)/111$$

$$= 75/111, \text{ or } 0.6757, \text{ or } 67.57\%$$

Remark: This same result may also be obtained by using the marginal total for males (75) as the numerator and the total number of subjects (111) as the denominator.

Probability Computations Using R

A number of useful functions in R are available for probability computations. These are illustrated in Example 5.9.

■ **Example 5.9:** The special R functions factorial(), choose(), sample(), and prod() in probability computations

(a) **The function** factorial()

An epidemiologist is testing the effects of five new cancer drugs to be given *sequentially* to a group of case subjects. How many sets of experiments (test sequences) are required to test all possible permutations?

For each case subject, the test sequence is

Drug1, Drug2, Drug3, Drug4, Drug5.

Clearly, there are five options for Drug1, leaving

4 options for Drug2,
3 options for Drug3,
2 options for Drug4, and
1 option for Drug5.

Thus, the total number of test sequences is $5 \times 4 \times 3 \times 2 \times 1$, or factorial 5 (5 factorial), usually written as 5! Now, 5! = 120.

The following R code segment shows that functions from the package base are available for such calculations:

```
> install.packages("base")
> library("base")
> factorial(5) # Outputting:
[1] 120
> lfactorial(5) # This is the natural log of 5!
[1] 4.787492
> lovg(factorial(5)) # This is the same as lfactorial(5).
[1] 4.787492
```

Hence, the epidemiology investigator should plan for 5! = 120 sequences of tests.

(b) The function choose()
Going back to the family planning of Mr. and Mrs. Smith, if they prefer to have 2 girls and 2 boys, in how many ways (the orders of the births of the girls and boys) can this occur?
By enumeration using Table 5.1:
Sample space: All possible combinations of having 4 children: G = girl, B = boy

Case #:	1	2	3	4	5	6	7	8	9	10	11	12	13	14	15	16
1st child	G	G	G	G	B	G	G	G	B	B	B	G	B	B	B	B
2nd child	G	G	G	B	G	G	B	B	B	G	G	B	G	B	B	B
3rd child	G	G	B	G	G	B	G	B	G	B	G	B	B	G	B	B
4th child	G	B	G	G	G	B	B	G	G	G	B	B	B	B	G	B

One can see that the number of cases with 2 G and 2 B is 6: Cases #6, #7, #8, #9, #10, and #11.
Using combinatorics, the answer is

$$^nC_r = n!/r! \, (n-r)!$$

$$= [n(n-1)\cdots(n-r+1)(n-r)!]/[x \, (x-1)\cdots 1][(n \, r)!]$$

$$= [n(n-1)\cdots(n-r+1)]/[x(x-1)\cdots 1]$$

Here, $n = 4$ and $x = 2$, so $^nC_r = {}^4C_2 = 4 \times 3/2 \times 1 = 12/2 = 6$, confirming the result by counting.
Again, the following R code segment shows that functions from the package base are available for these calculations:

```
> install.packages("base")
> library("base")
> choose(4, 2) # Outputting:
[1] 6
> lchoose(4, 2) # This is the natural log of 4C₂
[1] 1.791759
> log(choose(4, 2)) # This is the same as lchoose(4, 2)
[1] 1.791759
```

(c) The function sample()
Random sampling, with and without replacement, is a crucial step in the process of epidemiologic investigation of health characteristics of a population. Sampling must be done because it is simply not practical to test the whole population due to the large number of individuals in that population.
Suppose that, in a city of population of 1 million, each citizen is designated with a number, from 1 to 1,000,000. For biostatistical testing, a health worker would like to randomly select (without replacement) 3 representative sets of case subjects, each with 5 people. How can this be done?

Solution:
The function sample(), from the package base, may be used. The usage of this function (see its CRAN documentation) takes the following form for sampling with-

$$\text{sample}(x, \text{size}, \text{replace} = \text{FALSE}, \text{prob} = \text{NULL})$$

where:

x = a positive integer (say, 1)

size = a nonnegative integer giving the number of items in the whole population from which to choose

replace = FALSE means sampling without replacement; this is the default value
  replace = TRUE does sampling with replacement

prob = a vector of probability weights for obtaining the elements of the vector being sampled (this may be omitted)

The following R code segment executes the requisite computations:

```
> install.packages("base")
> library("base")
> # The default behavior of sample() is sampling without replacement;
> # this means that, each sampled person will not be selected more than once.
> # To obtain 3 representative sets of 5 case subjects each, the following
> # computation will be executed 3 times:
> sample(1:1000000, 5) # Outputting the first set of 5 case subjects:
[1] 503512 33035 363755 527424 904495
> sample(1:1000000, 5) # Outputting the second set of 5 case subjects:
[1] 853246 286220 211121 393481 842452
> sample(1:1000000, 5) # Outputting the third set of 5 case subjects:
[1] 644293 870071 163122 153612 348948
```

Remarks:

1. To randomly sample *with* replacement, the command is

   > sample(x, size, replace = TRUE).

2. For large populations, sampling without replacement is tolerated. For relatively small populations, one may choose to sample *with* replacement.

3. The function sample() is suitable for random sampling. For other, more restrictive sampling modes (such as *balanced cluster sampling, balanced stratification sampling, balanced two-stage sampling, multistage sampling, minimal support sampling, multinomial sampling, pivotal sampling, Poisson sampling, random systematic sampling, systematic sampling*, etc.), consult the CRAN documentation for the package sampling.

(d) The function prod()

Out of a patient population of 20 people, the health worker is preparing groups of 4 each for further clinical testing. How many groups may be combined, without concerning the order of testing within each group?

Solution:

This is an elementary problem in combinatorics: determining the number of possible combinations (without ordering) of groups of 4 from a total population of 20. The answer is $^{20}C_4$, which is given by

Rather than evaluating this expression by longhand methods, one may use the function prod() in the package base. The usage of this function (see its CRAN documentation) takes the following form:

> prod(..., na.rm = FALSE)

for which the arguments are as follows:

= a numeric or complex or logical vector

na.rm = logical. Should missing values be removed?

In R, computing $^{20}C_4$ may be performed in one of the following ways, using the code segments indicated.

1. In one step:
   ```
   > prod(20:1)/{prod(4:1)*prod((20 - 4):1)} # 20!/{4!(20 4)!
   [1] 4845
   ```
2. First, compute each of the three factorials; and then combine the results:
   ```
   > prod(20:1) # 20!
   [1] 2.432902e+18
   > prod(4:1) # 4!
   [1] 24
   > prod((20 - 4):1) # (20 4)!
   [1] 2.092279e+13
   > 2.432902e+18/(24*2.092279e+13) # Combining the three factorials
   [1] 4845
   ```
   Hence, from a population of 20 people, combination groups of 4 may be formed in 4,845 ways.

Remarks:

1. The result applies for combinations of groups of 4 case subjects each and is expressed as $^{20}C_4$.
2. If ordering of members of each group is taken into account, then the possible number of 4-member groups is: $^{20}P_4 = 20!/(20 - 4)!$

The following code segment may be used to compute the value of $^{20}P_4$:

```
> prod(20:1)/prod((20 4):1) # Outputting:
[1] 116280
```

This result may also be obtained by the following combinatoric considerations:

(i) To constitute a group of 4, there are 4 positions to be filled: _ _ _ _.
(ii) The first position may be filled by any one of the original 20 people.
(iii) The second position by any of the remaining 19,
(iv) The third position by any of the remaining 18, and
(v) The fourth and last position by any of the remaining 17.
(vi) Hence, the total number of such possible permutation groups is

$$20 \times 19 \times 18 \times 17 = 116,280$$

which is $^{20}P_4$.

Applications of Probability Theory to Health Sciences

Chapter 2, on research and design in epidemiology and public health, showed that applications of probability concepts and theories are widely used, especially for making decisions on diagnostic criteria in clinical medicine and for health screening tests in preventive medicine. Epidemiologists and clinicians would benefit from enhancement of their quantitative ability to effectively predict the absence or presence of a particular disease through test results (negative or positive) and the status of critical symptoms (absence or presence). Moreover, these health professionals would be interested in information with respect to the likelihood of negative or positive test results, and the likelihood of the absence or presence of special symptoms in case subjects with and without particular diseases.

The Chapter 2 discussion of Bayesian biostatistics in epidemiology indicated that the results of such screening tests are not always infallible. A particular testing procedure may yield false positives or false negatives, as shown in Table 5.3.

Applying the theory of probability, one may respond to the following four questions when attempting to evaluate the applicability and usefulness of test results and diagnostic status in assessing whether a case subject has some specific disease:

1. If a case subject does not have the disease, **what is the probability** of obtaining a negative test result (or the absence of a symptom)?
2. If a case subject does have the disease, **what is the probability** of obtaining a positive test result (or the presence of a symptom)?
3. If the screening test shows a negative result, or the diagnostic test shows the absence of a symptom, **what is the probability** that the case subject does not have the disease?
4. If the screening test shows a positive result, or the diagnostic test shows the presence of a symptom, **what is the probability** that the case subject does have the disease?

THE APPROACH USING PROBABILITY THEORY

For a large sample of n case subjects, one obtains the result shown in Table 5.4.

Table 5.4 shows the status of these n case subjects with respect to a particular disease resulting from a diagnostic screening test for identifying persons who

TABLE 5.3   A 2×2 Decision Table Showing the Four Possible Outcomes From a Standard Dichotomous Clinical Testing Process

Outcomes representing an error are in bold italic typeface.

TEST DECISION	STATE OF THE SAMPLE POPULATION	
	PATIENT IS INFECTED	PATIENT IS NOT INFECTED
Positive	True Positive	*False Positive*
Negative	*False Negative*	True Negative

TABLE 5.4   Screening Test Results of *n* Subjects Cross-Classified According to Disease Status

TEST RESULTS	DISEASE		
	PRESENT (D)	ABSENT (D̲)	TOTAL
Positive (T)	p	q	$p + q$
Negative (T̲)	r	s	$r + s$
Sum	$p + r$	$q + s$	n

have the disease. The cell entries represent the number of case subjects belonging to the categories defined by row and column headings. Thus, p is the number of case subjects who do have the disease and whose test result was positive, and q is the number who do not have the disease and whose test was also positive. From the information in this table, one may derive various probability estimates.

For example:

To answer Question (1): Note that the conditional probability estimate is

$$P(\underline{T}/\underline{D}) = s/(q + s) \tag{5.1-13}$$

This ratio is an estimate of the **specificity** of the diagnostic screening test. More specifically, the *specificity* of a screening test or of a diagnostic symptom is the probability of a negative test result (or the absence of a symptom), given the true absence of the disease.

To answer Question (2): The probability for a positive test for case subjects who indeed have the disease is given by

$$P(T \mid D) = p/(p + r) \tag{5.1-14}$$

This ratio is an estimate of the **sensitivity** of the diagnostic screening test. More specifically, the *sensitivity* of a screening test or of a diagnostic symptom is the probability of a positive test result (or the presence of a symptom), given the true presence of the disease.

To answer Question (3): Calculate the conditional probability:

$$P(D \mid T) = p/(p + q) \tag{5.1-15}$$

This ratio is an estimate of the probability that the subject has the disease, given that the screening test result was positive or the requisite symptom was present. It is called the **predictive value positive** of the diagnostic screening test or of a symptom. The *predictive value positive* of a screening test or of a symptom is the probability that a case subject has the disease, given that the subject has a positive screening test result or has the requisite symptom.

To answer Question (4): Calculate the conditional probability:

$$P(\underline{D} \mid \underline{T}) = s/(r + s) \tag{5.1-16}$$

This ratio is an estimate of the **predictive value negative** of the diagnostic screening test or of a symptom. The *predictive value negative* of a test or a symptom is the probability that a case subject does not have the disease, given that the subject has a negative screening test result or does not have the requisite symptom.

AN APPROACH USING BAYES'S THEOREM

Bayes's theorem, which may be used to derive the sensitivity and specificity of screening tests, may also be used to obtain the predictive value estimates (positive and negative). In the notation of Table 5.4, the following statement gives the predictive value positive of a diagnostic screening test or symptom:

$$P(D \mid T) = \frac{P(T \mid D)P(D)}{P(T \mid D)P(D) + P(T \mid \underline{D})P(\underline{D})} \tag{5.1-17}$$

The basis of this equation may be found in the multiplication rule for probabilities:

$$P(A \cap B) = P(B)\,P(A \mid B), \text{ if } P(B) \neq 0 \tag{5.1-7B}$$

or

$$P(A \mid B) = P(A \cap B)/P(B), \text{ if } P(B) \neq 0$$

Hence, the conditional probability

$$P(T \mid D) = P(T \cap D)/P(D), \text{ if } P(D) \neq 0$$

may be expressed as

$$P(T \mid D)\,P(D) = P(T \cap D) = P(D \cap T)$$

so that the numerator of Equation (5.1-17) represents $P(D \cap T)$. One can see that the denominator represents simply $P(T)$, since $P(D) + P(\underline{D}) = 1$. The latter may be established more formally as follows.

The events represented by $P(D \cap T)$ and $P(\underline{D} \cap T)$ are mutually exclusive; that is, they have zero intersection. Using the addition rule, Equation (5.1-8), one may write:

$$P(T) = P(D \cap T) + P(\underline{D} \cap T) \tag{5.1-18}$$

Now, by the multiplication rule:

$$P(D \cap T) = P(T \mid D)\,P(D) \tag{5.1-19A}$$

and

$$P(\underline{D} \cap T) = P(T \mid \underline{D})\,P(\underline{D}) \tag{5.1-19B}$$

Finally, substituting Equations (5.1-19A) and (5.1-19B) into Equation (5.1-18), we get:

$$P(T) = P(T \mid D)\,P(D) + P(T \mid \underline{D})\,P(\underline{D}) \tag{5.1-20}$$

which is the denominator of the right side of Equation (5.1-13).

Remarks:

1. The numerator of Equation (5.1-13) is equal to the sensitivity × rate (prevalence) of the disease.

2. The denominator of Equation (5.1-13) is equal to the sensitivity × rate of the disease + (1 – sensitivity) × (1 – rate of the disease).
3. These relationships allow the predictive value positive to be calculated from the sensitivity, specificity, and rate of the disease.
4. Another way to express Bayes's theorem, analogous to Equation (5.1-17), is

$$P(\underline{D} \mid \underline{T}) = \{P(\underline{T} \mid \underline{D})\, P(\underline{D})\} / \{P(\underline{T} \mid \underline{D})\, P(\underline{D}) + P(\underline{T} \mid D)\, P(D)\} \tag{5.1-21}$$

which permits one to calculate an estimate of the probability that a case subject who is *negative* on the screening test (or has no symptom) does *not* have the disease—which is the predictive value negative of a diagnostic screening test or a symptom.

In illustrative Example 5.10 (Daniel, 2005), Bayes's theorem is used to compute a predictive value positive of a diagnostic screening test.

■ **Example 5.10:** Screening for Alzheimer's Disease

A team of clinical epidemiologic investigators plan to evaluate a proposed diagnostic screening procedure for Alzheimer's disease (AD). The test procedure was undertaken with

(a) a random sample of 900 case subjects who had AD, and
(b) an independent random sample of 1000 case subjects without symptoms of the disease.

These two samples were drawn from populations who were at least 65 years old. The results are summarized in Table 5.5.

Solution:
The estimate of the sensitivity of the screening test may be obtained by using Table 5.4 and Equation (5.1-14):

$$P(T|D) = p/(p + r) \tag{5.1-14}$$

$$= 872/(872 + 28)$$

$$= 872/900$$

$$= 0.9689$$

TABLE 5.5 **Summary of Results for Alzheimer's Disease Diagnostic Screening Test**

TEST RESULTS	ALZHEIMER'S DISEASE DIAGNOSIS		
	YES (D)	NO (D)	TOTAL
Positive (T)	872	10	882
Negative (T)	28	990	1,018
Total	900	1,000	1,900

The specificity of the test may be calculated by using Table 5.4 and Equation (5.1-13):

$$P(\underline{T}/\underline{D}) = s/(q + s) \qquad (5.1\text{-}13)$$

$$= 990/(10 + 990)$$

$$= 990/1000$$

$$= 0.9900$$

To calculate the predictive value positive of the test (i.e., to estimate the probability that a case subject who is positive on the screening test does have AD), one draws from Table 5.5:

$$P(T|D) = 872/900 = 0.9689$$

$$P(T|\underline{D}) = 10/1000 = 0.0100$$

Substituting these values in Equation (5.1-17), we get:

$$P(D|T) = \frac{P(T|D)P(D)}{P(T|D)P(D) + P(T|\underline{D})P(\underline{D})} \qquad (5.1\text{-}17)$$

$$= \frac{(0.9689)P(D)}{(0.9689)P(D) + (0.0100)P(\underline{D})} \qquad (5.1\text{-}22)$$

Now, $P(D)$, the rate of AD in the relevant general population, has been estimated to be 11.3% (Daniel, 2005), or

$$P(D) = 0.1130$$

If one accepts this value for $P(D)$, then

$$P(\underline{D}) = 1 \; P(D) = 1 - 0.1130 = 0.8870$$

Hence,

$$P(D|T) = \frac{(0.9689)P(D)}{(0.9689)P(D) + (0.0100)P(\underline{D})} \qquad (5.1\text{-}17)$$

$$= \frac{(0.9689)(0.1130)}{(0.9689)(0.1130) + (0.0100)(0.8870)}$$

$$= 0.1095/0.1184$$

$$= 0.9248, \text{ or } 92.48\%$$

Remarks:

1. The predictive value positive of the screening test is more than 92%, a very high value, indicating that the test is reliable.
2. Equation (5.1-22) shows that the predictive value positive of the test depends on the rate of the disease in the population under investigation: case subjects who are 65 years or older. Because the two independent samples of the test were taken from two different populations, one has to obtain an independent estimate of $P(D)$.

Typical Summary Statistics in Biostatistics: Confidence Intervals, Significance Tests, and Goodness of Fit

In biostatistics, **summary statistics** are often used to summarize a set of observations, so as to express the largest amount as succinctly as possible. Biostatisticians may describe the observations as:

- A measure of location, or *central tendency*, such as the median, mean, or mode
- A measure of biostatistical dispersion, such as the confidence level, variance, standard deviation (SD), or range
- A measure of the shape of the distribution, such as normalcy, skewness, or kurtosis
- A measure of biostatistical dependence, such as a correlation coefficient, regression coefficients, or the like, if more than one variable is measured
- Visual summary biostatistics often give a biostatistical and visual overview of a sample, using a histogram and/or dot, box, mean, percentile, and SD plots to present data in a visually meaningful, graphic manner.

A common collection of order statistics used as summary statistics is the **five-number summary**, which is a descriptive biostatistic that provides information about a set of observations. It consists of the five most important sample percentiles:

1. The sample minimum
2. The lower quartile or **first quartile**
3. The median
4. The upper quartile or **third quartile**
5. The sample maximum

The following is an example of summary statistics using R.

■ **Example 5.11:** Summary Statistics Using R

Calculate the five-number summary in the R programming language using the function fivenum(). When applied to a vector, the function summary() displays the five-number summary *together* with the mean (which is not itself a part of the summary):

```
> x <- c(1, 2, 3, 4, 5, 6, 7, 8, 9, 10) # The first 10 natural numbers
> fivenum(x) # Outputting: the five-number summary
[1] 1.0 3.0 5.5 8.0 10.0
> summary(x) # Outputting: the summary statistics
   Min. 1st Qu.  Median    Mean 3rd Qu.    Max.
   1.00    3.25    5.50    5.50    7.75   10.00
> # Trying with another set of numbers:
> x <- rnorm(1000)    # Considering 1000 numbers drawn at random from
>                     # the standard normal distribution
> fivenum(x)
[1] -3.5289989 -0.6730484 0.0056094 0.6482582 3.0345093
> summary(x)
   Min. 1st Qu.  Median    Mean 3rd Qu.    Max.
```

```
> hist(x, freq=F) # Outputting the histogram (only) in Figure 5.1.
> curve(dnorm(x), add=T) # Outputting the curve (only) in Figure 5.1.
>
```

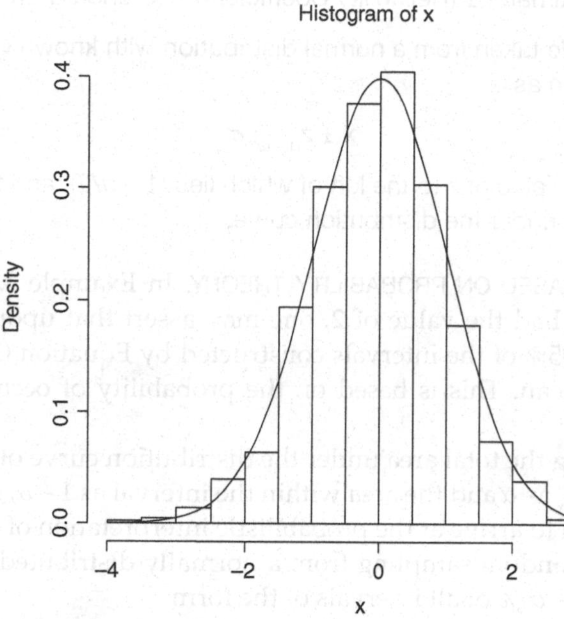

Histogram of x

FIGURE 5.1 Distribution of 1,000 numbers randomly drawn from the standard normal distribution: using functions hist() and curve().

CONFIDENCE INTERVAL (CI)

Example 5.12 shows a probabilistic interpretation of confidence intervals (CIs).

■ **Example 5.12:** Probabilistic Interpretation of CI

A biomedical scientist, who was investigating the average level of an enzyme E in a specific population, approached a random sample of 100 individuals, determined the enzyme level in each subject, and calculated a sample mean of $\underline{x}$ = 25 units. It was known that the enzyme levels are approximately normally distributed with a variance of 400 units. How may the population mean enzyme level μ be computed?

Solution:
The approximate 95% CI for μ is

$$\underline{x} \pm 2\sigma_{\underline{x}} = 25 \pm 2\sqrt{(400/100)} = 25 \pm 4 = [21, 29]$$

In calculating this CI, note that the interval contains:

(a) The point estimate of μ as its center.
(b) The factor 2, arising from the standard normal distribution, showing the number of standard errors (SEs) that lie approximately within 95% of the possible value of x.

(c) The component σ_x is the standard error or standard deviation of the sampling distribution of $\underline{x}$.

Thus, in general, an interval estimate is represented as

$$\text{Estimator} \pm (\text{Reliability Coefficient}) \times (\text{Standard Error}) \qquad (5.1\text{-}23)$$

Hence, for a sample taken from a normal distribution with known variance, the interval for μ may be written as

$$x \pm z_{(1 - \alpha/2)}\sigma_x \qquad (5.1\text{-}24)$$

where $z_{(1 - \alpha/2)}$ is the value of z to the left of which lies $(1 - \alpha/2)$, and to the right of which lies $\alpha/2$ of the area under the distribution curve.

INTERPRETATION BASED ON PROBABILITY THEORY. In Example 5.12, where the reliability coefficient had the value of 2, one may assert that upon repeated random sampling, about 95% of the intervals constructed by Equation (5.1-24) will include the population mean. This is based on the probability of occurrence of different values of $\underline{x}$.

By designating the total area under the distribution curve of x that is outside of the interval $\mu \pm 2\sigma_x$ as α and the area within the interval as $1 - \alpha$, one may generalize this interpretation to arrive at the probabilistic interpretation of CI as follows.

By repeated random sampling from a normally distributed population with a known SD, $100(1 - \alpha)\%$ of all intervals of the form

$$x \pm z_{(1 - \alpha/2)}\alpha_{\underline{x}} \qquad (5.1\text{-}25)$$

will ultimately include the population mean μ.

The quantity $(1 - \alpha)$, which is 0.95 in this case, is the **confidence coefficient** (or **confidence level**), and the interval $x \pm z_{(1 - \alpha/2)}\sigma_x$ is the *CI* for μ. When $(1 - \alpha) = 0.95$, the interval is called the "95% CI for μ." In Example 5.12, the biomedical researcher may state that she is 95% confident that the population mean is between 21 and 29. This is the practical interpretation of Equation (5.1-24).

REMARKS ON CI

1. **A practical interpretation**
    When sampling is randomly taken from a normally distributed population with a known SD, one may be $100(1 - \alpha)\%$ confident that the computed interval $x \pm z_{(1 - \alpha/2)}\sigma_x$ contains the true population mean μ.
    The more exact value of z is 1.96, instead of 2, corresponding to a confidence coefficient of 0.95. Commonly used confidence coefficients are 0.90, 0.95, and 0.99, for which the reliability factors are 1.645, 1.96, and 2.58, respectively.

2. **Quantiles, Median, and CI**
    The inverse of the cumulative distribution function (cdf) is called the **quantile function**. The **p-quantile** is the value such that there is a probability p of achieving a value equal to or less than that value. The **median** is defined as the 50%-quantile.
    For the calculation of CI, theoretical quantiles are used. Thus, for n normally distributed observations with mean μ and SD σ, the average x is normally dis-

A 95% CI for μ may be obtained as

$$\underline{x} + \sigma/\sqrt{n} \times N_{0.025} \leq \mu \leq \underline{x} + \sigma/\sqrt{n} \times N_{0.975} \qquad (5.1\text{-}26)$$

where $N_{0.025}$ is the 2.5%-quantile in the normal distribution.

For example: For $\sigma = 10$, in a study where 6 case subjects were tested and an average of 75 units was found, one may compute the quantiles and CI using the following R code segment:

```
> xbar <- 75
> sigma <- 10
> n <- 6
> # Quantiles and CI computation:
> sem <- sigma/sqrt(n) # sem = standard error of the mean
> sem
[1] 4.082483
> xbar + sem * qnorm(0.025)
[1] 66.99848
> xbar + sem * qnorm(0.975)
[1] 83.00152
```

Hence, a 95% CI for μ is [66.99848, 83.00152], or [70, 83] approximately.

Notes:

1. If the normal distribution is symmetric, then $N_{0.025} = N_{0.975}$.
2. One may express the CI as $\underline{x} \pm (\sigma/\sqrt{n})\, N_{0.975}$.
3. The quantile may be expressed as $\Phi^1(0.975)$, where Φ is the cdf of the normal distribution, pnorm().
4. Another application of quantiles is through the use of quantile-versus-quantile (Q–Q) plots, which may be used to test whether a dataset may be assumed to have come from a given distribution. The R function qqnorm() may be used for such graphic displays.

■ **Example 5.13:** Q–Q plots of randomly generated datasets

Consider:

1. A set of 10 randomly generated numbers, and show its Q–Q plot.
2. Repeat the procedure for a set of 10,000 numbers.

Solution:
The following code segments provide the required Q–Q plots:

```
> x1 <- rnorm(10)
> x1 # For a small dataset, print it out and take a look at it!
[1] 1.1076094 1.6250114 −0.2617057 −1.8640710 −0.7168488
[6] 0.5900851 −0.9575308 −1.3772980 0.8060826 −1.8170715
> qqnorm(x1) # Outputting: Figure 5.2(A).
> x2 <- rnorm(10000)
```

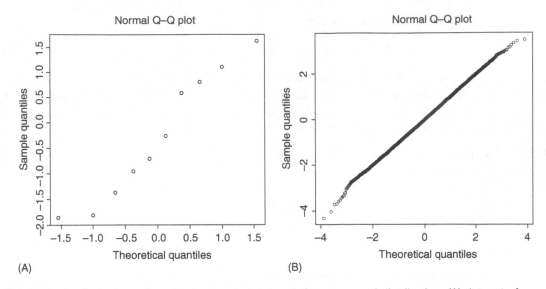

FIGURE 5.2 Q–Q plots of randomly sampled datasets from a normal distribution: (A) dataset of 10 points; (B) dataset of 10,000 points.

3. **One- and Two-Sample *t*-Tests for CI**

   In biostatistical analysis of real data, more often than not, both the population mean μ and the SD σ are *not* known. From the practical viewpoint, it had been considered that a reasonable approach would be to make some estimates of these vital parameters, while retaining the concept of a normal distribution for all variables. This approach includes:

   - Using sample mean $\underline{x}$ as an estimate for the true mean μ
   - Using sample SD s for the true SD σ
   - Using the t distribution instead of the normal distribution
   - Instead of the critical values of $z_{\alpha/2}$ in a normal distribution, using the larger critical values of $t_{\alpha/2}$ values from the t distribution

   If a given t distribution is close to a normal distribution (this is the essential assumption), then the distribution of the variable t defined by

   $$t = (\underline{x} - \mu)/(s/\sqrt{n}) \tag{5.1-27}$$

   is a t distribution for samples of size n.

   This distribution, also known as the Student's t distribution, may be used to find the critical value $t_{\alpha/2}$. The number of degrees of freedom (DFs) is $(n - 1)$, representing the number of *freely assignable* means to n case subjects. In practice, it is expected that $n > 30$.

   A number of data testing procedures have been developed. One of the most common is the **one-sample *t*-test**, which assumes that the datasets come from normal distributions. For the one-sample case, the data $x_1, x_2, x_3, ..., x_n$ are assumed to be independent results of random variables with distribution $N(\mu\sigma^2)$; that is, the normal distribution with mean μ and variance σ^2. The null hypothesis to be tested is $\mu = \mu$

One can then estimate the parameters μ and σ by the following empirical relations:

$$\mu \approx \underline{x} \text{ and } \sigma \approx s \tag{5.1-28}$$

In this approach, the essential concept is that the **standard error of the mean (SEM)**, describing the variation of the average of n random values with mean μ and variance σ^2, is

$$SEM = \sigma/\sqrt{n} \tag{5.1-29}$$

This implies that if the test were repeated a number of times and the average computed each time, these averages would form a distribution somewhat narrower than that of the original distribution. For normally distributed data, it is expected that there is a 95% probability that the data will be within a range of $(\mu \pm 2\sigma)$. One would further expect that $\underline{x}$ should be within 2 SEM of it. In practice, one calculates:

$$t = (\underline{x} - \mu_0)/SEM \tag{5.1-30}$$

and then checks to see if this computed parameter lies within an acceptance region, outside of which t should fall with probability equal to a predetermined significance level. This level is commonly taken to be 5%, corresponding to approximately the interval [2, 2]. The values for the acceptance region may be found as quantiles in the t distribution tables with $(n-1)$ DFs.

Acceptance Criteria:

- If t lies outside the acceptance region, then the null hypothesis is rejected at the predetermined significance level.
- One may also calculate the p-value (the probability of obtaining a value larger than the observed t-value) and, if the p-value is less than the significance level, reject the null hypothesis.
- A **one-sided t-test** is done if there is additional information such that the additional data would only cause μ to exceed μ_0. In such a case, one may then decide that the null hypothesis should be rejected only if t should fall in the upper tail of the distribution.

SIGNIFICANCE LEVELS

In biostatistical tests, one must decide which values go into the rejection region and which go into the nonrejection region (this latter is not necessarily the same as the acceptance region). This decision is based on the preferred **significance level** α, which specifies the area under the distribution curves of the test statistic that is above the values on the horizontal axis as constituting the **rejection region**.

Hypothesis tests are also called **significance tests**, and a computed value of the test statistic falling within the rejection region is called **significant**. Thus, the significance level α is the probability of rejecting a true null hypothesis.

Usually, small values of α are chosen to make the probability of rejecting a true null hypothesis small. Frequently, the chosen values of α are 0.01, 0.05, and 0.10, with 0.05 being the most common.

Review the discussion in Chapter 2 on the concept of biostatistical significance, and consider the following examples on the calculations of significance levels in biostatistical analysis.

■ **Example 5.14:** Significance levels for two-sample tests for normal populations (Verzani, 2005)

The first Food and Drug Administration (FDA)–supported antiretroviral drug used in the care of HIV-infected case subjects was azidothymidine (AZT). The normal dosage was 300 mg twice daily. Health researchers knew that higher dosages often caused more adverse side effects, but they wondered if they were also more effective. Back in 1900, an epidemiologic study compared varying doses at the 300-, 600-, and 1500-mg levels. The investigation found that higher dosages had elevated levels of toxicity; they also noted, somewhat more unexpectedly, that lower dosages might be equally effective.

The p24 antigen stimulates immune responses. Measurement of the p24 levels for the 300-mg and 600-mg groups is given by the simulated data in Table 5.6.

Solution:
First, a null hypothesis is set up. Then it is tested at specified significance levels.

Let μ_{300} be the mean of the 300-mg group and μ_{600} be the mean of the 600-mg group.

One may test the null hypotheses (H_0: $\mu_{300} = \mu_{600}$, H_A: $\mu_{300} \neq \mu_{600}$) with a t-test. Before testing, check to see whether the assumption of a common variance and normality is appropriate by inspecting two density plots.

The following R code segment will perform these tasks:

```
> # Inputting the two datasets: x300 and x600:
> x300 <- c(284, 279, 289, 292, 287, 295, 285, 279, 306, 298)
> x600 <- c(298, 307, 297, 279, 291, 335, 299, 300, 306, 291)
> plot(density(x300)) # Outputting: Figure 5.3(A).
> lines(density(x600), lty=2) # Outputting: Figure 5.3(B).
> t.test(x300, x600, var.equal=TRUE) # Now, do the t-test, outputting:
```

Two Sample t-test
data: x300 and x600
t = −2.034, df = 18, p-value = 0.05696
alternative hypothesis: true difference in means is not equal to 0
95 percent confidence interval:
−22.1584072   0.3584072
sample estimates:
mean of x   mean of y
**   289.4   300.3**

TABLE 5.6   Levels of p24 in Milligrams for Two Treatment Populations

DOSAGE					p24 LEVEL					
300 mg	284	279	289	292	287	295	285	279	306	298

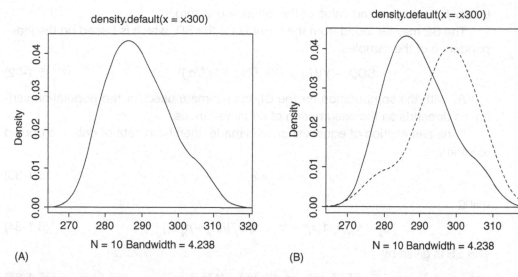

FIGURE 5.3 Density plots for comparing variances and shapes of the 300-mg dosage (solid) and the 600-mg dosage (dashed).

```
># Repeat the t-test, without assuming the same variances
> t.test(x300, x600)
```
Welch Two Sample t-test
data: x300 and x600
t = −2.034, df = 14.509, p-value = 0.06065
alternative hypothesis: true difference in means is not equal to 0
95 percent confidence interval:
−22.3557409   0.5557409
sample estimates:
mean of x   mean of y
289.4   300.3

Remarks:

1. For the equal variance test, the p-value is .05696 for the two-sided t-test. This implies a possible difference in the mean values, but it is not statistically significant at the 0.05 significance level. It may be concluded that this dataset is consistent with an assumption of no mean difference.
2. The test statistic is t = −2.034.
3. For the case without the assumption of equal variances, the same test statistic (as the equal variance case) is obtained: t = −2.034. This agreement is in accord with the theoretical model, as follows:

    Algebraically, if two samples are independent with normally distributed populations, as X and Y estimate μ_x and μ_y, respectively, the value of $(\underline{X} - \underline{Y})$ may be considered a good estimate for $(\mu_x - \mu_y)$. One may use this assumption to form a test statistic.

    Both sample means have normally distributed sampling distributions, and hence a natural test statistic T would be

Under H_0, the expected value of the difference is zero.

The SE may be found from the formula for the SD, which is based on the independence of the samples:

$$SD(\underline{X} - \underline{Y}|H_0) = \sqrt{\{(\sigma_x^2/n_x) + (\sigma_y^2/n_y)\}} \tag{5.1-32}$$

As with the computation for the CI, the estimate used for the population variances depends on the assumption of equal variances.

If the assumption of equal variance is made, then both sets of data are pooled to estimate

$$\sigma = \sigma_x = \sigma_y \tag{5.1-33}$$

using

$$s_p = \sqrt{[\{(n_x\ 1)s_x^2 + (n_y - 1)\ s_y^2\}/(n_x + n_y\ 2)]} \tag{5.1-34}$$

The SE is given by

$$SE(\underline{X} - \underline{Y}) = s_p\sqrt{\{(1/n_x) + (1/n_y)\}} \tag{5.1-35}$$

Under these conditions, T has a t distribution with $(n - 2)$ DFs.

If the population variances are *not* assumed to be equal, then one may estimate σ_x by s_x, and σ_y by s_y to obtain

$$SE(\mu_x - \mu_y) = \sqrt{\{(s_x^2/n_x) + (s_y^2/n_y)\}} \tag{5.1-36}$$

Thus, with the assumption of equal variances, Equations (5.1-35) and (5.1-36) show that when the two samples are the same size, their SEs are mathematically identical.

4. The *p*-value increased from .05696 to .06065, as the DFs decreased from 18 to 14.509.

Many additional tests, such as the Wilcoxon {stats}, and the pairwise.wilcox. test {stats}, are available in the CRAN site upon prompting by
> ??wilcoxon

GOODNESS OF FIT

A **goodness-of-fit** (**GoF**) test, used on a given dataset, statistically assesses the hypothesis that the frequency distribution of the data conforms to, or "fits," some particular distribution. In biostatistics, the GoF of a model shows how well the model fits a set of observations. Summary measures of GoF typically consist of the discrepancy between *observed* values and the values *expected* under the model. Such measures may be used in statistical hypothesis testing for several purposes, including:

- To test for normality of the dataset or the residuals
- To test whether outcome frequencies follow a specified distribution (see discussion of Pearson's chi-squared test later in this subsection)
- To test whether two samples are drawn from identical distributions (see discussion of the Kolmogorov–Smirnov [KS] test later in this section)
- In the analysis of variance (ANOVA), to test whether one of the components into which the variance is partitioned may be a lack-of-fit sum of squares (among

Typically, in epidemiologic investigations, one wishes to test whether or not a sample of observed values of some specific variable(s) is compatible with the hypothesis that the sample was drawn from a normally distributed population of values. This test procedure generally consists of putting the observed data into mutually exclusive class intervals and noting the frequency of occurrence of the values in each class. Next, using one's knowledge of normal distributions, one determines the frequencies for these classes that could be expected if the sample had come from a normal distribution. If the disagreement is such that it could have occurred owing to chance, one may conclude that the observed sample may indeed have come from a normal distribution. Similarly, GoF tests may be performed in investigations in which the hypothesized distribution is the binomial distribution, the multinomial distribution, the Poisson distribution, and so on.

From the theory of probability, a number of methodologies have been developed for GoF testing. These methodologies are presented here, and followed with examples to illustrate details of GoF hypothesis testing using these methods within the R environment.

PEARSON'S CHI-SQUARE DISTRIBUTION FOR GOF TEST. For populations that are normally distributed, with variance σ^2, randomly select independent samples of size n, and calculate the sample variance s^2, where

$$s^2 = [\sum x_i^2 (\sum x_i)^2/n]/(n-1) \qquad (5.1\text{-}37)$$

for each sample. The sample statistic χ^2, where

$$\chi^2 = (n-1)s^2/\sigma^2 \qquad (5.1\text{-}38)$$

has a distribution called the **chi-square distribution**, has the following special properties:

- This distribution is based on the number of DFs, which is usually taken as $(n-1)$ unless special conditions prevail.
- This distribution is not symmetrical, and the values cannot be negative; it can only be zero or positive.
- As DF increases, this distribution approaches a normal distribution.

The **test statistic** for the chi-squared test is

$$X^2 = \sum [(O_i - E_i)^2/E_i] \qquad (5.1\text{-}39)$$

where O_i is the observed frequency for the ith class of the variable of interest, and E_i is the expected frequency for the ith class of the variable of interest (if the null hypotheses H_0 were true).

The quantity X^2 is a measure of the extent to which, in any situation, pairs of observed and expected frequencies agree. The nature of X^2 is that:

(a) When there is a *perfect* **agreement** between observed and expected frequencies, it is *zero*, and H_0 must be accepted.
(b) When there is a **close agreement** between observed and expected frequencies, it is *small* (and the p-value is large).
(c) When there is a **poor agreement** between observed and expected frequencies,

In general, the calculated value of X^2 is compared with the tabulated value of $(k - r)$ DF, where k is the number of classes for which observed and expected frequencies are available, and r is the number of constraints or restrictions imposed on the given comparison. Thus, a restriction is imposed when one forces the sum of the expected frequencies to equal the sum of the observed frequencies. Additional restrictions are imposed for each parameter that is estimated from the observed sample.

The decision then is whether to reject the null hypothesis H_0 if X^2 is greater than or equal to the tabulated χ^2 for the chosen value of α.

Tables of critical values of the χ^2 distribution are available in standard texts and on the Internet.

THE PEARSON'S CHI-SQUARED TEST IN THE R ENVIRONMENT. The R function chisq. test(), in the CRAN package stats, performs chi-squared contingency table tests and GoF tests. Its usage format is

```
chisq.test(x, y = NULL, correct = TRUE,
          p = rep(1/length(x), length(x)), rescale.p = FALSE,
          simulate.p.value = FALSE, B = 2000)
```

for which the arguments are:

x	A numeric vector or matrix. x and y can also both be factors.
y	A numeric vector; ignored if x is a matrix. If x is a factor, then y should be a factor of the same length.
correct	A logical label indicating whether to apply continuity correction when computing the test statistic for 2×2 tables: one-half is subtracted from all $\lvert O\,E \rvert$ differences. No correction is done if simulate.p.value = TRUE.
p	A vector of probabilities of the same length as x. An error is given if any entry of p is negative.
rescale.p	A logical scalar; if TRUE, then p is rescaled (if necessary) to sum to 1. If rescale.p is FALSE, and p does not sum to 1, an error is given.
simulate.p.value	A logical label indicating whether to compute p-values by Monte Carlo simulation.
B	An integer specifying the number of replicates used in the Monte Carlo test.

The following example illustrates the use of the chisq.test() function.

■ **Example 5.15:** GoF Test for the Normal Distribution (Daniel, 2005, Verzani, 2005)

An epidemiologic research group collected the inpatient occupancy data on 250 U.S. hospitals over a 12-month period and reported the ratio of daily census to the number of beds maintained. The sample data were expressed in terms of the distribution of percentages, as shown in Table 5.7.

Show whether these data provide reasonably sufficient evidence to show that the sample did or did not come from a normally distributed population.

TABLE 5.7 Summary of Results of Hospital Occupancy Study

INPATIENT OCCUPANCY RATIO	NUMBER OF HOSPITALS
0.0 to 39.9	16
40.0 to 49.9	18
50.0 to 59.9	22
60.0 to 69.9	51
70.0 to 79.9	62
80.0 to 89.9	55
90.0 to 99.9	22
100.0 to 109.9	4
Total	250

Solution:

Begin by assuming that the dataset available for biostatistical analysis is a simple, random sample.

Hypothesis (H_0): In the population from which this sample was taken, inpatient occupancy ratios are normally distributed.

Test Statistic: $$X = \sum_{i=1 \text{ to } k} [(O_i E_i)^2/E_i] \tag{5.1-37}$$

This is the chi-squared statistic, in which O_i and E_i are the observed and expected frequencies, respectively, for the ith class of the dataset.

If H_0 is true, then the test statistic is distributed as chi-square with $(k - r)$ DFs.

Decision Rule: H_0 will be rejected if the calculated value of X^2 is equal to or greater than the critical value of chi-square, or the p-value is very small.

Computations: As the mean and variance of the hypothesized distribution are not known, the sample data will be used to estimate these parameters. The estimates of these parameters are needed to calculate the frequency that would be expected in each class when the hypothesis is true. For each of the 8 classes, the median of each will be used to represent the class; the medians of the 8 classes are 20, 45, 55, 65, 75, 85, 95, and 105.

The following R code segments are used to undertake the computations:

```
> x <- c(16, 18, 22, 51, 62, 55, 22, 4) # Inputting the frequencies
> x # Checking
[1]    16     18     22     51     62     55     22     4
> p1 <- c(20, 45, 55, 65, 75, 85, 95, 105) # Inputting data
> p1 # Checking
[1]    20     45     55     65     75     85     95     105
> p <- p1/sum(p1) # Normalizing
> p # Checking
```

```
[1] 0.03669725    0.08256881    0.10091743    0.11926606
[5] 0.13761468    0.15596330    0.17431193    0.19266055
> n <- sum(x) # Summing the frequencies
> n # Checking
[1] 250
> chi2 <- sum( (x - n*p)^2 / (n*p) ) # Computing the X² statistic
> chi2 # Outputting the X² statistic
[1] 100.7709
> pchisq(chi2, df = 8 - 1, lower.tail = F) # Outputting the p-value
[1] 7.476817e-19
>
> # An alternate computation:
> chisq.test(x, p=p)
    Chi-squared test for given probabilities
data: x
X-squared = 100.7709, df = 7, p-value < 2.2e-16
```

Biostatistical Decision and Conclusion: The probability of obtaining a value of X^2 to allow the hypothesis H_0 to be true is minute: $p \approx 0$. Thus, the dataset is mostly unlikely to be normally distributed, and one should seek another explanation.

THE CHI-SQUARED TEST OF INDEPENDENCE FOR GOF. Chapter 2 introduced the use of a two-way contingency table to clarify the relationship between the variables. In particular, one may be concerned whether the levels of one variable affect the distribution of the other variable. Often the question arises as to whether they are independent random variables. As an illustration, consider the following situation (Verzani, 2005).

In California, a survey of carseat-belt use investigated the relationship between the use of a seat belt by a parent and by a child. The result of the survey is given in Table 5.8.

While the data show some dramatic differences and important correlations between the relationships and actions, from a biostatistical viewpoint, one needs a significance test—starting with a probability mode, the associated test statistic, and the null and alternate hypotheses that are to be tested to reach a decision and yielding a GoF concept of the model. Such an approach may be applied to any similar four-way decision situation.

The Probability Model: The sampling model is that each car follows a given probability that is recorded in some specific cell. These probabilities do not change, and the outcome of one does not affect the distribution of another; thus, they form an iid sequence. Consider a multinomial model for the dataset.

TABLE 5.8   Survey of Car Seat-Belt Use in California

	CHILD	
PARENT	BUCKLED	UNBUCKLED
Buckled	56	8

Let

n_r = The number of rows in the table (the number of levels of the row variable)

n_c = The number of columns in the table

X_{ij} = A random variable recording the frequency of the (i,j) cell

p_{ij} = The cell probability for the ith row and jth column

Denote the marginal probabilities by p_i^r and p_j^c, where:

$$p_j^r = p_{i1} + p_{i2} + \cdots + p_{in_j} \tag{5.1-38}$$

and

$$p_j^c = p_{j1} + p_{j2} + \cdots + p_{jn_i} \tag{5.1-39}$$

Null Hypothesis: The column variables are independent of the row variables. That is,

$$H_0: p_{ij} = p_i^r \, p_j^c \tag{5.1-40}$$

In other words, the hypotheses are:

H_0: The variables are independent.

H_A: The variables are not independent.

After the p_{ij} values are estimated so as to calculate the "expected" counts, the χ^2 statistics

$$\chi^2 = \sum [(Observed - Expected)^2 / Expected] \tag{5.1-41}$$

may be used. The data are used to estimate the marginal probabilities (see Section 5.1), and the assumption of independence is used to estimate the p_{ij}.

For this example, the marginal probabilities are obtained by the marginal distributions of the data, resulting in Table 5.9.

From Table 5.9, it is easy to see that:

■ The estimate for p_1^r = P(Parent is Buckled) = p_1^r = 64/82
■ The estimate for p_2^r = P(Parent is Unbuckled) = p_2^r = 18/82
■ The estimate for p_1^c = P(Child is Buckled) = p_1^c = 58/82
■ The estimate for p_2^c = P(Child is Unbuckled) = p_2^c = 24/82

Having calculated these estimates, one may use the null hypothesis H_0 to find the estimate:

$$p_{ij} = p_i^r \, p_j^c \tag{5.1-40}$$

For the data on hand, the resultant estimates are obtained as shown in Table 5.10.

TABLE 5.9 Marginal Distribution for Survey of Car Seat-Belt Use in California

PARENT	CHILD		
	BUCKLED	UNBUCKLED	MARGINAL
Buckled	56	8	64
Unbuckled	2	16	18

TABLE 5.10 Estimated Marginal Probabilities for Survey of Car Seat-Belt Use in California

PARENT	CHILD		
	BUCKLED	UNBUCKLED	MARGINAL
Buckled	(64/82)(58/82)	(64/82)(24/82)	(64/82)
Unbuckled	(18/82)(58/82)	(18/82)(24/82)	(18/82)
Marginal	58/82	24/82	82/82

Using this table, one may calculate the expected amounts in the ijth cell with np_{ij}, that is, e_{ij}, which is written as R_iC_j/n, where R_i is the row sum and C_j the column sum:

$$e_{ij} = R_iC_j/n \qquad (5.1\text{-}42)$$

and the χ^2 statistic may now be expressed as

$$x^2 = \sum_{i=1\,to\,n_r} \sum_{i=1\,to\,n_c} \left[\left(Y_{ij} - n\underline{p}_{ij} \right)^2 \Big/ n\underline{p}_{ij} \right] \qquad (5.1\text{-}43)$$

By the hypothesis of multinomial data and the independence of the variables, the sampling distribution of χ^2 will be the chi-squared distribution with $(n_r - 1)(n_c - 1)$ DFs, because by subtracting 1 DF from $n_r \cdot n_c - 1$ for each estimated parameter, and since there are $n_r - 1 + n_c + 1$ parameters, the value for the DF is

$$n_r \cdot n_c - 1 - (n_r - 1 + n_c + 1) = n_r \cdot n_c - n_r - n_c + 1 = (n_r - 1)(n_c - 1)$$

In the R environment, the following procedure may be followed for a chi-squared test for the independence of two categorical variables:

- When the data are summarized in a matrix or table in the variable x, the test is done by the test function chisq.test().
- When the data are summarized and stored in two variables x and y where the ith entries match up, the test function is chisq.test(x, y).
- The data are first summarized using table(), as in chisq.test(table(x, y)).

The null and alternate hypotheses are not specified, as they are the same for each test. When the expected counts in some cells are too small to use the chi-squared distribution to represent the sampling distribution of χ^2, adding the argument simulate.p.value=TRUE will return a p-value estimate using a Monte Carlo simulation.

The following example illustrates the use of R for this problem.

■ **Example 5.16:** GoF Test Using the Pearson's χ^2 Test of Independence (Verzani, 2005)

Using the data from Table 5.8, the survey of car-seat-belt use in California, perform a GoF test using R.

Solution:
The following R code segments may be used to first create a table by using the function rbind() to combine rows (see Chapter 3 on computations in vectors and simple graph-

```
> seatbelt.usage.in.california <- rbind( c(56,8), c(2,16) )
> seatbelt.usage.in.california # Outputting:
     [,1]  [,2]
[1,]  56    8
[2,]   2   16
> chisq.test(seatbelt.usage.in.california) # Outputting:
```

Pearson's Chi-squared test with Yates' continuity correction
data: seatbelt.usage.in.california
X-squared = 35.9953, df = 1, p-value = 1.978e^{-09}

Biostatistical Decision and Conclusion: The computed p-value, 1.978e^{-09}, is small, is not significant, and therefore is consistent with the observation that the two variables are *not* independent.

THE CHI-SQUARED TEST OF HOMOGENEITY FOR GoF. In investigating the effectiveness of a drug treatment, research epidemiologists are often called upon to assess a clinical trial in which each case subject is randomly allocated to one of two groups: either a treatment group or a placebo group. To biostatistically analyze the results, the following approaches are available:

(A) If the results are recorded numerically, a t-test may be used to test whether any differences in sample means are significant.

(B) If the results are noted categorically, the following procedure shows that the χ^2 statistic may be used to check whether the distributions of the results are the same. A research study conducted at the Stanford University Medical Center (SUMC) is used here to illustrate this approach (Verzani, 2005).

SUMC investigated whether the antidepressant Celexa can be effective in modifying compulsive shopping behavior. In that study, 24 case subjects (who were known compulsive shoppers) participated: 12 were given a daily dose of Celexa for 7 consecutive days, and 12 were given a placebo. At the end of this treatment, all the subjects were surveyed to assess whether their desires to shop had been reduced. From the preliminary report, simulated data were developed; they are shown in Table 5.11.

To formulate this investigation as a significance test, one may use the following hypotheses:

H_0: The two distributions are the same.
H_A: The two distributions are different.

and the χ^2 statistics may be used. Because the expected amounts are not fully specified in H_0, that amount must be determined.

TABLE 5.11   Data on the Effect of Celexa for Reducing Compulsive Shopping

	MUCH WORSE	WORSE	SAME	MUCH IMPROVED	VERY MUCH IMPROVED
Celexa	0	2	2	5	2
Placebo	0	2	8		

The test procedure is as follows. In the data table, let

▪ The random variable be the **column** variable, and
▪ The category that breaks up the data be the **row** variable.
▪ For row i of the table, let p_{ij} be the probability that the random variable (the study result) will be in the jth level of the random variable.

We can then rephrase the hypotheses as

H_0: $p_{ij} = p_j$ for all rows i
H_A: $p_{ij} \neq p_j$ for some i, j

Let n_i be the number of counts in each row; then the expected amount in the (i, j) cell under H_0 should be $n_i p_j$. The value of p_j in H_0 has to be estimated because it is not specified. Under the hypothesis H_0, all the data in the jth column are binomial with n and p_j; thus, an estimator for p_j would be the column sum divided by n; that is, C_j/n.

Under these circumstances, the expected number in the (i, j) cell would be given by

$$e_{ij} = n_i p_j = R_i C_j / n \tag{5.1-44}$$

This is exactly the same formula as the χ^2 test of independence, Equation (5.1-42).

In spite of the differences in the hypotheses, the test statistic and its sampling distribution under null hypothesis H_0 are the **same** as the test of independence; hence, the chi-squared significance tests of homogeneity and independence are identical in practice and implementation.

GoF TESTS FOR CONTINUOUS DISTRIBUTIONS. Recall that when testing whether sampled data was taken from a normal distribution, one makes a histogram or a quantile plot of the data, then visually inspects the result. For a sampled continuous dataset, one may, using a significance test, compare the dataset with a theoretical one. This is the approach for GoF tests for continuous distributions.

For categorical data, it was shown that the chi-squared test may be applied. One may extend this technique by "binning": just as one does when constructing histograms, one chooses some bins and counts the number of data points in each bin. In this way, the data may be considered categorical, and the test may be used for GoF.

However, in practice, it has been found that, for continuous distributions, an approach that improves results is the **KS test**: Let X_1, X_2, X_3, ..., X_i, ..., X_n be a random sample from a continuous distribution.

Let $f(x)$ be the probability distribution density function (pdf), and X be some other random variable with this density.

The cdf for X is $F(x) = P(X \leq x)$, or the area to the left of x under the density curve of X.

The cdf may be similarly defined when X is discrete: It is calculated from the pdf by summing: $P(X \leq x) = \sum_{y \leq x} f(y)$.

For a sample X_1, X_2, X_3, ..., X_i, ..., X_n, the **empirical distribution** is the distribution obtained by sampling from the data points. The "probability that a number randomly selected from a sample is $\leq x$" is the number of data points in the sample $\leq (x/n)$. Using the notation $F_n(x)$ for this probability:

$$F_n(x) = \#\{i: X_i \leq x\} / n \tag{5.1-45}$$

Here, $F_n(x)$ is the *empirical cumulative distribution function* (ecdf).

In the R environment, $F_n(x)$ may be plotted using the function ecdf(), in the package stats, similar to the function density(), for which the return value may be plotted in a new figure using the function plot(), or it may be added to the existing plot using the function lines(). The following example illustrates the use of R for this application.

■ **Example 5.17:** Comparing a sample of 15 points from a normally distributed population to the theoretical distribution by showing both sample and theoretical densities and cdfs.

Solution:

The following R commands may be used:

```
> x1 <- rnorm(15)
> x1
```

[1]	−0.63573743	−0.14453713	−0.57131893
[4]	−1.76854783	1.41941167	−1.47808847
[7]	0.99010104	−0.06643542	0.25797379
[10]	−0.62145348	−0.77645263	0.31534275
[13]	−0.96369367	−1.15635521	−1.08556058

```
> plot(density(x1), main="Densities") # Plotting densities
> curve(dnorm(x), add=TRUE, lty=2) # Add Normal curve
> # Outputting: Figures 5.4(A) and 5.4(B).
> plot(ecdf(x1), main="C.d.f.s") # Plotting Cdf point values
> curve(pnorm(x), add=TRUE, lty=2) # Add Cdf curve
> # Outputting: Figures 5.5(A) and 5.5(B).
```

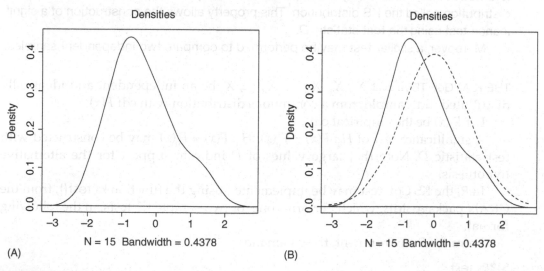

(A) (B)

FIGURE 5.4 For a sample size of 15 from a normally distributed population: (A) sample density; (B) theoretical density

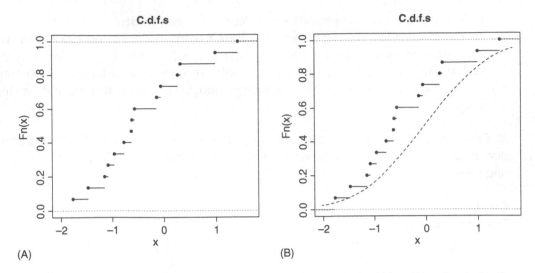

FIGURE 5.5 For a sample size of 15 from a normally distributed population: (A) estimated cdf; (B) theoretical cdf.

Remarks:

- The foregoing example shows that if the sampled data are from a population with the normal distribution, the distribution and cdf of the dataset will be close to the normal distribution and the cdf of the normal distribution.
- Similarly, if the data are from a population with cdf F, one may expect that F_n is close to F in some way. What does "close" mean in this context?
- Given two different functions of x, the separation D between them may be defined as

$$D = \text{maximum of } |F_n(x) - F(x)| \qquad (5.1\text{-}46)$$

It turns out that, with the only assumption that F is continuous, D has a known sampling distribution called the KS distribution. This property allows the construction of a significance test using the test statistic D.

Moreover, a similar test may be performed to compare two independent samples.

THE K–M GoF TEST. Let $X_1, X_2, X_3, \ldots, X_i, \ldots, X_n$ be an independent and identically distributed (iid) sample from a continuous distribution with cdf $F(x)$.

Let $F_n(x)$ be the empirical cdf.

A significance test of $H_0: F(x) = F_0(x)$, $H_A: F(x) \neq F_0(x)$ may be constructed with test statistic D. Note that large values of D indicate support for the alternative hypothesis.

In R, the KS GoF test may be implemented using the function ks.test(), from the CRAN package stats, which performs one- or two-sample KS tests, in the following format.

From the R environment, the command

```
> ?ks.test
```

provides the following information on the documentation of the function.

ks.test(), in the CRAN package stats[1]:
ks.test(x, y, ..., alternative = c("two.sided", "less", "greater"),
       exact = NULL)

Arguments:

x	A numeric vector of data values.
y	Either a numeric vector of data values or a character string naming a cdf or an actual cdf such as pnorm. Only continuous cdfs are valid.
...	Parameters of the distribution specified (as a character string) by y.
alternative	Indicates the alternative hypothesis and must be one of "two.sided" (default), "less", or "greater". You can specify just the initial letter of the value, but the argument name must be given in full. See "Details" for the meanings of the possible values.
exact	NULL or a logical label indicating whether an exact *p*-value should be computed. See "Details" for the meaning of NULL. This is not available in the two-sample case for a one-sided test, or if ties are present.

Details:

- If y is numeric, a two-sample test of the null hypothesis that x and y were drawn from the same *continuous* distribution is performed.
- Alternatively, y can be a character string naming a continuous (cumulative) distribution function, or another such function. In this case, a one-sample test is carried out of the null to see whether the distribution function that generated x is distribution y with parameters specified by ... .
- The presence of ties should always be taken as a warning because continuous distributions do not generate them. If the ties arose from rounding, the tests may be approximately valid, but even modest amounts of rounding can have a significant effect on the calculated statistic.
- Missing values are silently omitted from x and (in the two-sample case) y.
- The possible values "two.sided", "less", and "greater" of alternative specify the null hypothesis that the true distribution function of x is equal to, not less than or not greater than, the hypothesized distribution function (one-sample case) or the distribution function of y (two-sample case), respectively. This is a comparison of cdfs, and the test statistic is the maximum difference in value, with the statistic in the "greater" alternative being $D^+ = max[F\_x(u) - F\_y(u)]$. Thus, in the two-sample case, alternative = "greater" includes distributions for which x is stochastically *smaller* than y (the cdf of x lies above and hence to the left of that for y), in contrast to t.test or wilcox.test.
- Exact *p*-values are not available for the two-sample case if one-sided or in the presence of ties. If exact = NULL (the default), an exact *p*-value is computed if the sample size is less than 100 in the one-sample case *and there are no ties;* and if the product of the sample sizes is less than 10,000 in the two-sample case.

Otherwise, asymptotic distributions are used whose approximations may be inaccurate in small samples. In the one-sample, two-sided case, exact p-values are obtained as described in Marsaglia, Tsang, and Wang (2003) (but not using the optional approximation in the right tail, so this can be slow for small p-values). The formula of Birnbaum and Tingey (1951) is used for the one-sample, one-sided case.

■ If a single-sample test is used, the parameters specified in … must be prespecified and not estimated from the data. There is some more refined distribution theory for the KS test with estimated parameters (Durbin, 1973), but that is not implemented in ks.test.

Value:
A list with class "htest" having the following components:

statistic	The value of the test statistic
p.value	The p-value of the test
alternative	A character string describing the alternative hypothesis
method	A character string indicating what type of test was performed
data.name	A character string giving the name(s) of the data

Remarks:
For the current application, the function ks.test() may be used as ks.test(x, y), where x and y store the data. One- and two-sample tests are available (Conover, 1971).

The following example illustrates the use of R for this application.

■ **Example 5.18:** The Shapiro–Wilk (SW) GoF test for normality

Use the SW test for GoF, in R, to assess the following datasets for normality:

(a) A dataset of 1,000,000 points randomly selected from a normal distribution with mean 0 and SD 10
(b) A dataset of 1,000 points from a continuous uniform distribution

Solution:
The following R code segments may be used.

To generate the dataset from a *normal distribution*, one may use the function rnorm():

```
> x <- rnorm(1000, mean = 0, sd = 10)
> shapiro.test(x)
```

Shapiro–Wilk normality test
data: x
W = 0.9979, p-value = 0.2445

Remarks: The p-value, 0.2445, is not statistically significant. Thus, there is no evidence that the dataset is not normally distributed. H_0 cannot be rejected.

The probability density function of the *continuous uniform distribution* is

$$f(x)\begin{cases} \dfrac{1}{b-a} & \text{for } a \le x \le b \\ 0 & \text{for } x < a \text{ or } x > b \end{cases} \qquad (5.1\text{-}47)$$

The values of $f(x)$ at the two boundaries a and b do not affect the values of the integrals of $f(x)\,dx$ over any interval, nor of $x\,f(x)\,dx$ or any higher moment. They may be chosen to be zero, or to be $1/(b-a)$. The probability density function and the cdf of this distribution are shown in Figures 5.6(A) and (B), respectively.

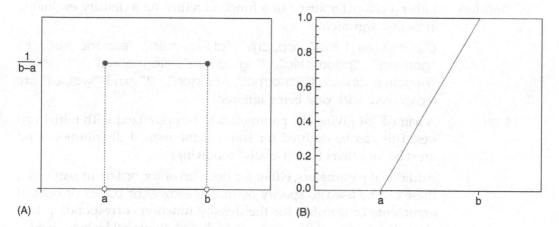

FIGURE 5.6   The uniform distribution function: (A) probability density function; (B) cumulative distribution function.

```
> z <- runif(1000) # Generating 1000 uniformly distributed data points
> shapiro.test(z) # Applying the SW GoF test for normality
> # Outputting:
Shapiro–Wilk normality test
data: z
W = 0.9516, p-value < 2.2e – 16
```

Remarks: The *p*-value is very small—less than 2.2×10^{16}. Hence, there is poor agreement between the observed values and normality. H_0 must be rejected.

Notes:

1. In applying the *t*-test, it was assumed that the observed dataset was sampled from a normally distributed population.
2. For data that have failed a test for normalcy, the *t*-test may still be used because
    (a) for small samples, the *t*-test may still be applicable because the distribution of the *t*-statistic is robust to small changes in the normalcy assumption of the parent distribution, and
    (b) for large samples, the central limit theorem may apply, validating the use of the *t*-test.

USING THE FUNCTION fitdistr() TO FIND PARAMETER VALUES. R Documentation of fitdistr {MASS}

Maximum Likelihood Fitting of Univariate Distributions

Description:

Maximum likelihood fitting of univariate distributions, allowing parameters to be held fixed if desired.

Usage:

fitdistr(x, densfun, start, ...)

Arguments:

x	A numeric vector of length at least one containing only *finite* values.
densfun	Either a character string or a function returning a density evaluated at its first argument.
	Distributions "beta", "cauchy", "chi-squared", "exponential", "f", "gamma", "geometric", "log-normal", "lognormal", "logistic", "negative binomial", "normal", "Poisson", "t", and "weibull" are recognized, with case being ignored.
start	A named list giving the parameters to be optimized with initial values. This can be omitted for some of the named distributions and must be for others (see "Details" following).
	Additional parameters, either for densfun or for optim. In particular, these can be used to specify bounds via lower or upper or both. If arguments of densfun (or the density function corresponding to a character-string specification) are included, they will be held fixed.

Details:

■ For the normal, log-normal, geometric, exponential, and Poisson distributions, the closed-form maximum likelihood estimators (MLEs and exact SEs) are used, and start should not be supplied.

■ For all other distributions, direct optimization of the log-likelihood is performed using optim. The estimated SEs are taken from the observed information matrix, calculated by a numerical approximation. For one-dimensional problems, the Nelder–Mead method is used; for multidimensional problems, the BFGS[2] method is used, unless arguments named lower or upper are supplied (when L-BFGS-B is used) or method is supplied explicitly.

■ For the "t" named distribution, the density is taken to be the location–scale family with location m and scale s.

■ For the following named distributions, reasonable starting values will be computed if start is omitted or only partially specified: "cauchy", "gamma", "logistic", "negative binomial" (parametrized by mu and size), "t", and "weibull". Note that these starting values may not be good enough if the fit is poor: in particular, they are not resistant to outliers unless the fitted distribution is long-tailed.

■ There are print, coef, vcov, and logLik methods for class "fitdistr".

---

[2] The BFGS (Broyden–Fletcher–Goldfarb–Shanno) algorithm in statistics for multidimensional

Value:

An object of class "fitdistr", a list with four components:

estimate   the parameter estimates

sd   the estimated standard errors

vcov   the estimated variance–covariance matrix

loglik   the log-likelihood

The following example illustrates the use of R for this application.

■ **Example 5.19:** Use a pseudo-random number generator in R to obtain samples of pseudo-random normally distributed numbers, and a GoF check for normalcy using the function fitdistr(). Vary the sample sizes from 10 to 1,000,000, in multiples of 10, and check the variations of the parameter SD with respect to sample sizes.

Solution:

The following R code segments may be used:

```
> # Starting with a sample size of 1,000,000, and vary in steps of multiples of 10:
> x <- rnorm(1000000, mean=0, sd=10)
> fitdistr(x, "normal")
```

```
      mean          sd
   -0.00503      9.99917
   (0.01000)    (0.00707)
>
> x <- rnorm(100000, mean=0, sd=10)
> fitdistr(x, "normal")
```

```
     mean         sd
  -0.0337       9.9641
  (0.0315)     (0.0223)
>
> x <- rnorm(10000, mean=0, sd=10)
> fitdistr(x, "normal")
```

```
     mean         sd
   0.00829      9.90678
  (0.09907)    (0.07005)
>
> x <- rnorm(1000, mean=0, sd=10)
> fitdistr(x, "normal")
```

```
     mean        sd
    0.279       9.888
   (0.313)     (0.221)
>
```

```
> x <- rnorm(100, mean=0, sd=10)
> fitdistr(x, "normal")
      mean        sd
     0.263     8.335
    (0.834)   (0.589)
>
> x <- rnorm(10, mean=0, sd=10)
> fitdistr(x, "normal")
      mean        sd
     -5.76     6.80
    (2.15)    (1.52)
> # The results are summarized in Table 5.12.
> # Plotting out these results:
> x <- c(6.80, 8.335, 9.888, 9.90678, 9.9641, 9.99917)
> y <- c(10, 100, 1000, 10000, 100000, 1000000)
> plot(y, x, ann=FALSE) # Setting ann=FALSE to inhibit annotations
> lines(y, x, col="red") # Adding a red line through the points
> title(main="GoF Test: Checking for SD=10 in a rnorm with +
> SD=10", xlab="Sample Size", ylab="Standard Deviation")
> # Outputting: Figure 5.7.
```

Remarks:

■ Figure 5.7 is a plot of the variation of the computed SDs with respect to the sample sizes, with a curve connecting the calculated values. It shows that as the sample sizes increase (to infinity), the SD asymptotically approaches the theoretical value of 10.

■ The outputs of the function fitdistr() included SEs in parentheses. These are used to give CIs for the estimates. These SEs and the corresponding 95% CIs (sd ± 1.96 × SE), have been calculated and are listed in Table 5.12.

■ The computed results support the use of the function fitdistr() to estimate parameters for known distributions and as a GoF test for these parameters.

TABLE 5.12 Using Function fitdistr() **to Find the SD in a Normal Distribution**

SAMPLE SIZE n	PREDICTED sd BY fitdistr()	SE	CI =(sd ± 1.96 × SE)
	10.00000 (Theoretical)	0	(10.00000–10.00000)
1000000	9.99917	0.00707	(9.99210–10.00624)
100000	9.9641	0.0223	(9.94180–9.98640)
10000	9.90678	0.07005	(9.83670–9.97680)
1000	9.888	0.221	(9.66700–10.10900)
100	8.335	0.589	(7.74600–8.92400)

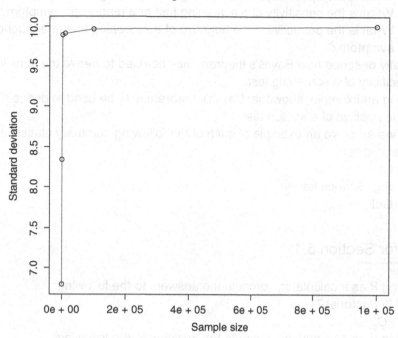

FIGURE 5.7 Using fitdistr() to check the SD in a normal distribution.

Further information on the R applications for GoF testing may be found in the updated CRAN package gof.

Review Questions for Section 5.1

1. (a) What is probability?
   (b) What is classical probability?
2. (a) Name and describe the three basic properties of probability.
   (b) What is the probability for complement events?
3. (a) Define the following, giving an example of each:
      (i) Conditional probability
      (ii) Joint probability
   (b) What is
      (i) the multiplication rule for probabilities?
      (ii) the addition rule for probabilities?
4. (a) What is marginal probability?
   (b) Give an example of this concept.
5. The following special R functions may be conveniently used in probability computations: factorial(), choose(), sample(), and prod(). Give an example of each of these functions as used for computing applications in probability applications.
6. In a 2 × 2 decision table showing the four possible outcomes from a standard dichotomous clinical testing process, what four questions must be addressed before

7. (a) What is the specificity of a screening test or a diagnostic symptom?
   (b) What is the sensitivity of a screening test or a diagnostic symptom?
   (c) What is the predictive value negative of a screening test or a diagnostic symptom?

8. Briefly describe how Bayes's theorem may be used to derive the sensitivity and specificity of a screening test.

9. Using an example, show that Bayes's theorem may be used to derive the predictive value positive of a screen test.

10. Define and give an example of each of the following summary statistics used in biostatistics:
    (a) CI
    (b) Significance levels
    (c) GoF

Exercises for Section 5.1

1. Using R as a calculator, compute the answers to the following:
   (a) 7! (factorial 7)
   (b) $^9C_5$

2. Using R as a calculator, compute the answers to the following:
   (a) Sampling, without replacement, 2 sets of 10 representative random numbers from a population of 2 million case subjects
   (b) Out of a patient population of 30 people, the health worker is preparing groups of 5 each for further clinical testing. How many groups may be combined, without concern for the order of testing within each group?

3. (a) With respect to the R function fivenum(), what is meant by the five-number summary in R?
   (b) From the set of the first 100 natural numbers, {1, 2, 3, ..., i, ..., 100}, use the R function summary() to obtain the summary statistics after obtaining the five-number summary for this set.

4. (a) What is meant by the Q–Q plot of a set of numbers?
   (b) Using the R function qqnorm(), obtain the Q–Q plot for a set of 1,000 normally distributed, randomly generated numbers.

5. *A one-sample t-test.*
   The daily calorie intake of 11 case subjects, in kilojoules (kJ), are 5,261, 5,674, 5,968, 6,275, 6,345, 6,587, 6,909, 7,021, 7,183, 8,251, and 8,650.
   (a) Compute some summary biostatistics for this dataset.
   (b) The recommended daily energy intake is 7,725 kJ. Assuming that this dataset is part of a normal distribution, calculate the mean (μ) of the dataset and compare it with the recommended daily energy intake value.

6. *A one-sample Wilcoxon signed-rank test.*
   (a) For the dataset in Exercise 5, use R to compute a one-sample Wilcoxon signed-rank test.
   (b) Compare the results with those from the one-sample *t*-test. Comment on these two results.

7. *An exercise in the calculation of significance tests.*

   (This exercise is based on a discussion by Dalgaard [2002, pp. 96ff.].)

   In the package ISwR is a data frame thuesen that consists of measurements of blood.glucose versus short.velocity for 24 case subjects. The following R code segment is used to obtain a linear model object lm to represent these two variables, followed by an analysis of the significance level of the model correlation.

   The complete R computation procedure is as follows:

```
> install.packages("ISwR")
> library(ISwR)
```
Attaching package: 'ISwR'

The following object(s) are masked from 'package:survival': lung
```
> ls("package:ISwR")
```

[1]	"alkfos"	"ashina"	"bcmort"	"bp.obese"
[5]	"caesar.shoe"	"coking"	"cystfibr"	"eba1977"
[9]	"energy"	"ewrates"	"fake.trypsin"	"graft.vs.host"
[13]	"heart.rate"	"hellung"	"IgM"	"intake"
[17]	"juul"	"juul2"	"kfm"	"lung"
[21]	"malaria"	"melanom"	"nickel"	"nickel.expand"
[25]	"philion"	"react"	"red.cell.folate"	"rmr"
[29]	"secher"	"secretin"	"stroke"	"tb.dilute"
[33]	"thuesen"	"tlc"	"vitcap"	"vitcap2"
[37]	"wright"	"zelazo"		

```
> data(thuesen)
> attach(thuesen)
> thuesen
```

	blood.glucose	short.velocity
1	15.3	1.76
2	10.8	1.34
3	8.1	1.27
4	19.5	1.47
5	7.2	1.27
6	5.3	1.49
7	9.3	1.31
8	11.1	1.09
9	7.5	1.18
10	12.2	1.22
11	6.7	1.25
12	5.2	1.19
13	19.0	1.95

14	15.1	1.28
15	6.7	1.52
16	8.6	NA
17	4.2	1.12
18	10.3	1.37
19	12.5	1.19
20	16.1	1.05
21	13.3	1.32
22	4.9	1.03
23	8.8	1.12
24	9.5	1.70

```
> lm(short.velocity ~ blood.glucose)
```

Call:
lm(formula = short.velocity ~ blood.glucose)
Coefficients:

(Intercept)	blood.glucose
1.09781	0.02196

```
> summary(lm(short.velocity ~ blood.glucose))
```

Call:
lm(formula = short.velocity ~ blood.glucose)
Residuals:

Min	1Q	Median	3Q	Max
−0.40141	−0.14760	−0.02202	0.03001	0.43490

Coefficients:

	Estimate	Std. Error	t value	Pr(>|t|)
(Intercept)	1.09781	0.11748	9.345	6.26e-09 ***
blood.glucose	0.02196	0.01045	2.101	0.0479 *

Signif. codes: 0 '***' 0.001 '**' 0.01 '*' 0.05 '.' 0.1 ' ' 1
Residual standard error: 0.2167 on 21 degrees of freedom (1 observation deleted due to missingness)
Multiple R-squared: 0.1737, Adjusted R-squared: 0.1343
F-statistic: 4.414 on 1 and 21 DF, p-value: 0.0479

```
> plot(blood.glucose, short.velocity) (Figure 5.8)
> abline(lm(short.velocity ~ blood.glucose)) (Figure 5.9)
>
```

With respect to the foregoing exercise in R computations:

(a) The tilde symbol (~) in the command > lm(short.velocity ~ blood.glucose) may be read as "described by." This command correlates the two variables short.velocity and blood.glucose. In this correlation, which component is

  (i) the *dependent* variable?

  (ii) the *independent* variable?

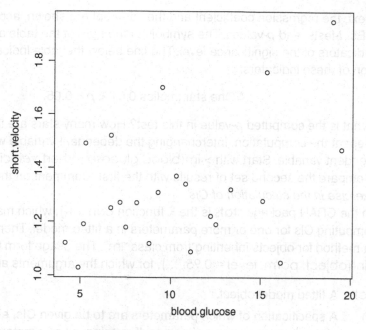

FIGURE 5.8 Scatter plot of data.

(b) Next, the basic extractor function summary() provides the information regarding the correlation. For a satisfactory correlation:

  (i) The average of the residuals is, by definition, zero. What is the median of the residuals?

  (ii) The maximum and minimum should be approximately equal in absolute value. What are the absolute values of the outputted maximum and minimum?

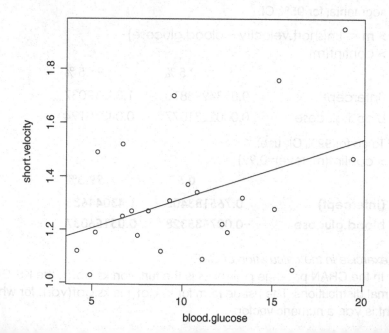

(c) Next, the regression coefficient and the intercept are shown, accompanied by SEs, *t*-tests, and *p*-values. The symbols to the right of the table are graphical indicators of the significance level. The line below the table indicates the definition of these indicators:

*One star implies $0.01 < p < 0.05$.

What is the computed *p*-value in this test? How many stars are there?

(d) Repeat the computation, interchanging the dependent variable with the independent variable. Start with > lm(blood.glucose ~ short.velocity)
Compare the second set of results with the first. Comment on the contrasts.

8. *An exercise in the calculation of CIs.*

In the CRAN package stats is the R function confint(), which may be used for computing CIs for one or more parameters in a fitted model. There is a default and a method for objects inheriting from class "lm". The usage form for confint() is confint(object, parm, level = 0.95, ...), for which the arguments are:

object   A fitted model object.

parm   A specification of which parameters are to be given CIs, either a vector of numbers or a vector of names. If missing, all parameters are considered.

level   The confidence level required.

          Additional argument(s) for methods.

confint() is a generic function. The default method assumes asymptotic normality. The default method can be called directly for comparison with other methods. For objects of class "lm", the direct formulas based on *t*-values are used.

(a) Compute the CI for the model object in Exercise 7 by the following R code segments, for 95% CI:

> m <- lm(short.velocity ~ blood.glucose)
> confint(m)

	2.5 %	97.5 %
(Intercept)	0.8534993816	1.34213037
blood.glucose	0.0002231077	0.04370194

(b) To go for 99% CI, use:
> confint(m, level=0.99)

	0.5%	99.5%
(Intercept)	**0.765183405**	**1.43044635**
blood.glucose	**−0.007635328**	**0.05156037**

>

9. *An exercise in the calculation of GoF.*

In the CRAN package pgirmess is the function ks.gof(), the KS GoF test for normal distributions. The usage form for ks.gof() is ks.gof(var), for which the argument is var, a numeric vector.

The following R code segment illustrates a simple GoF computation:

```
> install.packages("pgirmess")
> library(pgirmess)
> ls("package:pgirmess")
 [1] "CI                 classnum          cormat"
 [4] "correlog           date2winter       diag2edge"
 [7] "difshannonbio      dirProj           dirSeg"
[10] "distNNeigh         distNode          distSeg"
[13] "distTot            expandpoly        friedmanmc"
[16] "gps2gpx            kruskalmc         kruskalmc.default"
[19] "kruskalmc.formula  ks.gof            pairsrp"
[22] "pave               pclig             permcont"
[25] "PermTest           PermTest.glm      PermTest.lm"
[28] "PermTest.lme       piankabio         piankabioboot"
[31] "plot.correlog      polycirc          polycirc2"
[34] "postxt             print.clnum       print.correlog"
[37] "print.mc           print.PermTest    readGDALbbox"
[40] "readVista          rmls              rwhatbufCat"
[43] "rwhatbufCat2       rwhatbufNum       rwhatpoly"
[46] "Segments           selMod            selMod.list"
[49] "selMod.lm          shannon           shannonbio"
[52] "shannonbioboot     tabcont2categ     thintrack"
[55] "trans2pix          trans2seg         TukeyHSDs"
[58] "uploadGPS          val4symb          valchisq"
[61] "write.delim        writeGPX          writePRJ"
> # Let's try this on some normally distributed datasets:
> x<-rnorm(50) # Take a set of 50 randomly generated numbers
> x
 [1]  1.15482519  -0.05652142  -2.12936065   0.34484576  -1.90495545  -0.81117015
 [7]  1.32400432   0.61563685   1.09166896   0.30660486  -0.11015876  -0.92431277
[13]  1.59291375   0.04501060  -0.71512840   0.86522310   1.07444096   1.89565477
[19] -0.60299730  -0.39086782  -0.41622203  -0.37565742  -0.36663095  -0.29567745
[25]  1.44182041  -0.69753829  -0.38816751   0.65253645   1.12477245  -0.77211080
[31] -0.50808622   0.52362059   1.01775423  -0.25116459  -1.42999345   1.70912103
[37]  1.43506957  -0.71037115  -0.06506757  -1.75946874   0.56972297   1.61234680
[43] -1.63728065  -0.77956851  -0.64117693  -0.68113139  -2.03328560   0.50096356
[49] -1.53179814  -0.02499764
> ks.gof(x) # Outputting:
        One-sample Kolmogorov–Smirnov test
data: var
D = 0.0811, p-value = 0.8707
alternative hypothesis: two-sided
```

```
> ks.gof(blood.glucose) # Using the dataset from Exercise 8, outputting:
```
One-sample Kolmogorov–Smirnov test
data: var
D = 0.1148, p-value = 0.9097
alternative hypothesis: two-sided
Warning message:
In ks.test(var, "pnorm", mean(var), sd(var)):
ties should not be present for the Kolmogorov–Smirnov test
```
> x1 <- rnorm(10000) # Taking on a larger set of rnorm numbers:
> ks.gof(x1) # Outputting:
```
One-sample Kolmogorov–Smirnov test
data: var
D = 0.007, p-value = 0.718
alternative hypothesis: two-sided
```
> x2 <- rnorm(1000000) # For a still larger set of rnorm numbers:
> ks.gof(x2)
```
One-sample Kolmogorov–Smirnov test
data: var
D = 5e−04, p-value = 0.979
alternative hypothesis: two-sided

(a) What are the p-values obtained by this GoF test for a randomly generated and normally distributed set: 50, 100,000, and 1,000,000?
(b) Collect other sets of data, and use this simple procedure to test for normality.
(c) Increase the size of the datasets, and then repeat this test. How do the p-values vary progressively as the size of the datasets increases? Comment on the results.

10. gof: *Goodness-of-fit statistical software in* R.

A number of statistical software packages for computations in GoF analysis are available in the open-sourced R environment, available from the CRAN website (http://cran.r-project.org)

A typical contribution is:

cumres: calculating the cumulative residuals for generalized linear models (GLMs) within the package gof, which is developed as a GoF statistical software in R.

This software computes GoF measures for linear regression models lm(), including logistic and Poisson regression models, as well as generalized linear models glm(). These are illustrated as follows:

(i) the usage form of the class "lm" is
     cumres(model, …)
(ii) the usage form of the class "glm" is
     cumres(model,
           variable=c("predicted",colnames(model.matrix(model))),
           data=data.frame(model.matrix(model)),
           R=500, b=0, plots=min(R,50),
           seed=round(runif(1,1,1e9)),…)

in which the arguments are

model   Model object (lm or glm)
variable   List of variables to order the residuals after

R	Number of samples used in simulation
b	Moving average bandwidth (0 corresponds to infinity = standard cumulated residuals)
plots	Number of realizations to save for use in the plot routine
seed	Random seed
...	additional arguments

The computation returns as object of class "cumres".

A sample computation is shown in the following R code segment to illustrate the use of this GoF software, cumres(), to simulate a simple function: $f(x_1, x_2) = 10x_1 + x_2^2$, where both x_1 and x_2 are randomly generated, normally distributed independent variables:

```
> install.packages("gof")
> library(gof)
Loading 'gof' package...
Version : 0.8-1
> ls("package:gof")
[1] "cumres"
> sim1 <- function(n=100, f=function(x1,x2) {10+x1+x2^2},
+ sd=1, seed=1) {
+ if (!is.null(seed))
+ set.seed(seed)
+ x1 <- rnorm(n);
+ x2 <- rnorm(n)
+ X <- cbind(1,x1,x2)
+ y <- f(x1,x2) + rnorm(n,sd=sd)
+ d <- data.frame(y,x1,x2)
+ return(d)
+ }
> d <- sim1(100); l <- lm(y ~ x1 + x2,d)
> system.time(g <- cumres(l, R=100, plots=50))
user system elapsed
0.21 0.00 0.21
> g # Outputting:
Kolmogorov–Smirnov test: p-value = 0.32
Cramer–von Mises test: p-value = 0.36
Based on 100 realizations. Cumulated residuals ordered by predicted variable.
---

Kolmogorov–Smirnov test: p-value = 0.51
Cramer–von Mises test: p-value = 0.26
Based on 100 realizations. Cumulated residuals ordered by x1-variable.
---

Kolmogorov–Smirnov test: p-value = 0
Cramer–von Mises test: p-value = 0
Based on 100 realizations. Cumulated residuals ordered by x2-variable.
```

```
> plot(g) # Outputting: Figure 5.10.
> g1 <- cumres(l, c("y"), R=100, plots=50)
> g1 # Outputting:
```
Kolmogorov–Smirnov test: p-value = 0.26
Cramer–von Mises test: p-value = 0.32
Based on 100 realizations. Cumulated residuals ordered by predicted variable.

```
> plot(g1) # Outputting: Figure 5.11.
> g2 <- cumres(l, c("y"), R=100, plots=50, b=0.5)
> g2 # Outputting:
```
Kolmogorov–Smirnov test: p-value = 0.39
Cramer–von Mises test: p-value = 0.21
Based on 100 realizations. Cumulated residuals ordered by predicted variable.

```
> plot(g2) # Outputting: Figure 5.12.
>
```

(a) Consider the three plots for g, g1, and g2, respectively, shown in Figures 5.10, 5.11, and 5.12. What are the corresponding KS test p-values for these correlations?

(b) Inspect these three plots and note what happens as the p-values increase. Describe the graphical shapes of the corresponding correlation regressions.

(c) Of the three attempts to correlate, which provide the "best" correlation and the "worst" correlation? Why?

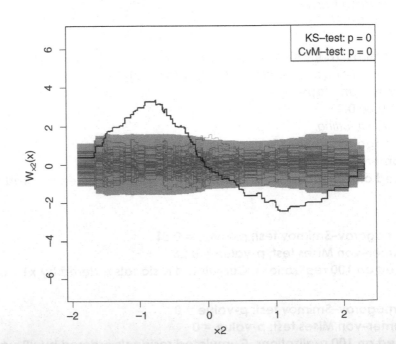

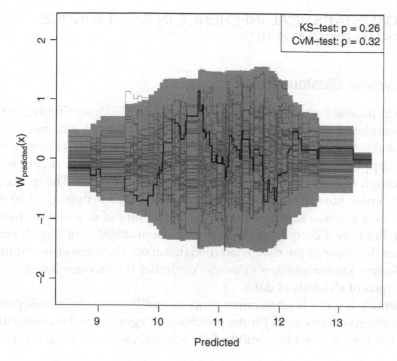

FIGURE 5.11 Plot of g1.

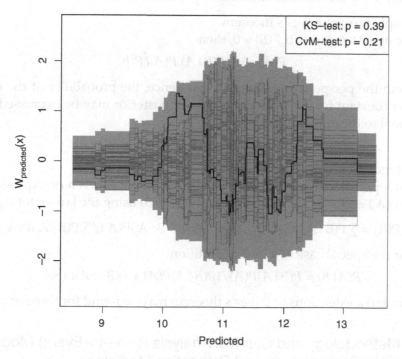

FIGURE 5.12 Plot of g2.

5.2 TYPICAL STATISTICAL INFERENCE IN BIOSTATISTICS: BAYESIAN BIOSTATISTICS

What Is Bayesian Biostatistics?

The term *Bayesian* refers to Thomas Bayes (1701–1761), an English mathematician who formulated a specific case of the theorem that bears his name.

Probability theory in the early 18th century arose to answer questions in gaming and to support applications in the new insurance business. A problem known as the question of *inverse probability* arose regarding the latter: The mathematicians of the time knew how to find the probability that, say, 5 people aged 50 would die in a given year out of a sample of 60 if the probability of any one of them dying was known. But they did not know how to find the probability of one 50-year-old dying based on the observation that 5 had died out of 60. The answer was found by Bayes. His solution, known as *Bayes's theorem*, underlies the modern Bayesian approach to the analysis of all kinds of data.

Scientific inquiry is an iterative process, and Bayesian inference provides a logical, quantitative framework for the process of integrating and accumulating information. It has been applied in a multitude of scientific, technological, and policy settings.

Bayes's Theorem in Probability Theory

One may view this seminal theorem in probabilistic terms.

- Simple form of Bayes's theorem
  For events A and B, if $P(B) \neq 0$, then

$$P(A \mid B) = P(B \mid A)\, P(A)/P(B) \qquad (5.2\text{-}1)$$

From the perspective of Bayesian inference, the probability of the existence of B is constant for all A_n models, and the posterior may be expressed as proportional to the numerator:

$$P(A_n \mid B) \; \alpha \; P(B \mid A_n)\, P(A_n) \qquad (5.2\text{-}2)$$

- Extended form of Bayes's theorem
  For a partitioning of the event space $\{A_i\}$, which is given or expressed in terms of $P(A_i)$ and $P(B \mid A_i)$, one may eliminate $P(B)$ using the law of total probability:

$$P(B) = \sum_j P(B \mid A_j)\, P(A_j) \Rightarrow P(A_i \mid B) = P(B \mid A_i)P(A_i)/\sum_j P(B \mid A_j)P(A_j) \qquad (5.2\text{-}3)$$

For the special case of a binary partition:

$$P(A \mid B) = P(B \mid A)P(A)/[P(B \mid A)P(A) + P(B \mid \neg A)P(\neg A)] \qquad (5.2\text{-}4)$$

Similarly, extensions of Bayes's theorem may be found for three or more events.

Bayesian Methodology and Survival Analysis (Time-to-Event) Models for Biostatistics in Epidemiology and Preventive Medicine

The application of Bayes's theorem in epidemiologic survival analysis is a seminal

methods. This approach is based on two sources: (1) the investigator's a priori belief in the characteristic of the survival function, when combined with (2) the data to form a **survival function**. This prior knowledge, which may be based on previous experiences with the behavior of similar processes as well as expert understanding, together contribute to an effective distribution for the **time-to-event** survival function.

The sample information is expressed in terms of a likelihood function. These two distinct sources of information are then combined by Bayes's theorem to produce the a posteriori distribution of the survival function, which is the distribution of the survival function for the given data.

In this approach, the parameters of the model are considered as random variables selected from the prior distribution. This prior distribution, a multivariate distribution on the parameters, is chosen to represent the investigator's a priori belief in the values of the parameters. They reflect the investigator's best estimates regarding the value of the parameters. The prior variance is a measure of the investigator's uncertainty in the prior means. In this analysis, the subject of interest is the survival function, also known as the *cumulative hazard function*.

BAYESIAN INFERENCE

Bayesian inference derives the *posterior probability* as a result of two antecedents: (a) a *prior probability* and (b) a likelihood function, which is derived from a probability model for the data to be observed. Bayesian inference then calculates the posterior probability according to Bayes's theorem:

$$P(A \mid B) = P(B \mid A) \, P(A)/P(B) \tag{5.2-1}$$

When applying Bayes's rule (another common name for Bayes's theorem), the evidence B corresponds to data that were not used in computing the prior probability. A represents any hypothesis whose probability may be affected by the observed data. (There may be competing hypotheses, and a decision will be made based on their relative probabilities.)

The interpretation of the factors in Bayes's theorem is as follows:

- $P(A \mid B)$, the **posterior**, is the probability of A *after* B is observed. This shows what the probabilities of different possible hypotheses are, given the observed evidence.
- $P(A)$, the **prior**, is the probability of A *before* B is observed. This reveals preconceived beliefs about how likely different hypotheses are.
- $P(A \mid B)$ is the **likelihood**. It indicates how likely it is that one will observe the evidence one actually observes, given a particular hypothesis; in other words, how compatible the evidence is with a given hypothesis.
- $P(B)$ is the **marginal likelihood** or "model evidence." This factor is the same for all possible hypotheses being considered. (This can be seen by the fact that the hypothesis A does not appear anywhere in the symbol, unlike for all the other factors.) This means that this factor does not enter into the determination of the relative probabilities of different hypotheses.

Note that only the factors $P(A)$ and $P(B \mid A)$ affect the value of $P(A \mid B)$ for different values of A. Both appear in the numerator, and hence the posterior probability

The posterior probability of a hypothesis is determined by a combination of the inherent likeliness of a hypothesis (the prior) and the compatibility of the observed evidence with the hypothesis (the likelihood).

Stated in a more concise and technical fashion: *Posterior is proportional to prior times likelihood.*

Note that Bayes's rule can also be written as follows:

$$P(A \mid B) = [P(B \mid A)/P(B)] \times P(A) \qquad\qquad (5.2\text{-}5)$$

The factor $[P(B \mid A)/P(B)]$ represents the impact of B on the probability of A. From a logical viewpoint, Bayes's theorem makes good sense. If the evidence does not match up with a hypothesis, one is unlikely to believe the hypothesis. However, if one thinks a hypothesis is extremely unlikely a priori, one is also unlikely to believe it even if the evidence does appear to match up.

For example, imagine that you have various hypotheses about the nature of a newborn baby. If you are presented with evidence in the form of a picture of a black-haired baby boy, you are likely to believe that the baby is indeed a boy and does indeed have black hair, and less likely to believe that the baby is actually a blonde-haired girl, as the evidence does not agree with this latter hypothesis. In contrast, if you are presented with evidence in the form of a picture of a baby dog, then you are unlikely to believe that the baby is actually a dog, as your prior belief in this hypothesis (that a human can give birth to a dog) is untenable.

Thus, Bayesian inference provides a systematic way of combining prior beliefs with new evidence, through the application of Bayes's theorem. This is in contradistinction to frequentist inference, which depends only on the evidence as a whole, with no reference to prior beliefs.

Bayes's theorem can also be applied iteratively and repeatedly. After observing some evidence, the resulting posterior probability can then be treated as a prior probability, and a *new* posterior probability computed from new evidence. This permits the Bayesian principles to be applied to various kinds of evidence, whether viewed all at once or over time. This procedure, called *Bayesian updating,* is widely used and computationally efficient.

SURVIVAL ANALYSIS

In clinical research and studies, an investigator often monitors the progress of case subjects under treatment from a specific point in time (such as when a drug treatment regimen is initiated or a critical surgical procedure is undertaken) until the occurrence and/or recurrence of some specific event (such as a cessation of critical symptoms or death). For example, a group of patients who have each had a first myocardial infarction (heart attack) are enrolled in a 2-year (January 1, 2011 through January 1, 2013) investigation to assess the effectiveness of two new competing drugs for the prevention of a second attack. The study commences when the first case subject, following the first heart attack, is enrolled in the program, and continues until each case subject experiences one of three events:

1. The event of interest (a heart attack),
2. Loss to follow-up, for reasons such as death from a cause other than a heart attack or ceasing study participation, or

For each case subject, the investigator records the duration (in years, months, days, etc.) elapsing between the point at which the case subject entered the study and at which the case subject experienced one of the terminating events. The time elapsing between enrollment and experiencing one of the events is the subject's **survival time**. The dataset of such survival times is the **survival data**.

Consider the following information on four case subjects in the study of heart-attack patients, case subjects A, B, C, and D:

- Case subject A entered the investigation on January 1, 2011, and had a heart attack on December 31, 2012.
- Case subject B entered the study on July 1, 2011, and moved out of town on December 31, 2011.
- Case subject C entered the investigation on September 1, 2011, and died on July 1, 2012 from a cause other than a heart attack.
- Case subject entered the program on August 1, 2011, and was still alive when the study program ended on December 31, 2012.

Hence:

- Case subject A's survival time is 24 months.
- Case subject B's survival time is 6 months. This is called a **censored survival time** because the terminating event was loss to follow-up rather than an event of interest.
- Case subject C's survival time is 9 months.
- Case subject D's survival time is 17 months. This is also a censored survival time.

The survival times for case subjects B and D are both referred to (more generally) as **censored data.**

The times spent in the study by these four case subjects are represented graphically in Figure 5.13.

In studies that compare the efficacies of two treatments, A and B, three items of information are of interest for each case subject:

1. Which treatment, A or B, did the case subject receive?
2. For what duration was the case subject observed?
3. Did the case subject experience the event of interest during the study, or was the case subject either alive at the end of the study or lost to follow-up?

In studies not concerned with comparative treatments or other special characteristics of the case subjects, only the latter two items are needed, With these three items of information, one may estimate the median survival time of the group receiving Treatment A, and compare that with the estimated median survival time of the group receiving Treatment B. Comparison of the two medians would provide critical information:

- Which treatment may delay for a longer period of time (on the average) the recurrence of the event of interest (in this example, the occurrence of another heart attack)?

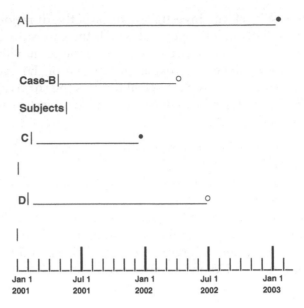

FIGURE 5.13   Four case subjects entering an epidemiologic study at different times with known (o) and censored (•) survival times.

■   What is the estimated probability that a case subject will survive for a specific period of time? The clinician conducting such a study might ask: "What is the probability that, after the first heart attack, a patient receiving Treatment A (or B) will survive for more than two years?"

The method used to address these types of questions, by using the information collected during a follow-up study, is called **survival analysis**.

SURVIVAL ANALYSIS USING THE KAPLAN–MEIER PROCEDURE.   The Kaplan–Meier (K–M) procedure, introduced by Kaplan and Meier (1958), consists of successive multiplication of individual estimated probabilities. It is also known as the **product-limit method** of estimating survival probabilities. The K–M procedure calls for computation of the proportions of case subjects in a sample who survive for various lengths of time. These sample proportions are then used as estimates of the probabilities of survival that one would expect to observe in the population represented by the sample. In essence, this process estimates a survivorship function. Frequency and probability distributions may then be constructed from observed survival times. These observed distributions may show evidence of conforming to some known theoretical distributions.

When the form of the sampled distribution is unknown, the estimation of a survivorship function may be accomplished by means of a nonparametric technique, such as the K–M procedure. Let:

n = the number of case subjects whose survival times are available

p_1 = the proportion of case subjects surviving at least the first time period (days, months, years, etc.)

p_2 = the proportion of case subjects surviving the second time period after having survived the first time period

p_3 = the proportion of case subjects surviving the third time period after having survived the second time period

p_k = the proportion of case subjects surviving the kth time period after having survived the $(k-1)$th time period

Using these proportions, we can relabel $p_1, p_2, p_3, \ldots, p_k$ as estimates of the probability that a case subject from the population represented by the sample will survive time periods 1, 2, 3, ..., k, respectively.

For any time period t, $1 \le t \le k$, one may estimate the probability of surviving the tth time period, p_t, as follows.

■ Number of case subjects surviving at least $(t-1)$ time periods:

$$p_t = \frac{\text{Number of case subjects who also survive the } t\text{th time period}}{\text{Number of case subjects alive at the end of time period } (t-1)} \tag{5.2-6}$$

Then the probability of surviving to time t, $S(t)$, is estimated by

$$\underline{S}(t) = \underline{p}_1 \times \underline{p}_2 \times \underline{p}_3 \times \cdots \times \underline{p}_t \tag{5.2-7}$$

THE K–M PROCEDURE USING R. R provides two functions that can be used in survival analysis:

1. The function survfit(), in the package survival
2. The function Surv(), also in the package survival

In R, the function survfit() creates survival curves from either a formula (e.g., K–M), a previously fitted Cox model, or a previously fitted accelerated failure time model. Its formal usage takes the following form:

> survfit(formula, ...)

in which the arguments are:

Formula	Either a formula or a previously fitted model
...	Other arguments specific to the chosen method

A *survival curve* is based on a tabulation of the number at risk and number of events at each unique death time. For further details, see the documentation for the appropriate method: either ?survfit.formula or ?survfit.coxph.

Also, in the R package survival, the function Surv() creates a *survival object*, typically as a response in a model formula. Its usage takes the following form:

> Surv(time, time2, event,
        type=c('right', 'left', 'interval', 'counting', 'interval2'), origin=0)

in which the arguments are:

time	For right-censored data, this is the follow-up time. For interval data, the first argument is the starting time for the interval.

event	The status indicator—normally 0 = alive, 1 = dead. Other choices are TRUE/FALSE (TRUE = death) or 1/2 (2 = death). For interval-censored data, the status indicators are 0 = right-censored, 1 = event at time, 2 = left-censored, 3 = interval-censored. Although unusual, the event indicator can be omitted, in which case all subjects are assumed to have had an event.
time2	Ending time of the interval for interval-censored or counting-process data only. Intervals are assumed to be open on the left and closed on the right [start, end]. For counting-process data, event indicates whether an event occurred at the end of the interval.
type	Character string specifying the type of censoring. Possible values are "right", "left", "counting", "interval", and "interval2". The default is "right" or "counting", depending on whether the time2 argument is absent or present, respectively.
origin	For counting-process data, this is the hazard function origin. This option was intended to be used in conjunction with a model containing time-dependent strata, so as to align the subjects properly when they cross over from one stratum to another, but it has rarely proven useful.
x	Any R object.

Application of the K–M procedure in the R environment is illustrated in the following examples.

■ **Example 5.20** Survival analysis using R in glioma radioimmunotherapy (Hastie & Tibshirani, 1990)

A *glioma* is a type of tumor that starts in the brain or spine (most commonly in the brain). It is so named because it arises from glial cells.

Treatment for brain gliomas depends on the location, the cell type, and the grade of malignancy. Often, treatment takes a combined approach, using surgery, radioimmunotherapy (RIT), and chemotherapy. The RIT is usually in the form of external beam radiation.

To assess the clinical effectiveness of loco-regional RIT, the survival times for case subjects from a control group and a treated group (the latter containing case subjects who were treated with a special therapy) may be biostatistically assessed by graphically plotting the K–M estimates of the respective survival times.

Using the glioma data file and applying the K–M procedure, compare results of the two groups of (Histology = Grade 3) case subjects: *Treated* and *Control*. Repeat the analysis for all Male subjects only.

Solution:
The following R code segments may be used:
```
> install.packages("survival") # First, install the survival package.
> library(survival) # Next, bring up the files in survival
```

Loading required package: splines
> install.packages("coin") # *Next, install the* coin *package.*
> library(coin) # *Then bring up the files in* coin.

Loading required package: mvtnorm
Loading required package: modeltools

Loading required package: stats4
> ls("package:coin") # *Inspecting the files in* coin *for* glioma:

[1] "alpha"	"alzheimer"	"ansari_test"
[4] "ansari_trafo"	"approximate"	"asat"
[7] "asymptotic"	"chisq_test"	"cmh_test"
[10] "consal_trafo"	"covariance"	"CWD"
[13] "dperm"	"exact"	"ExactNullDistribution"
[16] "expectation"	"f_trafo"	"fligner_test"
[19] "fligner_trafo"	"fmaxstat_trafo"	"friedman_test"
[22] "glioma"	"hohnloser"	"id_trafo"
[25] "independence_test"	"jobsatisfaction"	"kruskal_test"
[28] "lbl_test"	"logrank_trafo"	"maxstat_test"
[31] "maxstat_trafo"	"median_test"	"median_trafo"
[34] "mercuryfish"	"mh_test"	"neuropathy"
[37] "normal_test"	"normal_trafo"	"ocarcinoma"
[40] "of_trafo"	"oneway_test"	"photocar"
[43] "pperm"	"pvalue"	"qperm"
[46] "rotarod"	"spearman_test"	"sphase"
[49] "statistic"	"support"	"surv_test"
[52] "symmetry_test"	"trafo"	"treepipit"
[55] "variance"	"wilcox_test"	"wilcoxsign_test"

> attach(glioma) # *Bringing up the data frame* glioma
The following object(s) are masked from 'jasa':
age
> data(glioma) # *Getting the data frame* glioma *ready for analysis*
> glioma # *Taking an inside look at* glioma

	no.	age	sex	histology	group	event	time
1	1	41	Female	Grade3	RIT	TRUE	53
2	2	45	Female	Grade3	RIT	FALSE	28
3	3	48	Male	Grade3	RIT	FALSE	69
4	4	54	Male	Grade3	RIT	FALSE	58
5	5	40	Female	Grade3	RIT	FALSE	54
6	6	31	Male	Grade3	RIT	TRUE	25
7	7	53	Male	Grade3	RIT	FALSE	51
8	8	49	Male	Grade3	RIT	FALSE	61
9	9	36	Male	Grade3	RIT	FALSE	57
10	10	52	Male	Grade3	RIT	FALSE	57

11	11	57	Male	Grade3	RIT	FALSE	50
12	12	55	Female	GBM	RIT	FALSE	43
13	13	70	Male	GBM	RIT	TRUE	20
14	14	39	Female	GBM	RIT	TRUE	14
15	15	40	Female	GBM	RIT	FALSE	36
16	16	47	Female	GBM	RIT	FALSE	59
17	17	58	Male	GBM	RIT	TRUE	31
18	18	40	Female	GBM	RIT	TRUE	14
19	19	36	Male	GBM	RIT	TRUE	36
20	1	27	Male	Grade3	Control	TRUE	34
21	2	32	Male	Grade3	Control	TRUE	32
22	3	53	Female	Grade3	Control	TRUE	9
23	4	46	Male	Grade3	Control	TRUE	19
24	5	33	Female	Grade3	Control	FALSE	50
25	6	19	Female	Grade3	Control	FALSE	48
26	7	32	Female	GBM	Control	TRUE	8
27	8	70	Male	GBM	Control	TRUE	8
28	9	72	Male	GBM	Control	TRUE	11
29	10	46	Male	GBM	Control	TRUE	12
30	11	44	Male	GBM	Control	TRUE	15
31	12	83	Female	GBM	Control	TRUE	5
32	13	57	Female	GBM	Control	TRUE	8
33	14	71	Female	GBM	Control	TRUE	8
34	15	61	Male	GBM	Control	TRUE	6
35	16	65	Male	GBM	Control	TRUE	14
36	17	50	Male	GBM	Control	TRUE	13
37	18	42	Female	GBM	Control	TRUE	25

> # *Selecting the required sample for analysis:* Grade3 *in* histology
> g3 <-subset(glioma, histology == "Grade3") # *and naming it* g3
> g3 # *Checking* g3: *17 Grade 3 subjects out of 37 subjects are found*

	no.	age	sex	histology	group	event	time
1	1	41	Female	Grade3	RIT	TRUE	53
2	2	45	Female	Grade3	RIT	FALSE	28
3	3	48	Male	Grade3	RIT	FALSE	69
4	4	54	Male	Grade3	RIT	FALSE	58
5	5	40	Female	Grade3	RIT	FALSE	54
6	6	31	Male	Grade3	RIT	TRUE	25
7	7	53	Male	Grade3	RIT	FALSE	51

9	9	36	Male	Grade3	RIT	FALSE	57
10	10	52	Male	Grade3	RIT	FALSE	57
11	11	57	Male	Grade3	RIT	FALSE	50
20	1	27	Male	Grade3	Control	TRUE	34
21	2	32	Male	Grade3	Control	TRUE	32
22	3	53	Female	Grade3	Control	TRUE	9
23	4	46	Male	Grade3	Control	TRUE	19
24	5	33	Female	Grade3	Control	FALSE	50
25	6	19	Female	Grade3	Control	FALSE	48

```
>
> # Here comes the K-M procedure:
> # Obtain the Surv() object, then apply the function survfit(), and plot()
> plot(survfit(Surv(time, event) ~ group, data = g3),
+   main = "Grade III Glioma", lty = 2, col=c("red", "green"),
+   xlab = "Survival Time (months)",
+   ylab = "Probability Value",
+ )
> # Outputting the K-M curve: Figure 5.14.
```

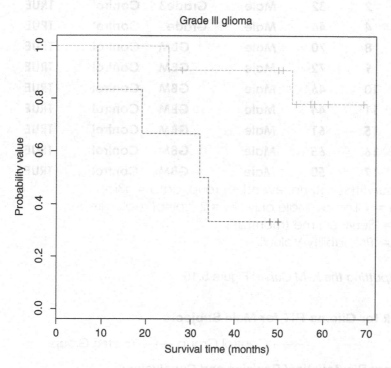

FIGURE 5.14 Bayesian survival analysis by the K–M procedure.

Using R for Glioma RIT for Grade 3 Subjects

To undertake the same analysis for all Male subjects only, the following R code segments may be used:

```
>
> g3m <- subset(glioma, sex == "Male")
> g3m # 21 Male subjects out of 37 subjects are found
```

	no.	age	sex	histology	group	event	time
3	3	48	Male	Grade3	RIT	FALSE	69
4	4	54	Male	Grade3	RIT	FALSE	58
6	6	31	Male	Grade3	RIT	TRUE	25
7	7	53	Male	Grade3	RIT	FALSE	51
8	8	49	Male	Grade3	RIT	FALSE	61
9	9	36	Male	Grade3	RIT	FALSE	57
10	10	52	Male	Grade3	RIT	FALSE	57
11	11	57	Male	Grade3	RIT	FALSE	50
13	13	70	Male	GBM	RIT	TRUE	20
17	17	58	Male	GBM	RIT	TRUE	31
19	19	36	Male	GBM	RIT	TRUE	36
20	1	27	Male	Grade3	Control	TRUE	34
21	2	32	Male	Grade3	Control	TRUE	32
23	4	46	Male	Grade3	Control	TRUE	19
27	8	70	Male	GBM	Control	TRUE	8
28	9	72	Male	GBM	Control	TRUE	11
29	10	46	Male	GBM	Control	TRUE	12
30	11	44	Male	GBM	Control	TRUE	15
34	15	61	Male	GBM	Control	TRUE	6
35	16	65	Male	GBM	Control	TRUE	14
36	17	50	Male	GBM	Control	TRUE	13

```
> plot(survfit(Surv(time, event) ~ group, data = g3m),
+ main = "Glioma - Male only", lty = 2, col=c("red", "green"),
+ xlab = "Survival Time (months)",
+ ylab = "Probability Value",
+ )
> # Outputting the K-M Curve: Figure 5.15.
```

Using R for Glioma RIT for Male Subjects

------- Control Group -------Treated Group

Summary Biostatistical Decision and Conclusion:
The computed K–M curves graphically show that the survival probability for the Treated group is higher than for the Control group. Figure 5.14 shows that for Grade III case subjects, at about 48 months (4 years), the survival probability for the Treated group is

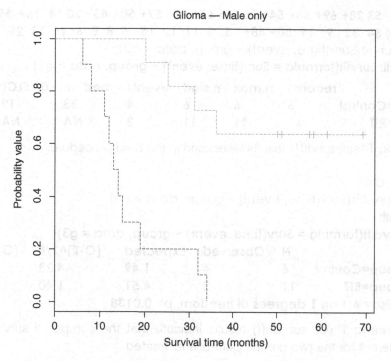

FIGURE 5.15   Bayesian survival analysis by the K–M procedure.

From Figure 5.15, a similar result is evident for the all-male sample. Thus, on the basis of the survival time analysis alone, it appears that glioma patients may derive considerable benefits from the RIT treatment; this indicates both the efficacy and effectiveness of the treatment.

However, the total population size is limited, and other tests may be used to support the tentative conclusion reached based on this K–M analysis.

Further Analysis:

A number of additional analyses may be undertaken in R to further investigate (and possibly lend support to) the preliminary conclusion, including survfit(), survdiff(), and surv-test(). Detailed descriptions of these classes of test may be obtained from the R environment, using the format (e.g., for survfit()): > ??survfit)

- survfit(), in the package survival, computes an estimate of a survival curve for censored data using either the K–M procedure or another method. For competing risks data, it computes the cumulative incidence curve.
- survdiff(), also in the package survival, tests if there is a difference between two or more survival curves using a special family of tests, or for a single curve against a known alternative.
- surv_test(), in the package coin, tests the equality of survival distributions in two or more independent groups.

The following are the respective results of these three classes of tests:

1.   survfit()

```
[1]   53 28+ 69+ 58+ 54+ 25 51+ 61+ 57+ 57+ 50+ 43+ 20 14  36+  59+  31  14  36
[20] 34  32  9  19 50+ 48+  8  8  11  12  15  5  8  8  6  14  13  25
> survfit(Surv(time, event) ~ group, data = g3)
Call: survfit(formula = Surv(time, event) ~ group, data = g3)
```

	records	n.max	n.start	events	median	0.95LCL	0.95UCL
group=Control	6	6	6	4	33	19	NA
group=RIT	11	11	11	2	NA	NA	NA

Remark: These survfit() results were used in the K–M procedure.

2. survdiff()

```
> survdiff(Surv(time, event) ~ group, data = g3)
Call:
survdiff(formula = Surv(time, event) ~ group, data = g3)
```

	N	Observed	Expected	(O-E)^2/E	(O-E)^2/V
group=Control	6	4	1.49	4.23	6.06
group=RIT	11	2	4.51	1.40	6.06

Chisq= 6.1 on 1 degrees of freedom, p= 0.0138

Remark: These survdiff() results indicate that the computed survival times are different for the two groups Control and Treated.

3. surv_test()

```
> surv_test(Surv(time, event) ~ group, data = g3)
        Asymptotic Logrank Test
data: Surv(time, event) by group (Control, RIT)
Z = 2.1711, p-value = 0.02992
alternative hypothesis: two.sided
```

Remark: These surv_test() results also indicate that the computed survival times are different for the two groups Control and Treated. This test may be applied for case subjects with GRADE4 (GBM = *glioblastoma multiforme*) glioma, as follows:

```
> g4 <-subset(glioma, histology == "GBM")
> surv_test(Surv(time, event) ~ group, data = g4,
+               distribution = "exact")
        Exact Logrank Test
data: Surv(time, event) by group (Control, RIT)
Z = 3.2215, p-value = 0.0001588
alternative hypothesis: two.sided
```

Remarks: The same difference is evident.

To test whether the new treatment is indeed superior for both groups of tumors simultaneously, the same test may be used by *stratifying* with respect to the tumor grading:

```
> surv_test(Surv(time, event) ~ group | histology,
+               data = glioma, distribution = approximate(B = 1000000))
        Approximative Logrank Test
```

group (Control, RIT)
stratified by histology
Z = 3.6704, p-value = 7.8e − 05
alternative hypothesis: two.sided

Remark: Once more, the computed results are consonant with the initial findings.

■ **Example 5.21:** Survival analysis using R: Applying the K–M procedure to an acute myelogenous leukemia (AML) data file

Survival analyses may be undertaken using the computational resources of the survival package.

(a) Use the survfit function and obtain a summary of the survival estimation.
(b) Compare and contrast the K–M procedure with the approach from the viewpoint of frequentist probability.

Solution:
Results of analyses using the K–M procedure may be applied using the following R code segment:

(a) Using the function summary():
> summary(leukemia.surv) # *Outputting:*
Call: survfit(formula = Surv(time, status) ~ x, data = aml)

x=Maintained

time	n.risk	n.event	survival	std.err	lower 95% CI	upper 95% CI
9	11	1	0.909	0.0867	0.7541	1.000
13	10	1	0.818	0.1163	0.6192	1.000
18	8	1	0.716	0.1397	0.4884	1.000
23	7	1	0.614	0.1526	0.3769	0.999
31	5	1	0.491	0.1642	0.2549	0.946
34	4	1	0.368	0.1627	0.1549	0.875
48	2	1	0.184	0.1535	0.0359	0.944

x=Nonmaintained

time	n.risk	n.event	survival	std.err	lower 95% CI	upper 95% CI
5	12	2	0.8333	0.1076	0.6470	1.000
8	10	2	0.6667	0.1361	0.4468	0.995
12	8	1	0.5833	0.1423	0.3616	0.941
23	6	1	0.4861	0.1481	0.2675	0.883
27	5	1	0.3889	0.1470	0.1854	0.816
30	4	1	0.2917	0.1387	0.1148	0.741
33	3	1	0.1944	0.1219	0.0569	0.664

| 45 | 1 | 1 | 0.0000 | NaN | NA | NA |

> leukemia.surv # *Outputting:*

Call: survfit(formula = Surv(time, status) ~ x, data = aml)

	records	n.max	n.start	events	median	0.95LCL	0.95UCL
x=Maintained	11	11	11	7	31	18	NA
x=Nonmaintained	12	12	12	11	23	8	NA

From a frequentist statistician viewpoint, a number of significance tests may be used to test the null hypothesis, such as

$$H_0 : F_1 = F_2,$$

in which F_1 and F_2 are the frequencies of occurrence for cases with and without censoring.

Empirical Survivor Function (esf): $S_n(t)$

Treating the data aml *as if there were no censoring,*

$$S_n(t) = \frac{Number\,of\,Observations > t}{n} = \frac{\#(t_i - t)}{n} \qquad (5.2\text{-}8)$$

In this equation, $S_n(t)$ is the proportion of patients still in remission after t weeks.

Let aml1 be the data subset of the Maintained group of aml. Then, on a timeline:

esf	Calculations:										
t	0	9	13	18	23	28	31	34	45	48	161
# (ti – t)	11	10	8	7	6	5	4	3	2	1	0
Sn(t)	11/11	10/11	8/11	7/11	6/11	5/11	4/11	3/11	2/11	1/11	0

The plot of this empirical survivor function (esf) function, $S_n(t)$ versus t, is shown in Figure 5.16.

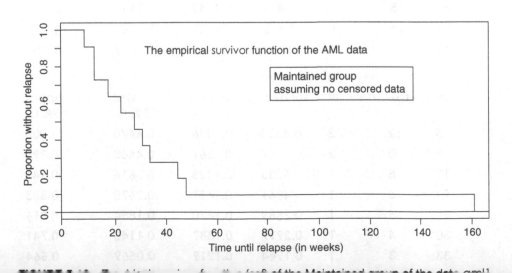

Remarks:

(a) The **esf** is a consistent estimator of the true survivor function $S(t)$. The exact distribution of $nS_n(t)$, for each fixed t, is binomial (n, p), where n = the number of observations and $p = P(T > t)$.

(b) From the central limit theorem, it follows that for each fixed t, $S_n(t)$ is approximately distributed as Normal $\{p, p(1 - p)/n\}$.

(c) The esf may be compared with the product-limit estimator of survival, commonly called the *Kaplan–Meier estimator (K–M estimator)*. The K–M curve is a right continuous step function that steps down only at an uncensored observation.

(d) A plot of the K–M curve for the aml1 data, together with the esf curve, is shown in Figure 5.17. The "+" on the K–M curve represents the survival probability at a censored time.

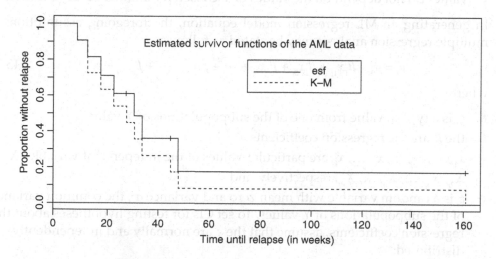

FIGURE 5.17 K–M and esf estimates of survival.

(e) Note the difference between the two curves: The K–M is always greater than or equal to esf. When there are no censored data values, K–M reduces to esf.

(f) The K–M curve does not reach down to zero, as the largest survival time (161+) is censored.

The "redistribute-to-the-right" algorithm considers a censored patient's potential contribution as being equally redistributed among all patients at risk of failure *after* the censored time.

Summary Biostatistical Decision and Conclusion:
Each of the two graphical displays, Figures 5.16 and 5.17, again shows that the esf results closely follow those of the K–M procedure. Although the latter shows a more realistic presentation, the conclusion drawn from both approaches would be in general agreement.

INTRODUCTION TO THE MULTIPLE LINEAR REGRESSION MODEL (DANIEL, 2005). In the multiple linear (ML) regression model, it is *assumed* that a linear relationship exists between some dependent variable Y and n independent variables: $X_1, X_2, X_3, ...,$

The X_i are also known as *explanatory variables* or *predictor variables*.
The following assumptions underlie ML regression analysis:

1. X_i are nonrandom fixed variables (this assumption is in contradistinction to the multiple correlation model). This condition means that any inferences drawn from sample data apply only to the set of X values observed, and *not* to other larger collections of Xs.
2. For each set of X_i values, there is a subpopulation of Y values. To construct the CI and to test hypotheses, the subpopulation must be known unless one may assume that these subpopulations of Y values are normally distributed. This assumption will be made in the first instance.
3. The variances of the subpopulations of Y are all equal.
4. The Y values are independent; that is, the values of Y chosen for one set of X values do not depend on the values of Y chosen for another set of X values.

In generating an ML regression model equation, the foregoing assumptions for multiple regression analysis may be stated as follows:

$$y_j = \beta_0 + \beta_1 x_{1j} + \beta_2 x_{2j} + \beta_3 x_{3j} + \cdots + \beta_i x_{ij} + \cdots + \beta_n x_{nj} + \varepsilon_j \qquad (5.2\text{-}9)$$

where

▪ y_j is a typical value from one of the subpopulations of Y values,
▪ the β_i are the regression coefficients,
▪ $x_{1j}, x_{2j}, x_{3j}, \ldots, x_{ij}, \ldots, x_{kj}$ are particular values of the independent variables $X_{1j}, X_{2j}, X_{3j}, \ldots, X_{ij}, \ldots, X_{nj}$ respectively, and
▪ ε_j is a random variable with mean zero and variance σ^2, the common variance of the subpopulations of Y values. To set CIs for testing hypotheses about the regression coefficients, assume that the ε_j are normally and independently distributed.

Estimates of the parameters $\beta_0, \beta_1, \beta_2, \beta_3, \ldots, \beta_j, \ldots, \beta_k$ of the ML regression model specified in Equation (5.2-9) may be obtained by the *method of least squares:* the sum of the squared deviations of the observed values of Y from the resulting regression surface in the minimized state.

SURVIVAL ANALYSIS USING THE COX REGRESSION MODEL (PROPORTIONAL HAZARDS). Regression techniques are available when the dependent measures consist of a mixture of either time-to-event data or censored time observations. The **Cox regression model**, also known as *proportional hazards*, is an approach in applied statistics used to account for the effects of continuous and discrete covariate (independent variable) measurements when the dependent variable is possibly censored time-to-event data. The model is also commonly applied to Bayesian survival analyses.

The hazard function, $h(t_i)$, describes the conditional probability that an event will occur at a time just exceeding t_i, conditional on having survived event-free until time t_i. This conditional probability, known as the **instantaneous failure rate** at time t_i, is written as $h(t_i)$. The regression model requires one to assume that the covariates have the effect of either increasing or decreasing the hazard for a particular case subject, as compared to some baseline value for the function.

Thus, in a typical clinical trial, one might measure n covariates on each of the case subjects, where there are $I = 1, 2, 3, \ldots, i, \ldots, n$ subjects, and $h_0(t_i)$ is the **baseline hazard function**. The regression model may now be written as

$$h(t_i) = h_0(t) \exp(\beta_1 z_{i1} + \beta_2 z_{i2} + \beta_3 z_{i3} + \cdots + \beta_i z_{ii} + \cdots + \beta_n z_{in}) \qquad (5.2\text{-}10)$$

The regression coefficients represent the changes in the hazard that results from the risk factor, z_{in}, that was measured. Recasting Equation (5.2-10) shows that the exponentiated coefficient represents the *hazard ratio*, or the ratio of the conditional probabilities of an event. This is the basis for calling this method the **proportional hazards regression**:

$$[h(t_i)/h_0(t)] = \exp(\beta_1 z_{i1} + \beta_2 z_{i2} + \beta_3 z_{i3} + \cdots + \beta_i z_{ii} + \cdots + \beta_n z_{in}) \qquad (5.2\text{-}11)$$

Estimation of the covariate effects, $\{\beta\}$, may best be achieved using statistical software, such as in the **R** environment.

THE COX REGRESSION MODEL (PROPORTIONAL HAZARDS) USING R. When applied to survival analysis, the Cox regression model is similar to linear models, lm, or generalized linear models, glm, in that it assumes linearity in the log-hazard scale. Models are then fitted using the maximization of the Cox likelihood (which is *not* a true likelihood function, although it may be used as one). Survival is then calculated as the product of conditional likelihoods of the observed time to event.

The procedure in R generally begins by computing the coxph objects, using the function coxph(), in the package survival. This class of objects is returned by the coxph class of functions to represent a fitted proportional hazards model. Objects of this class have methods for the functions print, summary, residuals, predict, and survfit.

Application of the Cox regression model (the proportional hazards) in the R environment is illustrated in the following example.

■ **Example 5.22:** Survival analysis using R: Applying the Cox regression model (the proportional hazards technique) to the ovarian cancer data file ovarian in the package survival

This example is taken from the package survival in the CRAN website[3] (entitled "cox. zph—Test the Proportional Hazards Assumption of a Cox Regression Model Fit (coxph)," dated February 15, 2012).

Solution:
The R function cox.zph() has the following usage form:

cox.zph(fit, transform="km", global=TRUE)

in which the arguments are:

fit	The result of fitting a Cox regression model using the function coxph().
transform	A character string specifying how the survival times should be transformed before the test is performed. Possible values are "km", "rank", "identity", or a function of one argument.

---

global   Asks whether a global chi-square test should be done in addition to the per-variable tests.

Moreover, an object of the class "cox.zph" has the following components:

table   A matrix with one row for each variable, and optionally a last row for the global test. Columns of the matrix contain the correlation coefficient between the transformed survival time and the scaled Schoenfeld residuals, a chi-square, and the two-sided p-value. For the global test, there is no appropriate correlation, so NA is entered into the matrix as a placeholder.

x   The transformed time axis.

y   The matrix of scaled Schoenfeld residuals. There will be one column per variable and one row per event. The row labels contain the original event times (for the identity transform, these will be the same as x).

call   The calling sequence for the routine.

The computations require the original x matrix of the Cox model fit. Thus, it saves time if the x=TRUE option is used in coxph. This function is usually followed by both a plot and a print of the result. The plot gives an estimate of the time-dependent coefficient beta(t). *If the proportional hazards assumption is true*, beta(t) will be *a horizontal line*. The printout gives a test for slope=0.

The Cox regression model may be applied using the following R code segment:

```
> install.packages("survival")
> library(survival)
```

Loading required package: splines

```
> ls("package:survival") # Looking for the data frame ovarian:
```

[1] "aareg"	"aml"	"attrassign"
[4] "basehaz"	"bladder"	"bladder1"
[7] "bladder2"	"cancer"	"cch"
[10] "cgd"	"clogit"	"cluster"
[13] "colon"	"cox.zph"	"coxph"
[16] "coxph.control"	"coxph.detail"	"coxph.fit"
[19] "dsurvreg"	"format.Surv"	"frailty"
[22] "frailty.gamma"	"frailty.gaussian"	"frailty.t"
[25] "heart"	"is.na.coxph.penalty"	"is.na.ratetable"
[28] "is.na.Surv"	"is.ratetable"	"is.Surv"
[31] "jasa"	"jasa1"	"kidney"
[34] "labels.survreg"	"leukemia"	"logan"
[37] "lung"	"match.ratetable"	"mgus"
[40] "mgus1"	"mgus2"	"nwtco"
[43] "ovarian"	"pbc"	"pbcseq"
[46] "pspline"	"psurvreg"	"pyears"
[49] "qsurvreg"	"ratetable"	"ratetableDate"
[52] "rats"	"ridge"	"stanford2"
[55] "strata"	"Surv"	"survConcordance"

[61] "survexp.us"	"survexp.usr"	"survfit"
[64] "survfitcoxph.fit"	"survobrien"	"survreg"
[67] "survreg.control"	"survreg.distributions"	"survreg.fit"
[70] "survregDtest"	"survSplit"	"tcut"
[73] "tobin"	"tt"	"untangle.specials"
[76] "veteran"		

> data(ovarian)

> ovarian # *Inspecting the data frame*:

	futime	fustat	age	resid.ds	rx	ecog.ps
1	59	1	72.3315	2	1	1
2	115	1	74.4932	2	1	1
3	156	1	66.4658	2	1	2
4	421	0	53.3644	2	2	1
5	431	1	50.3397	2	1	1
6	448	0	56.4301	1	1	2
7	464	1	56.9370	2	2	2
8	475	1	59.8548	2	2	2
9	477	0	64.1753	2	1	1
10	563	1	55.1781	1	2	2
11	638	1	56.7562	1	1	2
12	744	0	50.1096	1	2	1
13	769	0	59.6301	2	2	2
14	770	0	57.0521	2	2	1
15	803	0	39.2712	1	1	1
16	855	0	43.1233	1	1	2
17	1040	0	38.8932	2	1	2
18	1106	0	44.6000	1	1	1
19	1129	0	53.9068	1	2	1
20	1206	0	44.2055	2	2	1
21	1227	0	59.5890	1	2	2
22	268	1	74.5041	2	1	2
23	329	1	43.1370	2	1	1
24	353	1	63.2192	1	2	2
25	365	1	64.4247	2	2	1
26	377	0	58.3096	1	2	1

> attach(ovarian)
> fit <- coxph(Surv(futime, fustat) ~ age + ecog.ps,
+   data=ovarian)

```
> print(temp) # Displaying the results:
```

	rho	chisq	p
age	−0.243	0.856	0.355
ecog.ps	0.520	2.545	0.111
GLOBAL	NA	3.195	0.202

```
> plot(temp) # Plotting curves.
> # Outputting: Figure 5.18.
>
```

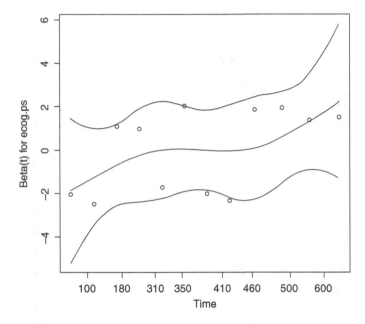

FIGURE 5.18 cox.zph() fitting: The plot gives an estimate of the time-dependent coefficient beta(t). If the proportional hazards assumption is true, beta(t) will be a horizontal line. The printout gives a test for slope = 0.

The Inverse Bayes Formula

The inverse Bayes formula (IBF) is an important statistical tool in distribution theory and Bayesian missing-data problems (examples can be seen in Tan, Tian, and Ng [2010], among others). Earlier in 1997, Ng provided a form of IBF essentially for product measurable space (PMS), and recognized that IBF is potentially useful in computing marginals and checking compatibility. Moreover, Tian and Tan (Ng & Tong, 2010) provided a form of modified IBF in nonproduct measurable space (NPMS) and gave some applications, extending the concept to the **generalized inverse Bayes formula (GIBF).**

In the Bayesian literature, one traditionally expresses the posterior distribution in terms of the prior distribution. In 1995, K. W. Ng introduced the point-wise **IBF** in order to emphasize its unconventional character, in that *the prior distribution may*

In standard Bayesian notation, one uses $\pi(\theta)$ to denote the prior probability density function (pdf) of parameter θ with support $S(\Theta)$; $L(y \mid \mu)$ to denote the likelihood function (i.e., the pdf of data, given the parameter) with support $S(Y \mid \theta)$; $p(\theta \mid y)$ to denote the posterior pdf with support $S(\Theta \mid Y)$ of parameter given the data; and $f(y)$ to denote the unconditional pdf for the data with support $S(Y)$. Both θ and y may be vectors.

Note that, in general, the projection of $S(Y \mid \theta)$ into $S(Y)$ is a subset:

$$S(Y \mid \theta) \subset S(Y) \tag{5.2-12A}$$

and the equality

$$S(Y \mid \theta) = S(Y) \tag{5.2-12B}$$

may hold for some θ.

With respect to integral or probability, the latter is essentially the same as when the complement of the projection of $S(Y \mid \theta)$ into $S(Y)$ is a set of measure zero. If the joint support $S(\theta, Y)$ equals the product space $S(\Theta) \times S(Y)$, then:

$$S(Y \mid \theta) = S(Y) \tag{5.2-13}$$

for all θ, and vice versa. A similar relationship holds true between $S(\Theta \mid y)$ and $S(\Theta)$.

From the joint pdf identity, $L(y \mid \theta)\pi(\theta) = p(\theta \mid y)f(y)$, the Bayes formula

$$p(\theta \mid y) = \pi(\theta)L(y \mid \theta) / \int_{S(\theta \mid y)} \pi(\theta)L(Y \mid \theta)d\theta \tag{5.2-14}$$

results by a substitution of $f(y)$, which is expressed as the integral of the joint pdf with respect to θ over $S(\Theta \mid y)$. One may rewrite this joint pdf identity as $\pi(\theta)L(y \mid \theta)/p(\theta \mid y) = f(y)$, where (θ, y) is in the joint support $S(\Theta, Y)$. Now, for any fixed θ, one may integrate both sides of the re-expressed joint pdf identity with respect to y over $S(Y \mid \theta)$ and obtain the prior pdf at θ:

$$\pi(\theta) = \int_{S(Y \mid \theta)} f(y)dy \left\{ \int_{S(Y \mid \theta)} \left[L(y \mid \theta)/p(\theta \mid y) \right] \right\}^{-1} \tag{5.2-15A}$$

$$\leq \left\{ \int_{S(Y \mid \theta)} \left[L(y \mid \theta)/p(\theta \mid y) \right] \right\}^{-1} \tag{5.2-15B}$$

where the equality holds if and only if $S(Y \mid \theta) = S(Y)$, or the complement of the projection of $S(Y \mid \theta)$ into $S(Y)$ is a set of measure zero.

In particular, under the so-called positivity assumption, where

$$S(\Theta, Y) = S(\Theta) \times S(Y) \tag{5.2-16}$$

one has

$$\pi(\theta) = \left\{ \int_{S(Y \mid \theta)} \left[L(y \mid \theta) / p(\theta / y) \right] dy \right\}^{-1} \tag{5.2-17}$$

The explicit form of Equation (5.2-17) was not found in the general literature of classical Bayesian statistics. This may be due to the tradition in the Bayesian literature

called Equation (5.2-17) the (pointwise) **IBF** to emphasize its unconventional character, in that *the prior distribution is expressed in terms of the posterior distribution*. In fact, it is the harmonic mean of $p(\theta \mid y)$ with respect to $L(y \mid \theta)$.

DERIVATIONS OF THREE FORMS OF THE INVERSE BAYES FORMULA (TAN, TIAN, & NG, 2010)

From the Bayes formula, one may derive three IBFs involving integration in the support of a random variable. To do so, it is necessary to consider two notions: the **product measurable space (PMS)** and the **nonproduct measurable space (NPMS)**.

Let two random variables (or vectors) (X, Y), taking values in the spaces $(\mathcal{X}, \mathcal{Y})$, respectively, be absolutely continuous with respect to some measure μ on the *joint* support:

$$S = S_{(X, Y)} = \{(x, y): f_{(X, Y)}(x, y) > 0, (x, y) \in (\mathcal{X}, \mathcal{Y})\} \qquad (5.2\text{-}18)$$

where $f_{(X, Y)}(x, y)$ denotes the joint probability density function (pdf) of (X, Y).

Now, denote the marginal and conditional pdfs of X and Y by $f_X(x)$, $f_Y(y)$, $f_{(X \mid Y)}(x \mid y)$, and $f_{(Y \mid X)}(y \mid x)$, respectively. Let

$$S_X = \{x: f_X(x) > 0, x \in \mathcal{X}\} \qquad (5.2\text{-}19)$$

and

$$S_Y = \{y: f_Y(y) > 0, y \in \mathcal{Y}\} \qquad (5.2\text{-}20)$$

denote the supports of X and Y, respectively.

If

$$S_{(X, Y)} = S_X \times S_Y \qquad (5.2\text{-}21)$$

then the measure μ is *product measurable*, and μ may be written as $\mu_X \times \mu_Y$; otherwise, it is *nonproduct measurable*.

The absolute continuous assumption allows consideration of a continuous variable (whose density is Lebesgue measurable) with a discrete variable (its probability mass function gives rise to a counting measure). To apply this concept, one may denote the conditional supports of $X \mid (Y = y)$ and $Y \mid (X = x)$ as follows:

$$S_{(X \mid Y)}(y) = \{x: f_{(X \mid Y)}(x \mid y) > 0, x \in \mathcal{X}\} \; \forall \, y \in S_Y \qquad (5.2\text{-}22)$$

$$S_{(Y \mid X)}(x) = \{y: f_{(Y \mid X)}(y \mid x) > 0, y \in \mathcal{Y}\} \; \forall \, x \in S_X \qquad (5.2\text{-}23)$$

In practice, one usually has

$$S_{(Y \mid X)}(x) \subseteq S_Y \; \forall \, x \in S_X \qquad (5.2\text{-}24)$$

and

$$S_{(X \mid Y)}(x) \subseteq S_X \; \forall \, y \in S_Y \qquad (5.2\text{-}25)$$

so that the joint pdf becomes

$$f_{(X \mid Y)}(x \mid y) f_Y(y) = f_{(Y \mid X)}(y \mid x) f_X(x), \; \forall \, (x, y) \in S_{(X, Y)} \qquad (5.2\text{-}26)$$

In PMSs, one has

$$S_{(Y\mid X)}(x) = S_Y, \forall\, x \in S_X \tag{5.2-27}$$

and

$$S_{(X\mid Y)}(x) = S_X \,\forall\, y \in S_Y \tag{5.2-28}$$

Hence, from Equation (5.2-26), one obtains by division:

$$f_Y(y) = \left[f_{(Y\mid X)}(y\mid x) / f_{(X\mid Y)}(x\mid y) \right] f_X(x), \forall\, x \in S_X, \text{and } \forall\, y \in S_Y \tag{5.2-29A}$$

Integrating the identity (5.2-29A) with respect to y, on support S_Y, one obtains:

$$\int f_Y(y)\,dy = \int \left\{ \left[f_{(Y\mid X)}(y\mid x) / f_{(X\mid Y)}(x\mid y) \right] f_X(x) \right\}$$

$$1 = \int \left\{ \left[f_{(Y\mid X)}(y\mid x) / f_{(X\mid Y)}(x\mid y) \right] f_X(x) \right\} dy$$

$$= f_X(x) \left\{ \int \left[f_{(Y\mid X)}(y\mid x) / f_{(X\mid Y)}(x\mid y) \right] dy \right\}$$

Because x and y are independent, one gets

$$f_X(x) = \left\{ \int_{S_Y} \left[f_{(Y\mid X)}(y\mid x) / f_{(Y\mid X)}(x\mid y) \right] dy \right\}^{-1}, \forall\, x \in S_x \tag{5.2-30A}$$

which is the pointwise IBF for $X(x)$.

The dual form of Equation (5.2-29A) is

$$f_X(x) = \left[f_{(X\mid Y)}(x\mid y) / f_{(Y\mid X)}(y\mid x) \right] f_Y(y), \forall\, x \in S_X, \text{and } \forall\, y \in S_Y \tag{5.2-29B}$$

whereas the dual form of Equation (5.2-30A) is

$$f_Y(y) = \left\{ \int_{S_X} \left[f_{(X\mid Y)}(x\mid y) / f_{(Y\mid X)}(y\mid x) \right] dx \right\}^{-1}, \forall\, y \in S_Y \tag{5.2-30B}$$

On substituting $f_Y(y)$ from Equation (5.2-30B) into Equation (5.2-29B), one obtains

$$f_X(x) = \left\{ \int_{S_X} \left[f_{(X\mid Y)}(x\mid y) / f_{(Y\mid X)}(y\mid x) \right] dx \right\}^{-1} \left[f_{(X\mid Y)}(x\mid y) / f_{(Y\mid X)}(y\mid x) \right], \forall\, (x,y) \in S_{(X,Y)}$$

$$= \left\{ \int_{S_X} \left[f_{(X\mid Y)}(x\mid y_0) / f_{(Y\mid X)}(y_0\mid x) \right] dx \right\}^{-1} \left[f_{(X\mid Y)}(x\mid y_0) / f_{(Y\mid X)}(y_0\mid x) \right]$$

$$\forall\, x \in S_X, \text{and } \forall \text{ arbitrarily fixed } y_0 \in S_Y \tag{5.2-31A}$$

which is the **functionwise IBF** for $X(x)$.

Finally, upon omitting the normalizing constant in Equation (5.2-31A), one obtains

$$f_X(x) \propto \left[f_{(X\mid Y)}(x\mid y_0) / f_{(Y\mid X)}(y_0\mid x) \right], \forall\, x \in S_X, \text{and } \forall \text{ arbitrarily fixed } y_0 \in S_Y \tag{5.2-32A}$$

Clearly, the corresponding dual forms of Equations (5.2-30A), (5.2-31A), and (5.2-32A) may be readily stated, for $f_Y(y)$, by interchanging $X(x)$ with $Y(y)$, as the corresponding IBFs for $Y(y)$:

$$f_Y(y) = \left\{ \int_{S_X} \left[f_{(X|Y)}(x \mid y) / f_{(Y|X)}(y \mid x) \right] dx \right\}^{-1}, \forall y \in S_Y \qquad (5.2\text{-}30B)$$

$$f_Y(y) = \left\{ \int_{S_Y} \left[f_{(Y|X)}(y \mid x_0) / f_{(X|Y)}(x_0 \mid y) \right] dy \right\}^{-1} \left[f_{(Y|X)}(y \mid x_0) / f_{(X|Y)}(x_0 \mid y) \right],$$

$$\forall\, y \in S_Y, \text{ and } \forall \text{ arbitrarily fixed } x_0 \in S_X \qquad (5.2\text{-}31B)$$

and

$$f_Y(y) \propto \left[f_{(Y|X)}(y \mid x_0) / f_{(X|Y)}(x_0 \mid y) \right], \forall y \in S_Y, \text{and } \forall \text{ arbitrarily fixed } x_0 \in S_X \quad (5.2\text{-}32B)$$

These are the corresponding **pointwise IBF** for $Y(y)$, **functionwise IBF** for $Y(y)$, and **sampling IBF** for $Y(y)$, respectively.

The following example illustrates the application of IBF for obtaining prior probabilities from posterior probabilities.

■ **Example 5.23:** An application of the inverse Bayes formula (Ng & Tong, 2010)

This example shows a direct application of the **pointwise IBF** for $Y(y)$, using Equation (5.2-30B) to obtain the prior probability of $f_Y(y)$ from the information available in the posterior probabilities of the system.

Consider the following conditional probability densities:

$$f_{X|Y}(x|y) = 1/2\sqrt{(1 - y^2)}$$

$$-\sqrt{(1 - y^2)} < x < \sqrt{(1 - y^2)}$$

$$-1 < y < 1$$

and

$$f_{Y|X}(y|x) = 1/2\sqrt{(1 - x^2)}$$

$$-\sqrt{(1 - x^2)} < y < \sqrt{(1 - x^2)}$$

$$-1 < x < 1$$

The support S_{XY} is the *interior* of the unit disk: with center (0, 0) and radius 1 unit. $f_{X|Y}(x|y)/f_{Y|X}(y|x)$ is defined only on S_{XY}, along the circumference of the unit disk.

To calculate $f_Y(y)$, consider a positive extension function of $f_{X|Y}(x|y)/f_{Y|X}(y|x)$ on the space $(-1, 1) \times (-1, 1)$. Set

$$u(x) = \sqrt{(1 - x^2)}, \text{ for } 1 < x < 1; \text{ and } v(y) = 1/\sqrt{(1 - y^2)}, \text{ for } 1 < y < 1$$

Then, $r(x, y) = u(x) \, v(y)$ may be considered as representing $f_{X|Y}(x|y)/f_{Y|X}(y|x)$ on the space $(-1, 1) \times (-1, 1)$. Moreover, applying the pointwise IBF by using Equation (5.2-30B), we get

$$f_Y(y) = \left\{\int_{S_X}\left[f_{(X|Y)}(x|y) / f_{(Y|X)}(y|x)\right]dx\right\}^{-1}, \forall\, y \in S_Y \qquad (5.2\text{-}30\text{B})$$

$$f_Y(y) = \left[\int_{-1}^{1} u(x)\,v(y)\,dx\right]^{-1}$$

$$= \left[\int_{-1}^{1}\sqrt{(1-x^2)} \,/ \sqrt{(1-y^2)}\,dx\right]^{-1}$$

$$= 2\sqrt{(1-y^2)}\,/\,\pi, \text{ for all } -1 < y < 1, \text{ as required}$$

■ **Example 5.24:** An application of the posterior distribution simulation using R

Within the currently available CRAN packages, there are application packages that use posterior simulation to obtain Bayesian inference. For example, the function MCMCregress(), in the package MCMCpack, uses Markov Chain Monte Carlo for Gaussian linear regression.

This function MCMCregress() generates a sample from the posterior distribution of a linear regression model with Gaussian errors using Gibbs sampling (with a multivariate Gaussian prior on the beta vector and an inverse gamma prior on the conditional error variance). The user must supply data and priors, and a sample from the posterior distribution is returned as an mcmc object, which can subsequently be analyzed with functions provided in the coda package.

Theoretical Background of the Application of the Function

MCMCregress()
MCMCregress() simulates from the posterior distribution using standard Gibbs sampling (a multivariate Normal draw for the betas, and an inverse Gamma draw for the conditional error variance). The simulation proper is performed in compiled C++ code to maximize efficiency; consult the coda documentation for a comprehensive list of functions that can be used to analyze the posterior sample.

The model takes the following form:

$$y_i = x'_I \beta + \varepsilon_i \qquad (5.2\text{-}33)$$

where the errors are assumed to be Gaussian, as follows:

$$\varepsilon_i \sim \mathcal{N}(0, \sigma^2) \qquad (5.2\text{-}34)$$

Assuming standard, semiconjugate priors:

$$B \sim \mathcal{N}(b_0, B_0^{-1}) \qquad (5.2\text{-}35)$$

and

$$\sigma^2 \sim \mathcal{G}amma(c_0/2, d_0/2) \qquad (5.2\text{-}36)$$

Note that only starting values for β are allowed because the simulation is done using Gibbs sampling with the conditional error variance as the first block in the sampler.

The value of the function MCMCregress() is an mcmc object that contains the posterior sample. This object can be summarized by functions provided by the coda package.

The R code for this example is

```
line <- list(X = c(-2,-1,0,1,2), Y = c(1,3,3,3,5))
posterior <- MCMCregress(Y~X, data=line, verbose=1000)
plot(posterior)
raftery.diag(posterior)
summary(posterior)
```

This example is run using the following R code segment:

```
> install.packages("MCMCpack")
> library(MCMCpack)
```

Loading required package: coda
Loading required package: lattice
Loading required package: MASS
##
Markov Chain Monte Carlo Package (MCMCpack)
Copyright (C) 2003-2012 Andrew D. Martin, Kevin M. Quinn, and Jong Hee Park
##
Support provided by the U.S. National Science Foundation
(Grants SES-0350646 and SES-0350613)
##

```
> ls("package:MCMCpack") # Noting the function MCMCregress()
```

[1] "BayesFactor"	"choicevar"	"ddirichlet"
[4] "dinvgamma"	"diwish"	"dnoncenhypergeom"
[7] "dtomogplot"	"dwish"	"HMMpanelFE"
[10] "HMMpanelRE"	"make.breaklist"	"MCbinomialbeta"
[13] "MCMCbinaryChange"	"MCMCdynamicEI"	"MCMCdynamicIRT1d"
[16] "MCMCfactanal"	"MCMChierEI"	"MCMChlogit"
[19] "MCMChpoisson"	"MCMChregress"	"MCMCirt1d"
[22] "MCMCirtHier1d"	"MCMCirtKd"	"MCMCirtKdHet"
[25] "MCMCirtKdRob"	"MCMClogit"	"MCMCmetrop1R"
[28] "MCMCmixfactanal"	"MCMCmnl"	"MCMCoprobit"
[31] "MCMCoprobitChange"	"MCMCordfactanal"	"MCMCpoisson"
[34] "MCMCpoissonChange"	"MCMCprobit"	"MCMCprobitChange"
[37] "MCMCquantreg"	"MCMCregress"	"MCMCSVDreg"
[40] "MCMCtobit"	"MCmultinomdirichlet"	"MCnormalnormal"
[43] "MCpoissongamma"	"mptable"	"plotChangepoint"
[46] "plotState"	"PostProbMod"	"procrustes"
[49] "rdirichlet"	"read.Scythe"	"rinvgamma"
[52] "riwish"	"rnoncenhypergeom"	"rwish"
[55] "SSVSquantreg"	"testpanelGroupBreak"	"testpanelSubjectBreak"
[58] "tomogplot"	"topmodels"	"vech"
[61] "write.Scythe"	"xpnd"	

```
> library(lattice)
> library(coda)
> library(MASS)
> line <- list(X = c(-2,-1,0,1,2), Y = c(1,3,3,3,5))
> posterior <- MCMCregress(Y~X, data=line, verbose=1000)
> # Outputting:
```

MCMCregress iteration 1 of 11000
beta =
  3.11989
  0.80906
sigma2 =   0.27278

MCMCregress iteration 1001 of 11000
beta =
  2.87038
  0.80699
sigma2 =   0.38403

MCMCregress iteration 2001 of 11000
beta =
  3.75130
  0.44314
sigma2 =   0.77820

MCMCregress iteration 3001 of 11000
beta =
  3.72461
  0.97119
sigma2 =   1.33523

MCMCregress iteration 4001 of 11000
beta =
  2.79921
  0.58334
sigma2 =   0.80892

MCMCregress iteration 5001 of 11000
beta =
  3.06049
  0.99932
sigma2 =   0.35595

MCMCregress iteration 6001 of 11000
beta =
  3.09242
  0.68169
sigma2 =   1.37335

```
MCMCregress iteration 7001 of 11000
beta =
   3.21538
   1.35860
sigma2 =   5.18619

MCMCregress iteration 8001 of 11000
beta =
   3.13608
   0.81812
sigma2 =   1.46922

MCMCregress iteration 9001 of 11000
beta =
   3.40301
   1.43191
sigma2 =   2.76159

MCMCregress iteration 10001 of 11000
beta =
   4.78574
   2.30508
sigma2 =   3.57808
```

> plot(posterior) # *Outputting several plots, summarized in* Figure 5.19.
> raftery.diag(posterior) # *Outputting:*

Quantile (q) = 0.025
Accuracy (r) = +/−0.005
Probability (s) = 0.95

	Burn-in (M)	Total (N)	Lower bound (Nmin)	Dependence factor (I)
(Intercept)	3	4374	3746	1.17
X	3	4374	3746	1.17
sigma2	2	3865	3746	1.03

> summary(posterior)

Iterations = 1001:11000
Thinning interval = 1
Number of chains = 1
Sample size per chain = 10000

1. **Empirical mean and standard deviation for each variable, plus standard error of the mean:**

	Mean	SD	Naive SE	Time-series SE
(Intercept)	3.013	0.5459	0.005459	0.005948
X	0.807	0.3873	0.003873	0.004647
sigma2	1.510	5.0969	0.050969	0.084921

2. Quantiles for each variable:

	2.5%	25%	50%	75%	97.5%
(Intercept)	2.04394	2.7552	3.0043	3.2483	4.083
X	0.05681	0.6287	0.8047	0.9769	1.562
sigma2	0.17091	0.3876	0.6837	1.3395	7.155

```
>
> line <- list(X = c(-2,-1,0,1,2), Y = c(1,3,3,3,5))
> line # Outputting:
$X
[1] -2 -1 0 1 2

$Y
[1] 1 3 3 3 5
> posterior <- MCMCregress(Y~X, data=line, verbose=1000)
> plot(posterior)
> # Outputting: Figure 5.19.
```

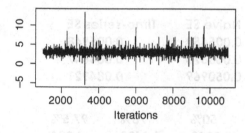

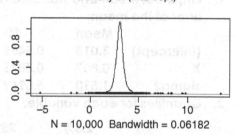

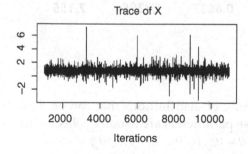

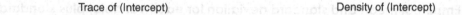

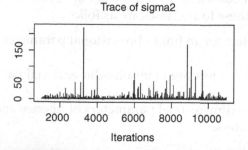

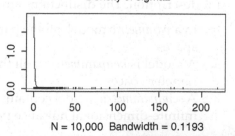

```
> raftery.diag(posterior) # Outputting:
Quantile (q) = 0.025
Accuracy (r) = +/-0.005
Probability (s) = 0.95
```

	Burn-in (M)	Total (N)	Lower bound (Nmin)	Dependence factor (I)
(Intercept)	3	4374	3746	1.17
X	3	4374	3746	1.17
sigma2	2	3865	3746	1.03

```
> summary(posterior) # Outputting:
Iterations = 1001:11000
Thinning interval = 1
Number of chains = 1
Sample size per chain = 10000
```

1. Empirical mean and standard deviation for each variable, plus standard error of the mean:

	Mean	SD	Naive SE	Time-series SE
(Intercept)	3.013	0.5459	0.005459	0.005948
X	0.807	0.3873	0.003873	0.004647
sigma2	1.510	5.0969	0.050969	0.084921

2. Quantiles for each variable:

	2.5%	25%	50%	75%	97.5%
(Intercept)	2.04394	2.7552	3.0043	3.2483	4.083
X	0.05681	0.6287	0.8047	0.9769	1.562
sigma2	0.17091	0.3876	0.6837	1.3395	7.155

```
>
```

Modeling in Biostatistics

In biostatistics, a *parametric model* is a family of distributions that can be described using a finite number of parameters. These parameters are usually collected to form a single n-dimensional parameter vector $\theta = (\theta_1, \theta_2, \theta_3, \ldots, \theta_i, \ldots, \theta_n)$.

Parametric models are contrasted with semiparametric, semi-nonparametric, and nonparametric models, all of which consist of an infinite set of "parameters" for description. The distinctions among these four classes are as follows:

- In a *parametric* model, all the parameters are in finite-dimensional parameter spaces.
- A model is *nonparametric* if all the parameters are in infinite-dimensional parameter spaces.
- A *semiparametric* model contains finite-dimensional parameters of interest and infinite-dimensional nuisance parameters.

■   A *semi-nonparametric* model has both finite-dimensional and infinite-dimensional unknown parameters of interest.

Among the modeling tools available in the CRAN packages, two important ones are selected for discussion here:

1.   The CRAN package grofit for estimating dose–response curves
2.   The CRAN packages gam (generalized additive model, gam[x]) by Hastie and Tibshirani (1990); and gamair[y] (Wood, 2006)

These models favor the *nonparametric* approach, use techniques derived from numerical analysis and approximation theory, and are generally applicable to all biostatistical applications. They are both readily adaptable to computations using R.

THE CRAN PACKAGE GROFIT FOR ESTIMATING DOSE–RESPONSE CURVES

The package grofit was developed to fit many growth curves obtained under different conditions in order to derive a conclusive dose–response curve. For instance, for a compound that may affect growth, grofit fits data to different parametric models using function gcFitModel(), and also provides a model-free spline fit using function gcFitSpline() to circumvent systematic errors that might occur with the application of parametric methods.

Also within the package grofit, the R functions drFitSpline() and drBootSpline() may be used to generate a table with estimates for **half maximal effective concentration (EC50)** and associated statistics. The term *half maximal effective concentration* (EC50) refers to the concentration of a drug, antibody, or toxicant that induces a response halfway between the baseline and maximum after some specified exposure time. It is commonly used as a measure of the potency of a drug.

The EC50 of a graded dose–response curve therefore represents the concentration of a compound at which 50% of its maximal effect is observed. The EC50 of a quantal dose–response curve represents the concentration of a compound where 50% of the population exhibits a response, after a specified exposure duration. It is also related to IC50, which is a measure of a compound's inhibition (50% inhibition). For competition binding assays, functional antagonist assays, and agonist/stimulator assays, EC50 is the most common summary measure of the dose–response curve. Responses to concentration typically follow a sigmoidal curve, increasing rapidly over a relatively small change in concentration. The **inflection point** at which the increase in effectiveness with increasing concentration begins to slow is the EC50. This can be determined mathematically by derivation of the best-fit line. Although relying on a graph for estimation is more convenient, it yields less precise and less accurate results.

Within the CRAN package grofit, the R function gcFitModel(x,y) may be used for general modeling tasks.

THE CRAN PACKAGES gam AND gamair

This subsection introduces GAM, the generalized additive model (Hastir & Tibshirani, 1990; Wood, 2006).[4]

Let Y be a response random variable and $X_1, X_2, X_3, \ldots, X_i, \ldots, X_n$ be a set of predictor variables. A regression procedure may be considered as a method for estimating how the value of Y depends on the values of $X_1, \ldots, X_n$. The standard linear regression model assumes that the expected value of Y has a linear form. The expected value of Y, $E[Y]$ is calculated as follows:

$$= f(X_1, X_2, X_3, \ldots, X_i, \ldots, X_n) \qquad (5.2\text{-}37A)$$

$$= \beta_0 + \beta_1 X_1 + \beta_2 X_2 + \beta_3 X_3 + \ldots + \beta_i X_i + \ldots + \beta_n X_n \qquad (5.2\text{-}37B)$$

Given a sample of values for Y and X, estimates of $\beta_0, \beta_1, \beta_2, \beta_3, \ldots, \beta_i, \ldots, \beta_n$ are usually obtained by the least squares method.

The additive model generalizes the linear model by modeling the expected value of Y as

$$E(Y) = f(X_1, X_2, X_3, \ldots, X_i, \ldots, X_n) \qquad (5.2\text{-}38A)$$

$$= s_0 + s_1(X_1) + s_2(X_2) + s_3(X_3) + \ldots + s_i(X_i) + \ldots s_n(X_n) \qquad (5.2\text{-}38B)$$

where $s_i(X)$, $i = 1, \ldots, n$ are smooth functions. These functions are to be estimated in a *nonparametric* approach.

GAM extends traditional linear models in another way, by allowing for a link between $f(X_1, \ldots, X_n)$ and the expected value of Y. This amounts to allowing an alternative distribution for the underlying random variation *besides just the normal distribution*. Although Gaussian models can be used in many statistical applications, there are types of problems for which they are not appropriate. The normal distribution may not be adequate for modeling categorical variables, discrete responses such as counts, or bounded responses such as proportions.

GAM consists of a **random component**, an **additive component**, and a **link function** relating these two components. The response Y, the random component, is assumed to have a density in the exponential family:

$$f_Y(y; \theta; \phi) = \exp\{[\{y\theta - b(\theta)\} / a(\phi)] + c(y, \phi)\} \qquad (5.2\text{-}39)$$

where θ is called the *natural parameter* and ϕ is the *scale parameter*. The normal, binomial, and Poisson distributions are all in this family. The quantity

$$\eta = s_0 + \sum_{i=1}^{n} s_i(X_i) \qquad (5.2\text{-}40)$$

where $s_1(\cdot), \ldots, s_n(\cdot)$ are smooth functions, defines the additive component. Finally, the relationship between the mean μ of the response variable and η is defined by a link function:

$$g(\mu) = \eta \qquad (5.2\text{-}41)$$

---

[4] Moulman, J.J. *Lecture 4: Generalized additive models*. (2008). Available at www.math.vu.nl/sto/

The most commonly used link function is the *canonical link,* for which

$$\eta = \theta \tag{5.2-42}$$

A combination of *backfitting* and *local scoring* algorithms is used in the actual fitting of the model.

GAM and GLMs can be applied in similar situations, but they serve different analytic purposes. GLMs emphasize estimation and inference for the parameters of the model, whereas GAM focuses on exploring data nonparametrically. The GAM model is fitted using a local scoring algorithm, which iteratively fits weighted additive models by backfitting. The backfitting algorithm is a Gauss–Seidel method for fitting additive models, with iterative smoothing of partial residuals. The algorithm separates the parametric from the nonparametric part of the fit, fitting the parametric part using weighted linear least squares within the backfitting algorithm.

The following example provides an elementary introduction to the GAM approach, using R in computation.

■ **Example 5.25:** An application of GAM to a simple linear model of two independent variables[4]

Let x_1 and x_2 be two independent predictor variables. The same treatment may be extended to n ($n > 2$) independent variables. Let y be the dependent outcome variable, and e be the error term. A linear model may then be written as

$$y = b_1 x_1 + b_2 x_2 + e \tag{5.2-43}$$

The objective of the modeling is to minimize the least squares loss function L defined by

$$L(b) = \| y\ b_1 x_1,\ b_2 x_2 \|^2 \tag{5.2-44}$$

A simple GAM seeks the model given by

$$L[f(x)] = \| y\ f_1(x_1) - f_2(x_2) \|^2 \tag{5.2-45}$$

where $f_1(x_1)$ and $f_2(x_2)$ are functions—specifically nonlinear transformations of x_1 and x_2.

The computation of these functions, $f_1(x_1)$ and $f_2(x_2)$, may now be undertaken using the following R code segment:

```
> n <- 100 # Considering 100 data points
> x1 <- scale(runif(n, 0, 1))
> x2 <- scale(runif(n, 0, 1))
> # The function runif(n, min=0, max=1) provides information about
> # the uniform distribution on the interval from min to max.
> # runif() generates random deviates.
> # The uniform distribution has density
> # f(x) = 1/(max – min)
> # for min ≤ x ≤ max.
> # scale() is a generic function whose default method centers and/or scales
```

```
> f <- x1**2 + x2**2
> e <- rnorm(n, 0, 0.1)
> # The function rnorm(n, mean, sd) randomly generates normally
> # distributed numbers with mean equal to mean, and standard deviation
> # equal to sd.
>
> y <- f + e
> a <- lm(y ~ cbind(x1,x2))
> yhat <- a$fitted.values
> mr2 <- cor(yhat,y)**2
> plot(yhat, y, main=c('multiple R2=',(round(mr2,digit=5))))
> # Outputting: Figure 5.20.
```

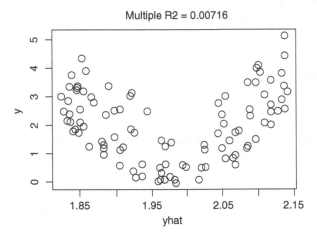

Multiple R2 = 0.00716

FIGURE 5.20 Linear model.

```
> # Now, for the GAM, the following computation will generate the functions
> # f1(x1) and f2(x2):
> # GAM step-by-step:
> xx1 <- x1
> xx2 <- x2
>
> plot((x1+x2),y, main='y as sum of x1 and x2')
> # Outputting Figure 5.21 GAM-1
> plot(x1,(y-x2), main='(y - x2) versus x1')
> # Outputting: Figure 5.22 GAM-2
> dev.copy2eps(file="plots1.eps")
>
> plot(xx1,(y-xx2),main='(y - f2(x2)) versus f1(x1)')
> # Outputting: Figure 5.23 GAM-3
```

```
> plot(xx2,(y-xx1),main='(y - f1(x1)) versus f2(x2)')
> # Outputting: Figure 5.24 GAM-4
> plot((xx1+xx2),y-(xx1+xx2),asp=1,main='Residuals')
> # Outputting: Figure 5.25 GAM-5

> plot(x1,xx1,main='Transformation of x1')
> lines(x1[order(x1)],xx1[order(x1)],col='red')
> # Outputting: Figure 5.26 GAM-6
> plot(x2,xx2,main='Transformation of x2')
> lines(x2[order(x2)],xx2[order(x2)],col='blue')
> # Outputting: Figure 5.27 GAM-7
```

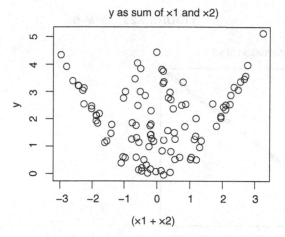

FIGURE 5.21 GAM-1.

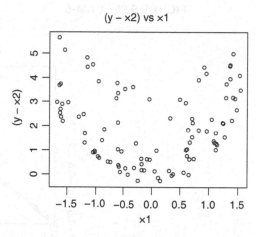

FIGURE 5.22 GAM-2.

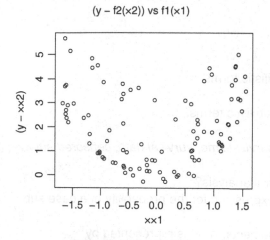

FIGURE 5.23 GAM-3.

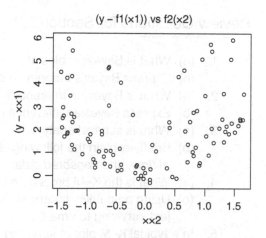

FIGURE 5.24 GAM-4.

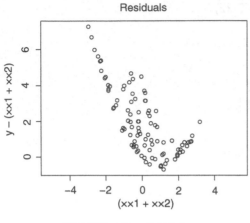

FIGURE 5.25   GAM-5.

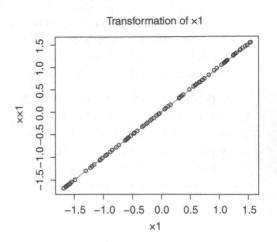

FIGURE 5.26   GAM-6.

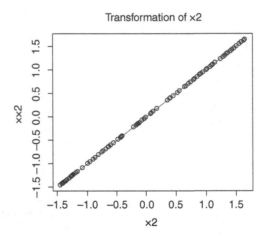

FIGURE 5.27   GAM-7.

Review Questions for Section 5.2

1. (a) What is Bayesian biostatistics?
   (b) Express Bayes's theorem in probabilistic terms.
2. (a) What is Bayesian inference?
   (b) Express Bayesian inference in probabilistic terms.
3. (a) What is survival analysis?
   (b) Briefly explain the following terms: *survival time*, *survival data*, *censored survival time*, and *censored data*.
4. (a) What is the K–M procedure in survival analysis?
   (b) Using probability theory, derive an expression for the probability of a case subject surviving to time *t*.
5. In a typical K–M plot of surviving case subjects, what is represented by
   (a) a vertical segment?
   (b) a horizontal segment?

6. (a) In survival analysis, what is the Cox regression model (also known as *proportional hazards*)?
   (b) In the Cox regression model, what is meant by *instantaneous failure rate, baseline hazard function*, and *proportional hazards regression*?

7. In the K–M procedure, explain the usages of the following R functions:
   (a) Surv()
   (b) survfit()
   (c) survdiff()
   (d) surv_test()

8. In the Cox regression model, explain the usages of the following R functions:
   (a) survfit()
   (b) coxph()
   (c) cox.zph()

9. (a) What is meant by the inverse Bayes formula (IBF)?
   (b) What are the advantages of using the IBF in biostatistical modeling?

10. (a) In the CRAN package grofit, which was developed for fitting growth curves, explain the usages of the following R functions: gcFitModel(), gcFitSpline(), and drBootSpline().
    (b) In the CRAN package gam, which was developed for generalized additive modeling, explain the usages of the R function gam() and the use of a gam.object.

Exercises for Section 5.2

1. A study by Gehan, reported by Daniel (2005), attempted to find the optimum dosage of the pain-killing drug lignocaine (LC), which was introduced by injection with propofol (PF) into the case subjects. A total of 310 case subjects were involved, and these case subjects were allocated to four categories according to the LC dosage:

   Group A = subjects receiving no LC

   Groups B, C, and D = subjects receiving 0.1, 0. 2, and 0.4 mg/kg LC mixed with PF, respectively

   The degree of pain experienced by the case subjects was categorized from 0 (no pain) to 3 (most severe). The following table records the case subjects cross-classified by dosage level and pain score:

	Pain Score	A	B	C	D	Total
			Group			Total
	0	49	73	58	62	242
	1	16	7	7	8	38
	2	8	5	6	6	25
	3	4	1	0	0	5
Total		77	77	86	71	76	310

(a) Compute the following probabilities and explain their meanings:
   (i) $P(2 \cap A)$
   (ii) $P(B \cup 3)$

(b) Is each of the following equations true? Why or why not?
   (i) $P(A \cap 3) = P(3 \cap A)$
   (ii) $P(1 \cup D) = P(D \cup 1)$
   (iii) $P(B \cap D) = 0$

2. In a clinical trial, the case subjects are divided into two groups (0 = Control, 1 = Treatment).[5] The probability that an adverse outcome will occur in the control group is $P0$, and in the treatment group is $P1$. These case subjects are placed alternately into the two groups, and their outcomes are independent. Using the theory of probability, Bayes's theorem, or another formula, show that the probability that the first adverse event will occur in the control group is

$$P0/(P0 + P1 - P0 \times P1)$$

Proof:
Define:
   ■ The sample space to consist of all possible infinite sequences of patient outcomes
   ■ Event E1—first subject (allocated to the control arm) suffers an adverse outcome
   ■ Event E2—first subject (allocated to the control arm) does not suffer an adverse outcome, but the second patient (allocated to the treatment arm) does suffer an adverse outcome
   ■ Event E0—neither of the first two subjects suffers an adverse outcome
   ■ Event F—first adverse event occurs on the control arm

To answer this question, you are required to find $P(F)$.

The events E1, E2, and E0 partition, so, by the theorem of total probability, $P(F) = P(F|E1)P(E1) + P(F|E2)P(E2) + P(F|E0)P(E0)$. Also, $P(E1) = P0$, $P(E2) = (1 - P0)\ P1$, $P(E0) = (1 - P0)\ (1 - P1)$, and $P(F|E1) = 1$, $P(F|E2) = 0$.

Finally, because after two nonadverse outcomes the allocation process effectively restarts, one has $P(F|E0) = P(F)$. Hence:

$$P(F) = (1 \times P0) + (0 \times (1 - P0)\ P1) + (P(F) \times (1 - P0)\ (1 - P1))$$

$$= P0 + (1 - P0)\ (1 - P1)\ P(F),$$

which may be rearranged to give $P(F) = P0/(P0 + P1 - P0\ P1)$, as required.

3. *The K–M procedure using* R.
   Using the following R code segment, the K–M procedure may be applied to the melanom dataset in the package ISwR:

```
> install.packages("survival")
> library(survival)
> ls("package:survival")
> install.packages("ISwR")
> library(ISwR)
> ls("package:ISwR")
```

[5] *Worked examples 1: Total probability and Bayes' theorem.* Available at www2.imperial.ac.uk/~ayoung/

```
> data(melanom)
> attach(melanom)
> melanoma
> names(melanom)
> survfit(Surv(days,status==1)~1,data=melanom)
> plot(survfit(Surv(days,status==1)~1,data=melanom))

> # Outputting: Figure 5.28.
> summary(survfit(Surv(days,status==1)~1,data=melanom))
```

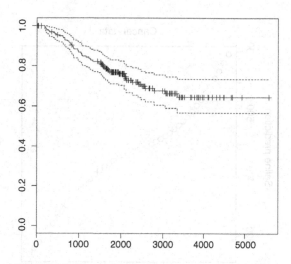

FIGURE 5.28   K–M plot for the melanom dataset.

(a) Describe, in your own words, the meaning and purpose of each of the R commands in the preceding code segment.
(b) Suggest alternative R commands that could achieve the same results.
(c) Enter the R environment and run the code segment to obtain Figure 5.28.
(d) Suggest R commands to add labels to the axes in, and a suitable title for, Figure 5.28.

4. *The Cox regression model (proportional hazards) using R.*
   Using the following R code segment, the Cox regression model procedure may be applied to the cancer dataset in the package survival:

```
> install.packages("survival")
> library(survival)
> ls("package:survival")
> data(cancer)
> attach(cancer)
> cancer
> lfit6 <- survreg(Surv(time, status)~pspline(age, df=2), cancer)
> plot(cancer$age, predict(lfit6), xlab="Age", ylab="Spline
+        prediction")
> title("Cancer Data")
```

```
> # Outputting: Figure 5.29.
> fit0 <- coxph(Surv(time, status) ~ ph.ecog + age, cancer)
> fit1 <- coxph(Surv(time, status) ~ ph.ecog + pspline(age,3),
+              cancer)
> fit3 <- coxph(Surv(time, status) ~ ph.ecog + pspline(age,8),
+              cancer)
> fit0
> fit1
> fit3
```

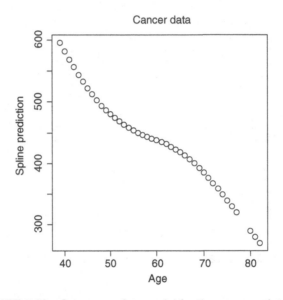

Cancer data

FIGURE 5.29   Cox regression model for the cancer dataset.

(a) Describe, in your own words, the meaning and purpose of each of the R commands in the preceding code segment.
(b) Suggest alternative R commands that could achieve the same results.
(c) Enter the R environment and run the code segment to obtain Figure 5.29.
(d) Following the command > ls("package:survival"): Is the dataset cancer included in the package survival?
(e) Following the command > cancer: How many cases are included in this dataset?

5. *More on the K–M procedure using* R.

Using the following R code segment, the K–M procedure may be applied to the heart dataset in the CRAN package survival. (Before generating plots, some preprocessing is performed to get this dataset in proper form for the event. history function. You need to create one line per subject and sort by time under observation, with those experiencing an event coming before those tied with censoring time.)

```
> install.packages("survival")
```

```
> ls("package:survival")
> data(heart)
> heart

> # Creation of the event.history version of the heart dataset (called heart.one):
> heart.one <- matrix(nrow=length(unique(heart$id)), ncol=8)
> for(i in 1:length(unique(heart$id)))

+ {
+    if(length(heart$id[heart$id==i]) == 1)
+    heart.one[i,] <- as.numeric(unlist(heart[heart$id==i, ]))
+    else if(length(heart$id[heart$id==i]) == 2)
+    heart.one[i,] <- as.numeric(unlist(heart[heart$id==i,][2,]))
+ }

> heart.one[,3][heart.one[,3] == 0] <- 2

> # Converting censored events to 2, from 0
> if(is.factor(heart$transplant))
+ heart.one[,7] <- heart.one[,7] - 1

> ## Getting back to correct transplantation coding
> heart.one <-
+        as.data.frame(heart.one[order(unlist(heart.one[,2]),
+        unlist(heart.one[,3])),])
> names(heart.one) <- names(heart)

> # Back to usual censoring indicator:
> heart.one[,3][heart.one[,3] == 2] <- 0

> # Note: transplant says 0 (for no transplants) or 1 (for one transplant)
> # and event = 1 is death, while event = 0 is censored.
> # Plot a single K–M curve from the heart data, first creating
> # a survival object
> heart.surv <- survfit(Surv(stop, event) ~ 1, data=heart.one,
+                       conf.int = FALSE)
> # Traditional K–M curve
> # postscript('ehgfig3.ps', horiz=TRUE)
> # omi <- par(omi=c(0,1.25,0.5,1.25))
> plot(heart.surv, ylab='estimated survival probability',
+                  xlab='observation time (in days)')
> title('Kaplan-Meier curve for Stanford data', cex=0.8)
```

> Outputting: Figure 5.30.

(a) Describe, in your own words, the meaning and purpose of each of the R commands in the preceding code segment.

(b) Suggest alternative R commands that could achieve the same results.

(c) Enter the R environment and run the code segment to obtain Figure 5.30.

6. *More on the Cox regression model using* R.

   Using the following R code segment, the Cox regression model procedure may

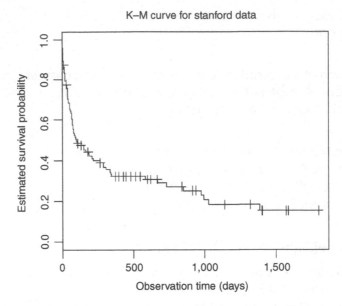

FIGURE 5.30 K–M survival plot for the cancer dataset.

the CRAN package survival. The program displays a graph of the scaled Schoenfeld residuals, along with a smooth curve, developed for a graphical test of proportional hazards:

```
> install.packages("survival")
> library(survival)
> ls("package:survival")
> data(veteran)
> attach(veteran)
> veteran
> vfit <- coxph(Surv(time,status) ~ trt + factor(celltype) +
+               karno + age, data=veteran, x=TRUE)
> temp <- cox.zph(vfit)
> plot(temp, var=5) # Look at the Karnofsky score; this is an old way of doing
   the plot.
> plot(temp[5]) # New way with subscripting:
> abline(0, 0, lty=3)

> # Add the linear fit as well:
> abline(lm(temp$y[,5] ~ temp$x)$coefficients, lty=4, col=3)
> title(main="VA Lung Study")
```

> *Outputting:* Figure 5.31.

(a) Describe, in your own words, the meaning and purpose of each of the R commands in the preceding code segment.

(b) Suggest alternative R commands that could achieve the same results.

(c) Enter the R environment and run the code segment to obtain Figure 5.31.

(d) Following the command > ls("package:survival"): Is the dataset veteran

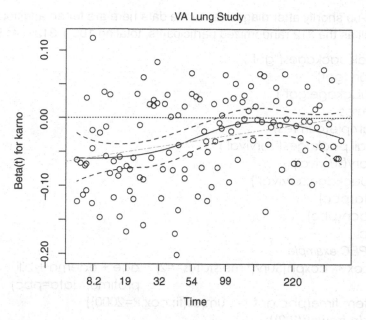

FIGURE 5.31 Cox regression model for the modified cancer dataset.

(e) Following the command > veteran: How many cases are included in this dataset?

(f) What is the green line in Figure 5.31?

7. *More on survival analysis: The Cox regression model, based on cumulative residues, using* R.

Using the following R code segment, apply the Cox regression model procedure, based on cumulative residues, to the Mayo Clinic pbc [primary biliary cirrhosis (PBC) or cirrhosis of the liver] dataset. These data were obtained from clinical trials in case subjects with PBC of the liver, conducted between 1974 and 1984. PBC is an autoimmune disease of the liver marked by the slow, progressive destruction of the small bile ducts within the liver. When these ducts are damaged, bile builds up in the liver and over time damages the tissue, which may lead to scarring, fibrosis, and cirrhosis. *Cirrhosis* is a consequence of chronic liver disease characterized by replacement of liver tissue by fibrosis, scar tissue, and regenerative nodules (lumps that occur as a result of a process in which damaged tissue is regenerated), leading to loss of liver function. Cirrhosis is most commonly caused by alcoholism, hepatitis B and C, and fatty liver disease, but also has many other possible causes. Some cases are idiopathic, (i.e., of unknown cause). Recent studies have shown that it may affect up to 1 in 3,000 people, and the gender ratio is at least 9:1 (female to male).

A total of 424 PBC patients, all referred to the Mayo Clinic during that 10-year interval, met eligibility criteria for the randomized placebo controlled trial of the drug D-penicillamine. The first 312 cases in the dataset participated in the randomized trial, and the data for these cases are largely complete. The additional 112 cases did not participate in the clinical trial but consented to have their basic mea-

follow-up shortly after diagnosis, so the data here are for an additional 106 cases, as well as the 312 randomized participants, totaling 106 + 312 = 418 cases:

```
> install.packages("gof")
> library(gof)
> ls("package:gof")
> cumres
> example(cumres)
> install.packages("survival")
> library(survival)
> ls("package:survival")
> data(pbc)
> attach(pbc)
> pbc
> ## PBC example
> fit.cox <- coxph(Surv(time,status==2) ~ age + edema + bili +
+                                          protime, data=pbc)
> system.time(pbc.gof <- cumres(fit.cox,R=2000))
> par(mfrow=c(2,2))
> plot(pbc.gof, ci=TRUE, legend=NULL)

> # Outputting: Figure 5.32.
```

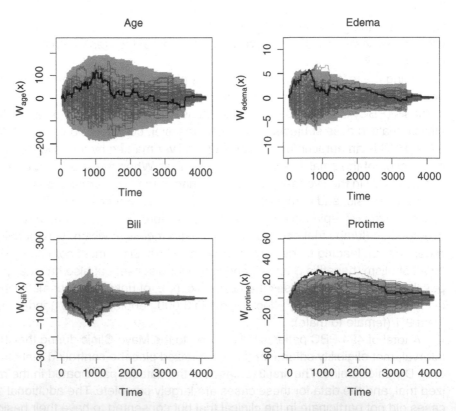

FIGURE 5.32 Survival modeling of the pbc dataset: the Cox regression model, based on

(a) Describe, in your own words, the meaning and purpose of each of the R commands in the preceding code segment.
(b) Suggest alternative R commands that could achieve the same results.
(c) Enter the R environment and run the code segment to obtain Figure 5.32.
(d) Following the command > ls("package:survival"): Is the dataset pbc included in the package survival?
(e) Following the command > pbc: How many cases are included in this dataset?

8. *An example of application of the inverse Bayes formula* (Ng & Tong, 2010)

One criticism of the Monte Carlo simulation technique for generating random samples from univariate and multivariate distributions concerns when to reject a selection. A recognized method is the Rubin proposal of a noniterative sampling procedure: the **sampling/importance resampling (SIR)** method. For simulation from a density defined in the unit interval, let r be a known positive integer, and $X \sim f(x)$, where:

$$f(x) = \pi \sin^r(\pi x)/B[\tfrac{1}{2}, (r+1)/q], 0 < x < 1 \qquad (5.2\text{-}46)$$

and B is the beta function.

Based on Equation (5.2-46), the following R code segment computes $f(x)$ when $r = 6$, for a skew beta density $B(x|2, 4)$, as the importance sampling density $g(x)$. Figure 5.33(A) shows the importance weight $w(x) = f(x)/B(x|2, 4)$. The algorithm sets $J = 200,000$ and $m = 20,000$ to obtain Figure 5.33(B), which shows that the histogram entirely recovers the target density function $f(x)$.

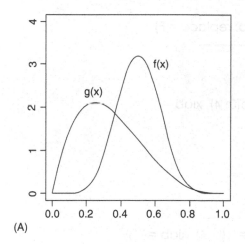
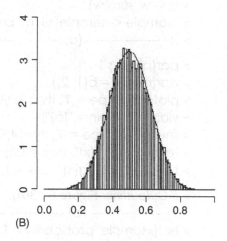

(A) (B)

FIGURE 5.33 Output of the SIR method for noniterative sampling.

Here is the requisite R code segment:

```
> J = 200000
> m = 20000
> # Function name: IBF2.2.SIR(J=200,000, m=20,000)

> # ************** Input ***************************
> # J = 200,000 is the sampling size in the SIR method
> # m = 20,000 is the resampling size in the SIR method
```

```
> # Aim: Plotting Figures 5.33(A) and 5.33(B)
> r <- 6
> a <- 2
> b <- 4
> x <- seq(0, 1, 0.01)
> x
```

[1]	0.00	0.01	0.02	0.03	0.04	0.05	0.06	0.07	0.08	0.09	0.10	0.11	0.12	0.13	0.14
[16]	0.15	0.16	0.17	0.18	0.19	0.20	0.21	0.22	0.23	0.24	0.25	0.26	0.27	0.28	0.29
[31]	0.30	0.31	0.32	0.33	0.34	0.35	0.36	0.37	0.38	0.39	0.40	0.41	0.42	0.43	0.44
[46]	0.45	0.46	0.47	0.48	0.49	0.50	0.51	0.52	0.53	0.54	0.55	0.56	0.57	0.58	0.59
[61]	0.60	0.61	0.62	0.63	0.64	0.65	0.66	0.67	0.68	0.69	0.70	0.71	0.72	0.73	0.74
[76]	0.75	0.76	0.77	0.78	0.79	0.80	0.81	0.82	0.83	0.84	0.85	0.86	0.87	0.88	0.89
[91]	0.90	0.91	0.92	0.93	0.94	0.95	0.96	0.97	0.98	0.99	1.00				

```
>
> cc <- (gamma(0.5) * gamma((r + 1)/2))/gamma(0.5 * r + 1)
> fx <- (pi * (sin(pi * x))^r)/cc
> gx <- dbeta(x, a, b)

> #---------------------------------------------------------
> xJ <- rbeta(J, a, b)
> w <- (sin(pi * xJ))^r/dbeta(xJ, a, b)
> p <- w/sum(w)
> xsample <- sample(xJ, m, prob = p, replace = F)
> #------------------ (a) ---------------------------

> par(pty = "s")
> par(mfrow = c(1, 2))
> plot(x, fx, type = "l", lty = 1, ylim = c(0, 4), xlab = "",
+ ylab = "", main = "(a)")
> lines(x, gx, type = "l", lty = 4)
> text(0.65, 3, "f(x)", cex = 1.8)
> text(0.22, 2.5, "g(x)", cex = 1.8)

> # Outputting: Figure 5.33(A).
> #------------------ (b) ---------------------------
> hist(xsample, probability = T, ylim = c(0, 4), xlab = " ",
+ breaks = seq(0, 1, 0.01), ylab = "", main = "(b)")
> lines(x, fx, type = "l", lty = 1) # Outputting: Figure 5.33(B).
```

(a) The target density $f(x)$, as defined by Equation (5.2-46), with $r = 6$ and $g(x) = B(x|2, 4)$.

(b) The histogram of $f(x)$ as obtained by using the SIR method, with $J = 200,000$ and $m = 20,000$.

(c) Describe, in your own words, the meaning and purpose of each of the R commands in the preceding code segment.

(d) Suggest alternative R commands that could achieve the same results.

(f) Repeat the computation for varying values of J (greater and less than 200,000) and m (greater and less than 20,000).

(g) How do these new results differ from the results of the first computation? Explain.

9. *Applying the function* with() *in the CRAN package* base.

The function with() evaluates an R expression in an environment constructed from data, possibly modifying the original data. Starting with the package gamair,[1] the following example uses a short R code segment to illustrate the simple applicability of gam modeling (from the package gamair). gam is used to model the average air temperature (in degrees Fahrenheit) in Cairo, Egypt, from January 1, 1995, to May 21, 2005 (Wood, 2006).

Usage:
data(cairo)

Format:
A data frame with 6 columns and 3,780 rows. The columns are:
- month   Month of year from 1 to 12
- day.of.month   Day of month, from 1 to 31
- year   Year, starting 1995
- temp   Average temperature (degrees Fahrenheit)
- day.of.year   Day of year from 1 to 366
- time   Number of days since January 1, 1995

Source: Wood (2006), pp. 321–324.

The R computation is based on data(cairo) with the statement:
(cairo,plot(time,temp,type="l")
The following R code segment may be used:

```
> install.packages("gamair") # Installing package gamair
> library(gamair)
> ls("package:gamair")
character(0)

> data(cairo)

> # The author was visiting this ancient Egyptian city at the time of writing
> # the first draft of this portion of the book!
> # Source: http://www.engr.udayton.edu/weather/citylistWorld.htm

> attach(cairo)

> cairo # Inspecting the data frame cairo

> # Outputting: A data frame with 6 columns and 3780 rows.
```

month	day.of.month	year	temp	day.of.year	time
1	1	1	1995	59.2	1	1
2	1	2	1995	57.5	2	2

3	1		3	1995	57.4		3	3
4	1		4	1995	59.3		4	4
5	1		5	1995	58.8		5	5

3790	5	17	2005	78.1	137	3790
3791	5	18	2005	79.9	138	3791
3792	5	19	2005	82.7	139	3792
3793	5	20	2005	83.5	140	3793
3794	5	21	2005	76.9	141	3794

```
>
> # The function with():
> ls("package:base")
```

| [1] "-" | "-.Date" | "-.POSIXt" | "!" |
| [5] "!.hexmode" | "!.octmode" | "!=" | "$" |

| [1169] "while" | "with" "with.default" "withCallingHandlers" |

[1197] "xtfrm.Surv" "xzfile" "zapsmall"

```
> # Listing 1199 files
> with

function (data, expr, ...)
UseMethod("with")
<bytecode: 06DB2644>
<environment: namespace:base>

> with(cairo,plot(time,temp,type="l"))
> # Outputting: Figure 5.34.
```

(a) Describe, in your own words, the meaning and purpose of each of the R commands in the preceding code segment.

(b) Suggest alternative R commands that could achieve the same results.

(c) Enter the R environment and run the code segment to obtain Figure 5.34.

(d) Following the command > ls("package:base"):

  (i) Is the function with() included in the package base?

  (ii) How many files are included in this package?

10. *More about* gam *(generalized additive models): The* R *function* vis.gam() *and visualization of* gam *objects.*

    The CRAN package mgcv (gcv = generalized cross validation) contains functions for generalized additive modeling and generalized additive mixed modeling. The term *GAM* is taken to include any GLM estimated by quadratically penalized (possibly quasi-) likelihood maximization. A Bayesian approach to confidence/credible interval calculation is provided. Linear functional (i.e., functions of functions) of smooths, penalization of parametric model terms, and linkage of smoothing parameters are all supported.

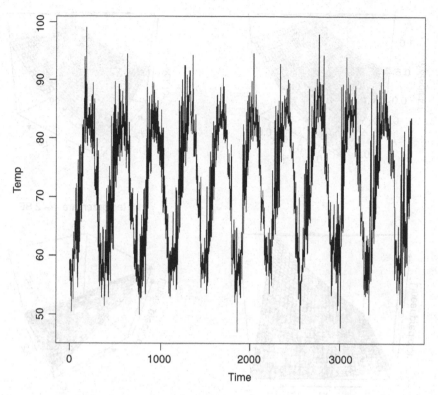

FIGURE 5.34   Generalized additive model gamair() for daily temperature data for Cairo, Egypt.

Consider the following R code segment:

```
> install.packages("mgcv")
> library(mgcv)
> help("mgcv-package")
> ls("package:mgcv")
> set.seed(0)
> n <- 200; sig2 <- 4
> x0 <- runif(n, 0, 1); x1 <- runif(n, 0, 1)
> x2 <- runif(n, 0, 1)
> y <- x0^2 + x1*x2 + runif(n,-0.3,0.3)
> g <- gam(y~s(x0,x1,x2))
> old.par <- par(mfrow=c(2,2))
> # display the prediction surface in x0, x1 ....
> vis.gam(g,ticktype="detailed",color="heat",theta=-35)
> vis.gam(g,se=2,theta=-35)
> # with twice standard error surfaces
> vis.gam(g, view=c("x1","x2"),cond=list(x0=0.75))
> # different view
> vis.gam(g, view=c("x1","x2"),cond=list(x0=.75), theta=210,
+       phi=40, too.far=.07)
```

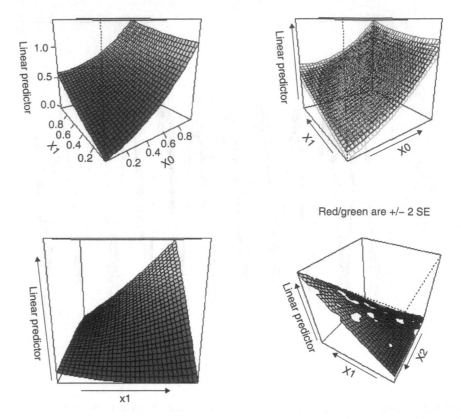

FIGURE 5.35 Contour plots of prediction and standard error surfaces using vis.gam().

```
>
> # ..... areas where there is no data are not plotted
>
> # contour examples....
> vis.gam(g, view=c("x1","x2"),plot.type="contour",color="heat")
> vis.gam(g, view=c("x1","x2"),plot.type="contour",
+           color="terrain")
> vis.gam(g, view=c("x1","x2"),plot.type="contour",color="topo")
> vis.gam(g, view=c("x1","x2"),plot.type="contour",color="cm")
> # Outputting: Figure 5.36.
>
> par(old.par)
> # Examples with factor and "by" variables:
> fac <- rep(1:4,20)
> x <- runif(80)
> y <- fac+2*x^2+rnorm(80)*0.1
> fac <- factor(fac)
```

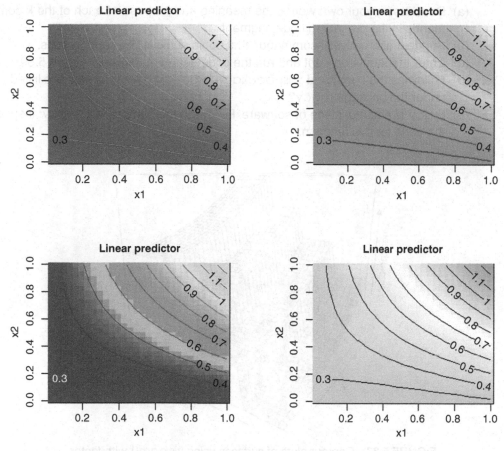

FIGURE 5.36 Contour plots of contour surfaces using vis.gam().

```
> b <- gam(y~fac+s(x))
> vis.gam(b,theta=-35,color="heat") # factor example
> # Outputting: Figure 5.37.
>
> z <- rnorm(80)*0.4
> y <- as.numeric(fac)+3*x^2*z+rnorm(80)*0.1
> b <- gam(y~fac+s(x,by=z))
> vis.gam(b,theta=-35,color="heat",cond=list(z=1))
> # "by" variable example

> # Outputting: Figure 5.38.
>
> vis.gam(b,view=c("z","x"),theta= 35)
> # plot against by variable

> # Outputting: Figure 5.39.
```

(a) Describe, in your own words, the meaning and purpose of each of the R commands in the preceding code segment.
(b) Suggest alternative R commands that could achieve the same results.
(c) Enter the R environment and run the code segment to obtain Figure 5.39.
(d) Following the command > ls("package:mgcv"): How many files are listed under the package mgcv?
(e) mgcv is a useful piece of software. Following the command > mgcv: Inspect the code for this function.

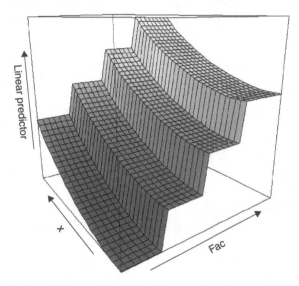

FIGURE 5.37   Contour plots of surfaces using vis.gam() with factor.

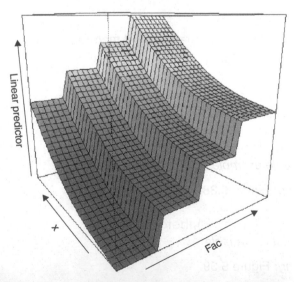

FIGURE 5.38   Contour plots of surfaces using vis.gam() "by" variables.

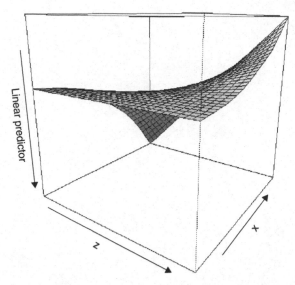

FIGURE 5.39   Contour plots of surfaces using vis.gam() against the "by" variable.

REFERENCES

Birnbaum, Z. W., & Tingey, F. H. (1951). One-sided confidence contours for probability distribution functions. *Annals of Mathematical Statistics, 22*(4), 592–596.

Conover, W. J. (1971). *Practical nonparametric statistics.* New York, NY: John Wiley & Sons. Pp. 295–301 (one-sample Kolmogorov test), 309–314 (two-sample Smirnov test).

Dalgaard, P. (2002). *Introductory statistics with R* (Statistics and Computing Series). New York, NY: Springer.

Daniel, W. W. (2005). *Biostatistics: A foundation for analysis in the health sciences* (7th ed.; Wiley Series in Probability and Statistics—Applied Probability and Statistics Section). New York, NY: John Wiley & Sons.

Durbin, J. (1973). *Distribution theory for tests based on the sample distribution function.* Philadelphia, PA: SIAM.

Hastie, T., & Tibshirani, R. (1990). *Generalized additive models.* London, UK: Chapman & Hall.

Kaplan, E. L., & Meier, P. (1958). Nonparametric estimation from incomplete observations. *Journal of the American Statistical Association, 53,* 457–481.

Kolmogorov, A. N. (1964). *Foundations of the theory of probability.* New York, NY: Chelsea Publishing.

Marsaglia, G., Tsang, W. W., & Wang, J. (2003). Evaluating Kolmogorov's distribution. *Journal of Statistical Software, 8*(18), 1–4. Retrieved from http://www.jstatsoft.org/v08/i18/

Ng, K. W., & Tong, H. (2010, November). *Inversion of Bayes formula and the measures of Bayesian information gain and pairwise dependence* (Research Report No. 477). Hong Kong, China: University of Hong Kong, Department of Statistics and Actuarial Science. Retrieved from http://lx2.saas.hku.hk/research/research-report-477.pdf

Tan, M. T., Tian, G-L., & Ng, K. W. (2010). *Bayesian missing data problems: EM, data augmentation, and noniterative computation.* Boca Raton, FL: Chapman & Hall/CRC.

Triola, M. M., & Triola, M. F. (2006). *Biostatistics for the biological and health sciences.* Boston, MA: Pearson/Addison Wesley.

Verzani, J. (2005). *Using R for introductory statistics.* Boca Raton, FL: Chapman & Hall/CRC.

Wood, S. N. (2006). *Generalized additive models: An introduction with R.* Boca Raton, FL: Chapman

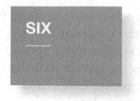

## SIX

Case–Control Studies and Cohort Studies in Epidemiology

INTRODUCTION

A **case–control study** is a class of epidemiologic observational study. An *observational study* is one in which the case subjects are not randomized to the exposed or unexposed groups, but rather are observed in order to determine both their exposure and their outcome status. The exposure status is thus not determined by the researcher.

The case–control study may be considered an observational epidemiologic study of people with the disease of interest—the **case** group—together with a suitable **control** group of persons without the disease (the *comparison group* or *reference group*). The investigation seeks the potential relationship of a suspected risk factor (or an attribute of the disease) by comparing the diseased and nondiseased subjects with regard to how frequently the risk factor is present in each of the two groups. A case–control study is frequently contrasted with cohort studies, wherein exposed and unexposed subjects are observed until they develop an outcome of interest.

A **cohort** is a group of people who share a common characteristic within a defined period (e.g., the members of the cohort underwent a certain medical procedure, were exposed to a drug, or were born in a certain period). For example, the group of people who were born in a particular period form a *birth cohort*: the Baby Boomers (those who were born after 1946 and before 1964) are one such group. The comparison group may be another cohort of subjects who have had little or no exposure to the substance under investigation, or may be the general population from which the cohort is drawn (but otherwise similar), and so on. Moreover, subgroups *within* the cohort may be compared with each other.

A **cohort study** is a form of longitudinal study (itself a type of observational study) used in epidemiologic investigations[1]. It is an analysis of risk factors undertaken by following a group of case subjects who do not have the disease and uses correlations to determine the absolute risk of a subject contracting the disease of interest. It is one of several types of clinical study designs and should be compared with a cross-sectional study. Cohort studies are generally concerned with the life histories of segments of populations, as well as the individual people who constitute these segments.

---

[1] Cohort studies in epidemiology: http://en.wikipedia.org/wiki/Cohort_study

Randomized controlled trials (RCTs) are considered a superior methodology in the hierarchy of evidence in therapy because they restrict the potential for any biases by randomly assigning one case-subject pool to an intervention and another subject pool to nonintervention (or a placebo). This minimizes the chance that the incidence of *confounding* variables will differ between the two groups. Cohort studies can be conducted either prospectively or retrospectively. A more detailed examination of RCTs is presented in Chapter 7.

6.1 THEORY AND ANALYSIS OF CASE–CONTROL STUDIES

Research and investigations in epidemiology and the health sciences make wide use of case–control studies. Such studies can identify factors that may contribute to a medical condition by comparing case subjects who have that disease/condition (the **cases**) with subjects who do not have the disease/condition but are otherwise similar (the **controls**).[2]

A practical advantage of the case–control study is that it is relatively inexpensive. Also, this type of study can be (and frequently is) undertaken by individual researchers, small teams, or single facilities.

Use of the case–control study has led to a considerable number of scientific advances and significant discoveries. In the annals of epidemiology, an outstanding success of this type of study was the demonstration of the relationship between the occurrence of lung cancer and the use of tobacco products by Richard Doll et al., who demonstrated a statistically significant association between the two in a large case–control study (Doll, Petro, Boreham, & Sutherland, 2004). Though opponents correctly point out that this type of study cannot by itself prove causation, the eventual results of cohort studies confirmed the causal link that the case–control studies had suggested: *tobacco smoking is a cause of about 87% of all lung cancer mortality in the United States.*

Advantages and Limitations of Case–Control Studies

Case–control studies tend to be less costly to carry out than prospective cohort studies, and they have the potential to be shorter in duration. Another advantage is the greater statistical power of this type of study in several situations; cohort studies often require a sufficient number of disease events to accrue before they can provide much information.

However, case–control studies are observational in nature and thus do not provide the same level of evidence as RCTs. The results may be confounded by various factors to the extent that they give answers that are the opposite of those of better studies. It may also be more difficult to establish the timeline of exposure to disease outcome in the setting of a case–control study than within a prospective cohort study design. In the latter, the exposure is ascertained before the case subjects are followed over time to ascertain their outcome status.

The most important drawback to case–control studies relates to the difficulty of obtaining reliable information about an individual's exposure status over time. Case–control studies are therefore placed low in the hierarchy of evidence. Nevertheless, many high-quality and reliable case–control studies have been carried out and have produced useful results.

Analysis of Case–Control Studies

Case–control studies were initially analyzed by testing whether there were significant differences between the proportion of exposed subjects among cases and controls. If the disease outcome of interest is rare, the odds ratio of exposure may be used to estimate the relative risk. Moreover, the odds ratio of exposure can be used to estimate the incidence rate ratio of exposure directly, without the need for the rare disease assumption.

The following is an example of a case–control study where R computations were used to analyze the datasets.

■ **Example 6.1:** A case–control study on the efficacy of BCG vaccination against tuberculosis (TB)

The Bacillus Calmette-Guerin (BCG) vaccine is widely used against tuberculosis (TB). Developed in the 1930s, it is made of a live, weakened strain of *Mycobacterium bovis*.

Colditz et al. (1994) reported data from 13 clinical trials of the BCG vaccine, each investigating its efficacy in the treatment of TB. The number of case subjects suffering from TB with or without BCG vaccination was recorded. The dataset also contains the values of two other variables for each study: the geographic latitude of the place where the study was undertaken and the year of publication. These two variables may be used to Investigate any heterogeneity among the studies.

Source of Dataset:
Colditz, G. A., Brewer, T. F., Berkey, C. S., Wilson, M. E., Burdick, E., Fineberg, H. V., & Mosteller, F. (1994). Efficacy of BCG vaccine in the prevention of tuberculosis: Meta-analysis of the published literature. *Journal of the American Medical Association, 271*(2), 698–702.

The following R code segment may be used to compute a case–control study based on the available dataset:

```
> install.packages("HSAUR")
> # Taken from A Handbook of Statistical Analyses Using R (Everitt & Hothorn, 2006)
> library(HSAUR)
Loading required package: lattice
Loading required package: MASS
Loading required package: scatterplot3d
Warning messages:
1: package 'HSAUR' was built under R version 2.13.2
2: package 'scatterplot3d' was built under R version 2.13.2
```

[1] "agefat"	"aspirin"	"BCG"	"birthdeathrates"
[5] "bladdercancer"	"BtheB"	"clouds"	"CYGOB1"
[9] "epilepsy"	"Forbes2000"	"foster"	"gardenflowers"
[13] "GHQ"	"heptathlon"	"HSAURtable"	"Lanza"
[17] "mastectomy"	"meteo"	"orallesions"	"phosphate"
[21] "pistonrings"	"planets"	"plasma"	"polyps"
[25] "polyps3"	"pottery"	"rearrests"	"respiratory"
[29] "roomwidth"	"schizophrenia"	"schizophrenia2"	"schooldays"
[33] "skulls"	"smoking"	"students"	"suicides"
[37] "toothpaste"	"voting"	"water"	"watervoles"
[41] "waves"	"weightgain"	"womensrole"	

```
> data(BCG)
# Dataset Format -
# A data frame with 13 observations on the following 7 variables:
# Study       An identifier of the study.
# BCGTB       The number of subjects suffering from TB after a BCG vaccination.
# BCGVacc     The number of subjects who were vaccinated with BCG.
# NoVaccTB    The number of subjects suffering from TB who did not receive
#             BCG vaccination.
# NoVacc      The total number of subjects without BCG vaccination.
# Latitude    Geographic position of the place the study was undertaken.
# Year        The year the study was undertaken.
> BCG # Inspecting the dataset
```

	Study	BCGTB	BCGVacc	NoVaccTB	NoVacc	Latitude	Year
1	1	4	123	11	139	44	1948
2	2	6	306	29	303	55	1949
3	3	3	231	11	220	42	1960
4	4	62	13598	248	12867	52	1977
5	5	33	5069	47	5808	13	1973
6	6	180	1541	372	1451	44	1953
7	7	8	2545	10	629	19	1973
8	8	505	88391	499	88391	13	1980
9	9	29	7499	45	7277	27	1968
10	10	17	1716	65	1665	42	1961
11	11	186	50634	141	27338	18	1974
12	12	5	2498	3	2341	33	1969
13	13	27	16913	29	17854	33	1976

```
> attach(BCG)
> boxplot(BCG$BCGTB/BCG$BCGVacc, # Two boxplots on BCG
+       BCG$NoVaccTB/BCG$NoVacc,
+       names = c("BCG Vaccination", "No BCG Vaccination"),
+       ylab = "Percent BCG cases")
> # Outputting Figure 6.1
```

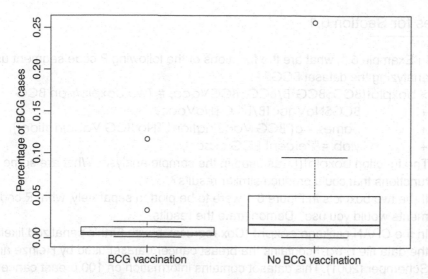

FIGURE 6.1 Boxplots for case–control study on the efficacy of BCG vaccination in preventing TB.

Biostatistical Decision and Conclusion: A comparison of the two boxplots in Figure 6.1 clearly shows that the percentages of TB cases for the group with no BCG vaccination are several times *higher* than for the group with BCG vaccination. Hence, a reasonable preliminary conclusion is that populations receiving BCG vaccination will be *less* likely to contract TB.

Remarks:

1. In the data frame BCG, the data information has been categorized in terms of seven variables: "Study", "BCGTB", "BCGVacc", "NoVaccTB", "NoVacc", "Latitude", and "Year".

2. This dataset lends itself to ready analysis using the function boxplot(), distinguishing the groups with BCG vaccination from the groups without the BCG vaccination:

   ```
   > boxplot(BCG$BCGTB/BCG$BCGVacc,
   +         BCG$NoVaccTB/BCG$NoVacc, ...
   ```

   The use of this function immediately provided the graphical representation of the dataset in Figure 6.1.

3. Thus, in the analysis of data from case–control studies, the preparation of the data frame is important to the direct analysis of the dataset.

4. Further boxplot()-type analyses may be undertaken with such datasets.

Review Questions for Section 6.1

1. (a) What is a case–control study?
   (b) Give an example of a case–control study in epidemiology or the health sciences.
2. What are the main limitations of a case–control study? Explain and give examples.
3. (a) Can a case–control study and a cohort study be undertaken simultaneously in epidemiology? If so, how? What are the advantages of this approach?

Exercises for Section 6.1

1. In Example 6.1, what are the functions of the following R code segment used in analyzing the dataset BCG?

```
> boxplot(BCG$BCGTB/BCG$BCGVacc, # Two boxplots on BCG
+          BCG$NoVaccTB/BCG$NoVacc,
+          names = c("BCG Vaccination", "No BCG Vaccination"),
+          ylab = "Percent BCG cases")
```

2. The function boxplot() was used in the sample analysis. What are some other R functions that could produce similar results?

3. If the two boxplots in Figure 6.1 were to be plotted separately, what R code segments would you use? Demonstrate the results.

4. In the CRAN package coxphf (Cox regression with Firth's penalized likelihood), the data file breast contains the breast cancer dataset used by Heinze and Schemper (2001). This dataset contains information on 100 breast cancer patients, including survival time, survival status, tumor stage, nodal status, grading, and cathepsin-D tumor expression.

   Describe what the following R code segment achieves for this dataset:

```
> data(breast)
> fit.breast <-
+          coxphf(data=breast,Surv(TIME,CENS)~T+N+G+CD)
> summary(fit.breast)
```

5. Execute the R code segment in Exercise 3. Comment on the results.

6. In the CRAN package survival, the data file bladder contains a clinical dataset with information on 340 case subjects.
   (a) Download this dataset.
   (b) Describe what the following R code segment achieves for this dataset:

```
# Fit a stratified model, clustered on patients
> bladder1 <- bladder[bladder$enum < 5, ]
> coxph(Surv(stop, event) ~ (rx + size + number) *
+          strata(enum) + cluster(id), bladder1)
```

7. Execute the R code segment in Exercise 5. Comment on the results.

6.2   THEORY AND ANALYSIS OF COHORT STUDIES

A **cohort** is a group of case subjects who share a common experience or characteristic (e.g., are exposed to a drug or vaccine or pollutant, or undergo a certain medical procedure, or are born) within a defined period. A group of people who were born on a given day, or in a particular period, form a **birth cohort**. The comparison group may be the general population from which the cohort is drawn, or it may be another cohort of persons thought to have had little or no exposure to the substance under investigation, but otherwise similar. Alternatively, subgroups within the cohort may be compared with each other.

Cohort study data can help determine risk factors for contracting new diseases because such a study is a longitudinal observation of the individual through time

study may provide evidence refuting the existence of a suspected association between cause and effect. In contrast, failure to refute a hypothesis strengthens confidence in that hypothesis. Prospective longitudinal cohort studies between disease and exposure thus help in the study of causal associations, though distinguishing true causality usually requires further corroboration from other sources.

Importantly, *the defined cohort cannot be a group of people who already have the disease.* The cohort must be identified before the appearance of the disease under investigation. The investigation follows, for a period of time, a group of case subjects who do not have the disease and notes who develops the disease.

Generally, cohort studies are expensive to conduct, are sensitive to attrition, and require extensive follow-up to generate useful data. However, the quality of the results from long-term cohort studies are substantially superior to those obtained from retrospective or cross-sectional studies. *Prospective cohort studies yield the most reliable results in observational epidemiology.* They enable a wide range of exposure–disease associations to be studied.

For example, some cohort studies track groups of children from birth, and record a wide range of information about them. The value of a cohort study often depends on the researchers' capacity to stay in touch with all members of the cohort; some studies have continued for decades.

An Important Application of Cohort Studies

An example of an epidemiologic question that can be answered by the use of a cohort study is: **Does exposure to X (say, smoking) associate with outcome Y (say, lung cancer)?**

Such a study would recruit a group of smokers and a group of nonsmokers (the unexposed group), follow them for a set period of time, and note differences in the incidence of lung cancer between the groups at the end of this time. The groups are *matched* in terms of many other variables, such as economic status and other health status, so that the variable being assessed, the **independent variable** (in this case, smoking) may be isolated as the cause of the **dependent variable** (in this case, lung cancer). In this example, a **statistically significant** increase in the incidence of lung cancer in the smoking group as compared to the nonsmoking group is evidence in favor of the hypothesis. However, rare outcomes, such as lung cancer, are generally not studied by using cohorts; instead, case–control studies are used.

Clinical Trials

A great deal of medical research undertakes shorter-term **clinical trial** studies. Such studies typically follow two groups of patients for a period of time and compare an endpoint or outcome measure between the two groups.

Randomized Controlled Trials

An RCT is a superior methodology in the hierarchy of evidence because it limits the

and another case-subject pool to a placebo, thus minimizing the chance that the incidence of confounding variables will differ between the two groups. However, it is sometimes not ethical or practical to perform an RCT to resolve a clinical question. For example, if one already has reasonable evidence that smoking causes lung cancer, persuading a group of nonsmokers to take up smoking in order to test this hypothesis would generally be considered unethical.

Cohort Studies for Diseases of Choice and Noncommunicable Diseases (Handysides & Landless, 2012)

In 2011, the United Nations Secretary General, addressing the global crises caused by the rapid growth of **noncommunicable diseases (NCDs)**—which are mostly preventable diseases—stated: "Our collaboration is more than a public health necessity. NCDs are a threat to development. NCDs hit the poor and vulnerable particularly hard, and drive them deeper into poverty" (Handysides & Landless, 2012). The outlook has been grim owing to the rapidly increasing incidence of NCDs worldwide, with poorer and emerging countries facing the greatest challenges.

Globally, although continuing efforts are being directed toward communicable and infectious diseases (such as malaria, TB, gastroenteritis, AIDS, HIV, etc.), the NCDs are increasing rapidly. They are both a major cause of preventable deaths and major contributors to loss of productivity and poverty. NCDs include:

- Heart diseases
- Stroke
- Cancer
- Chronic respiratory diseases
- Diabetes

These affect all communities and people. Their main risk factors are similar worldwide and are well known, including the use and effects of:

- Tobacco, in all its forms (including secondhand smoke)
- Alcohol, in all its forms
- Excessive salt and sugar in the diet
- Foods high in trans and saturated fats
- Obesity
- Physical inactivity

From the viewpoint of biostatistics, it is clear that the establishment of the cause-and-effect relationship between these risk factors and NCDs may be approached using cohort studies. Such a study would compare any cohorts who engaged in lifestyles that include one or more of the main risk factors previously listed, and compare their respective incidences of NCDs.

SOME WELL-KNOWN COHORT STUDIES

Two cohort studies that have been going on for more than 50 years are the Framingham Heart Study and the National Child Development Study (reported in the *International Journal of Epidemiology*). The latter study compares two cohorts: the "Millennium Cohort Study" (United States) and the "King's Cohort" (United Kingdom).

The largest cohort study in women is the Nurses' Health Study. Started in 1976, it is tracking more than 120,000 nurses and has been analyzed for many different conditions and outcomes.

The largest cohort study in Africa is the *Birth to Twenty* study, which began in 1990 and tracks a cohort of more than 3,000 children born in the weeks following Nelson Mandela's release from prison.

The Adventist Health Studies (AHS-1 and AHS-2) have enrolled between 30,000 and 100,000 case subjects.

In all these investigations, exposed and unexposed subjects are observed until they develop an outcome of interest. An insightful analytical approach is to use the tools of survival analysis (e.g., the Kaplan–Meier [K–M] procedure, the Cox regression model, or proportional hazards plots), all of which may be executed in the R environment (see Chapter 5). The following are some typical examples.

■ **Example 6.2:** Cohort studies using the Cox regression model and the K–M procedure to analyze a secondhand tobacco smoke dataset

Tammemagi, Neslind-Dudas, Simoff, and Kvale (2004) reported on the role of comorbidity and treatment for smoking and lung cancer survival of 1,155 case subjects. The sample consisted of 470 women (41%), 685 men (59%), 462 Blacks (40%), and 693 Whites (60%). The objective was to determine whether smoking independently predicts survival in patients with lung cancer or whether an existent effect is mediated through comorbidity and/or treatment.

Study Approach:
Cox proportional hazards analysis was used to study the cohort of 1,155 patients with lung cancer diagnosed at the Henry Ford Health System between 1995 and 1998, inclusive.

Results:
■ Adjusted for the baseline covariates of age, gender, illicit drug use, adverse symptoms, histology, and stage, the hazard ratio (HR) for smoking (current vs. former/never) was 1.37 (95% CIs [1.18, 1.59]; $p < .001$).
■ Adjusted for the baseline covariates and for 18 deleterious comorbidities, the HR for smoking was 1.38 (95% CIs [1.18, 1.60]; $p < .001$), indicating that the hazardous effect of smoking was not mediated by comorbidity. Current smoking was inversely associated with treatment (any surgery and/or chemotherapy and/or radiation therapy vs. none; odds ratio, 0.73; 95% CIs [0.55, 0.98]; $p = .03$).
■ Adjusted for baseline covariates, comorbidities, and treatment, the HR for current smoker versus former/never was 1.26 (95% CIs [1.08, 1.47]; $p = .003$), a decline of 30.7% that was explained by treatment (HR for any treatment vs. none: 0.40; 95% CIs [0.33, 0.48]; $p < .001$).

The median survival for current smokers was 0.76 years (95% CIs [0.67, 0.89]), and for former/never smokers was 1.01 years (95% CIs [0.89, 1.15]). See Figure 6.2.

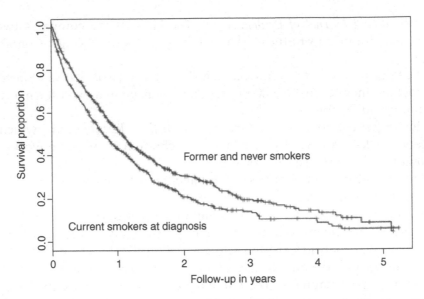

FIGURE 6.2 K–M survival plot for 1,155 case subjects with lung cancer, stratified by smoking status.

Conclusions:

Current smoking at diagnosis is an important independent predictor of shortened lung cancer survival. The fact that this effect was not explained by sociodemographic and exposure factors, adverse symptoms, histology, stage, comorbidity, and treatment suggests that it may be mediated through direct biological effects.

■ **Example 6.3:** Cohort study using Cox proportional regression model

In the CRAN package coxrobust, the function coxr() is available for efficiently and robustly fitting the Cox proportional hazards regression model in its basic form, where explanatory variables are time independent with one event per subject. The method is based on a smooth modification of the partial likelihood.

The approach is to maximize an objective function that is a smooth modification of the partial likelihood. Observations with excessive values of

$$\Lambda(T)exp(\beta'Z)$$

where:

Λ = the cumulated hazard,

β = vector of parameters and β' = transpose of β

Z = some explanatory variables, and

T = possibly censored survival time,

are down-weighted. Both Λ and β are iteratively robustly estimated.

Numerical results are supported by the function plot(), a graphical tool, which in a series of five graphs compares how well data are correlated by the estimated proportional hazards model with nonrobust (in black) and robust methods (in green):

- The first graph shows the standardized difference of two estimated survival functions, one using the Cox model and the other using the K–M estimator.
- The other four graphs show the same differences for four strata, defined by the quartiles of the estimated linear predictor.

Comparison of estimation results, along with analysis of the graphs, may yield very detailed information about the model fit.

Usage:

```
coxr(formula, data, subset, na.action, trunc = 0.95,
     f.weight = c("linear", "quadratic", "exponential"),
     singular.ok = TRUE, model = FALSE)
```

Arguments:

formula	A formula object, with the response on the left of a ~ operator and the terms on the right. The response must be a survival object as returned by the function Surv().
data	A data frame for interpreting the variables named in the formula, or in the subset.
subset	Expression saying that only a subset of the rows of the data should be used in the fit.
na.action	A missing-data filter function, applied to the model.frame after any subset argument has been used.
trunc	Roughly, a quantile of the sample $T_i exp(\beta'Z_i)$; determines the trimming level for the robust estimator.
f.weight	Type of weighting function; default is "quadratic".
singular.ok	logical value indicating how to handle collinearity in the model matrix. If TRUE, the program will automatically skip over columns of the X matrix that are linear combinations of earlier columns. In this case, the coefficients for such columns will be NA, and the variance matrix will contain zeros. For ancillary calculations, such as the linear predictor, the missing coefficients are treated as zeros.
model	A logical value indicating whether the model frame should be included as a component of the returned value.

The following R code segment may be used to compute a cohort study based on two available datasets:

1. lung—the lung cancer data at Mayo Clinic
2. veteran—the Veteran's Administration lung cancer data

```
> # Using lung, the lung cancer data at Mayo Clinic
> install.packages("coxrobust")
> library(coxrobust)
Loading required package: survival
Loading required package: splines
> ls("package:coxrobust")
[1] "coxr"    "gen_data"    "plot.coxr"    "print.coxr"
> data(lung)
```

```
> attach(lung)
> lung
```

	inst	time	status	age	Sex	ph.ecog	ph.karno	pat. karno	meal. cal	wt.loss
1	3	306	2	74	1	1	90	100	1175	NA
2	3	455	2	68	1	0	90	90	1225	15
3	3	1010	1	56	1	0	90	90	NA	15
4	5	210	2	57	1	1	90	60	1150	11
5	1	883	2	60	1	0	100	90	NA	0
224	1	188	1	77	1	1	80	60	NA	3
225	13	191	1	39	1	0	90	90	2350	-5
226	32	105	1	75	2	2	60	70	1025	5
227	6	174	1	66	1	1	90	100	1075	1
228	22	177	1	58	2	1	80	90	1060	0

```
> #use the lung cancer data at Mayo Clinic to
> #compare results of nonrobust and robust estimation
> result <- coxr(Surv(time, status) ~ age + sex + ph.karno +
+               meal.cal + wt.loss, data = lung)
> result # Outputting:
```

Call:
coxr(formula = Surv(time, status) ~ age + sex + ph.karno +
**   meal.cal + wt.loss, data = lung)**

Partial likelihood estimator

	coef	exp(coef)	se(coef)	p
age	1.25e-02	1.013	0.011686	0.2844
sex	−4.73e-01	0.623	0.197557	0.0166
ph.karno	−9.64e-03	0.990	0.0071260	1764
meal.cal	−8.96e-05	1.000	0.000245	0.7146
wt.loss	−2.82e-03	0.997	0.006989	0.6868

Wald test=11.6 on 5 df, p=0.0408

Robust estimator

	coef	exp(coef)	se(coef)	p
age	0.004927	1.005	0.013755	0.720210
sex	−0.839739	0.432	0.261861	0.001342
ph.karno	−0.033673	0.967	0.009986	0.000746
meal.cal	−0.000397	1.000	0.000336	0.236812
wt.loss	−0.008365	0.992	0.009398	0.373400

Extended Wald test=23.3 on 5 df, p=0.000292
> plot(result)
Waiting to confirm page change... # *Outputting* Figure 6.3.
>
> # *Outputting:* Figure 6.4.
>
Using veteran—*the Veteran's Administration lung cancer data*
> data(veteran)
> attach(veteran)
The following object(s) are masked from 'lung': age, status, time
> veteran

	trt	celltype	time	status	karno	diagtime	age	prior
1	1	squamous	72	1	60	7	69	0
2	1	squamous	411	1	70	5	64	10
3	1	squamous	228	1	60	3	38	0
4	1	squamous	126	1	60	9	63	10
5	1	squamous	118	1	70	11	65	10
133	2	large	133	1	75	1	65	0
134	2	large	111	1	60	5	64	0
135	2	large	231	1	70	18	67	10
136	2	large	378	1	80	4	65	0
137	2	large	49	1	30	3	37	0

> # *Use the Veteran's Administration Lung Cancer Data*
> # *to compare results of nonrobust and robust estimation*
> result <- coxr(Surv(time,status) ~ age + trt + celltype + karno
+   diagtime + prior, data = veteran)
> result
Call: coxr(formula = Surv(time, status) ~ age + trt + celltype + karno
+ diagtime + prior, data = veteran)
Partial likelihood estimator

	coef	exp(coef)	se(coef)	p
age	−0.008739	0.991	0.00931	3.48e-01
trt	0.289208	1.335	0.20757	1.64e-01
celltypesmallcell	0.855501	2.353	0.27517	1.88e-03
celltypeadeno	1.188162	3.281	0.30092	7.87e-05
celltypelarge	0.392164	1.480	0.28260	1.65e-01
karno	−0.032808	0.968	0.00551	2.64e-09
diagtime	0.000191	1.000	0.00913	9.83e-01
prior	0.007261	1.007	0.02323	7.55e-01

Wald test=62.2 on 8 df, p=1.71e-10
Robust estimator

	coef	exp(coef)	se(coef)	p
Age	−0.01184	0.988	0.01336	3.75e-01
Trt	0.20132	1.223	0.24286	4.07e-01
Celltypesmallcell	1.14056	3.129	0.43445	8.66e-03
Celltypeadeno	1.22137	3.392	0.49300	1.32e-02
Celltypelarge	0.20405	1.226	0.46553	6.61e-01
Karno	−0.04230	0.959	0.00687	7.26e-10
Diagtime	−0.00489	0.995	0.00981	6.18e-01
Prior	0.01335	1.013	0.03447	6.98e-01

Extended Wald test=62 on 8 df, p=1.9e-10
> plot(result)
Waiting to confirm page change. # *Outputting* Figure 6.5.
> # *Outputting:* Figure 6.6.

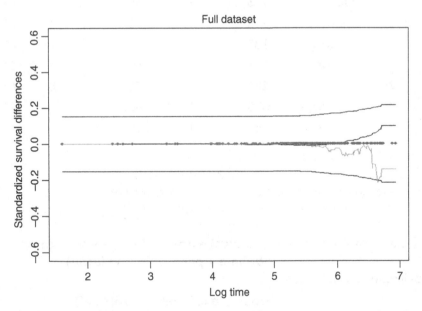

FIGURE 6.3 Cohort study using lung (the lung cancer data at Mayo Clinic). Standardized difference of two estimated survival functions, one via the Cox model and the other via the K–M estimator: nonrobust (black) and robust (green).

Cohort Studies and the Lexis Diagram[3] in the Biostatistics of Demography

Demographic biostatistics dealing with the study of human populations often make use of a **Lexis diagram** (named after economist Wilhelm Lexis). This two-dimensional diagram represents events (such as deaths or births) that happen to

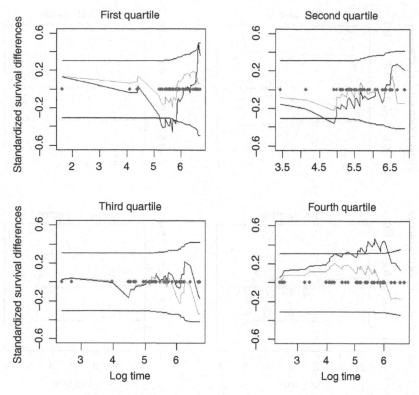

FIGURE 6.4 Cohort study using lung (lung cancer data at Mayo Clinic). Standardized difference of two estimated survival functions: one via the Cox model and the other via the K–M estimator. The four graphs show the same differences for four strata, defined by the quartiles of the estimated linear predictor: nonrobust (black) and robust (green).

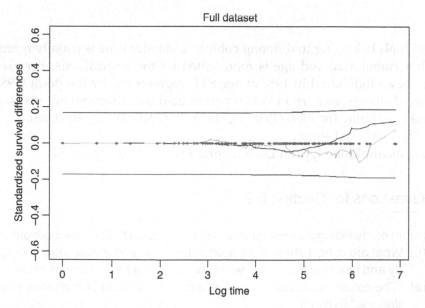

FIGURE 6.5 Cohort study using veteran (Veterans Administration lung cancer data). Standardized difference of two estimated survival functions: one via the Cox model and the other via the K–M

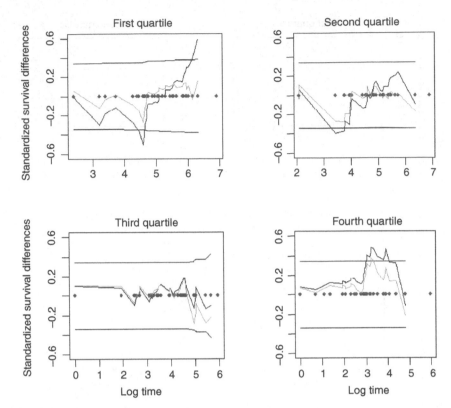

FIGURE 6.6   Cohort study using veteran (Veterans Administration lung cancer data). Standardized difference of two estimated survival functions: one via the Cox model and the other via the K–M estimator. The four graphs show the same differences for four strata, defined by the quartiles of the estimated linear predictor: nonrobust (black) and robust (green).

individuals belonging to different cohorts. Calendar time is usually represented on the horizontal axis, and age is represented on the vertical axis. For example, the death of an individual in 1988 at age 83 is represented by the point (1988, 83); the cohort of all persons born in 1937 is represented by a diagonal line starting at (1937, 0) and continuing through (1938, 1), (1939, 2), (1940, 3), ..., (2000, 63), ..., (2012, 75), ..., (2037, 100), and so on.

An example of a typical Lexis diagram is shown in Figure 6.7.

Review Questions for Section 6.2

1. (a) In epidemiologic investigations, what is a cohort? Give an example.
   (b) What are cohort studies, as used in research and investigations in epidemiology and health sciences? Give an example of a typical cohort study.
2. (a) "The cohort cannot be defined as a group of people who already have the disease." Explain.
   (b) "A cohort study may be a time-consuming task and may be very expensive to

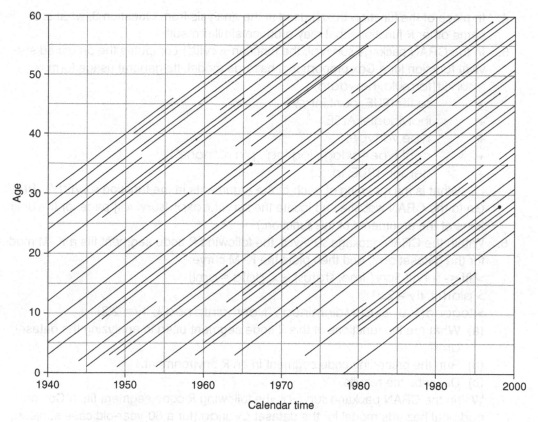

FIGURE 6.7   A typical Lexis diagram for demographic biostatistics.

3. (a) "Cohort studies are suitable for investigations in diseases of choice and non-communicable diseases." Explain.
    (b) Name five diseases that are suitable for investigation by cohort studies.
4. (a) Name five well-known examples of cohort studies, each involving thousands of case subjects.
    (b) Name two approaches in survival analysis that are suitable for cohort studies.
5. (a) What is a Lexis diagram?
    (b) "A Lexis diagram may be suitable for analysis in cohort studies." Explain.

Exercises for Section 6.2

1. In Example 6.3, what are the functions of the following R code segment used in analyzing the dataset lung?
    ```
    > result <- coxr(Surv(time, status) ~ age + sex + ph.karno +
    +                meal.cal + wt.loss, data = lung)
    ```
2. In place of the function coxr() used in the analysis, what are some other R functions that may produce similar results?
3. In Example 6.3, what are the functions of the following R code segment used in analyzing the dataset veteran?
    ```
    > result <- coxr(Surv(time, status) ~ age + trt + celltype + karno
    ```

4. In place of the function coxr() used in the analysis from Question 3, what are some other R functions that may produce similar results?

5. In the CRAN package survival, the function survfit() computes the predicted survival function for a Cox proportional hazards model. Its general usage form is

```
> survfit(formula, newdata,
+         se.fit=TRUE, conf.int=.95,
+         individual=FALSE,
+         type,vartype,
+         conf.type=c("log","log-log","plain","none"),
+         censor=TRUE, id, ...)
```

What is the meaning of each of the arguments in the function survfit()? (***HINT***: Go to the CRAN website and locate the survfit.coxph{survival} page for the definitions of the arguments of this function.)

6. Within the CRAN package survival, the following R code segment fits a K–M model for the dataset aml, and then plots the K–M curve:

```
> fit <- survfit(Surv(time, status) ~ x, data = aml)
> plot(fit, lty = 2:3)
> legend(100, .8, c("Maintained", "Nonmaintained"), lty = 2:3)
```

(a) What are the functions of this R code segment used in analyzing the dataset aml?

(b) Run the preceding code segment in an R environment.

(c) Describe the results.

7. Within the CRAN package survival, the following R code segment fits a Cox proportional hazards model for the dataset ovarian (for a 60-year-old case subject), and then plots the model curve:

```
> fit <- coxph(Surv(futime, fustat) ~ age, data = ovarian)
> plot(survfit(fit, newdata=data.frame(age=60)),
+       xscale=365.25, xlab = "Years", ylab="Survival")
```

(a) What are the functions of this R code segment used in analyzing the dataset ovarian?

(b) Run the preceding code segment in an R environment.

(c) Describe the results.

8. Within the CRAN package survival, the following R code segment fits a K–M model (for time to progression/death for patients with monoclonal gammopathy), for the dataset mgus1, and then plots the model competing risk curves for cumulative incidence:

```
> fit1 <- survfit(Surv(stop, event=='progression') ~1,
+                 data=mgus1, subset=(start==0))
> fit2 <- survfit(Surv(stop, status) ~1, data=mgus1,
+                 subset=(start==0), etype=event)
> # Competing Risks:
> # CI curves are plotted from 0 upward, rather than
> # from 1 downward
> plot(fit2, fun='event', xscale=365.25, xmax=7300,
+       mark.time=FALSE,
+       col=2:3, xlab="Years post diagnosis of MGUS")
```

```
> lines(fit1, fun='event', xscale=365.25, xmax=7300,
+       mark.time=FALSE, conf.int=FALSE)
> text(10, .4, "Competing Risk: death", col=3)
> text(16, .15,"Competing Risk: progression", col=2)
> text(15, .30,"KM:prog")
```

(a) What are the functions of this R code segment used in analyzing the dataset mgus1?

(b) Run the preceding code segment in an R environment.

(c) Describe the results.

9. The CRAN package survrec.

A migrating myoelectric complex [or migrating motor complex (MMC)] is a wave of bioelectric activity that sweeps through the intestines in a regular cycle during fasting. These complexes help trigger peristaltic waves, which facilitate movement of indigestible substances (fiber and foreign bodies) from the stomach, through the small intestine, past the ileocecal sphincter, and into the colon. The MMC originates in the stomach roughly every 80 minutes between meals and is responsible for the stomach rumbling experienced when hungry. The MMC lasts for approximately 15 minutes. It also serves to transport bacteria from the small intestine to the large intestine and to inhibit the migration of colonic bacteria into the terminal ileum. The MMC may be partially regulated by motilin; it is initiated in the stomach as a response to vagal stimulation and does not directly depend on extrinsic nerves.

In the CRAN package survrec, the function mlefrailty.fit() is a survival function estimator for correlated recurrence time data under a gamma frailty model using the maximum likelihood criterion. The resulting object of class survfitr may be plotted by the function plot.survfitr() before it is returned.

The usage form of this function mlefrailty.fit() is

```
mlefrailty.fit(x,tvals, lambda=NULL, alpha=NULL, alpha.min, alpha.max,
tol=1e-07, maxiter=500,alpha.console=TRUE)
```

for which the arguments are:

x	A survival recurrent event object.
tvals	Vector of times where the survival function can be estimated.
lambda	Optional vector of baseline hazard probabilities at t (see details in survrec package). Default is numdeaths/apply(AtRisk,2,-sum).
alpha	Optional parameter of shape and scale for the frailty distribution. If this parameter is unknown, it is estimated via an expectation-maximization (EM) algorithm. A seed is calculated to obtain the convergence of this algorithm (see details in survrec package).
alpha.min	Optional left bound of the alpha parameter; used to obtain a seed to estimate the alpha parameter. Default value is 0.5.
alpha.max	Optional right bound of the alpha parameter; used to obtain a seed to estimate the alpha parameter. Default value is the maximum of distinct times of events.

tol	Optional tolerance of the EM algorithm used to estimate the alpha parameter. Default is 10e – 7.
maxiter	Optional maximum number of iterations of the EM algorithm used to estimate the alpha parameter. Default is 500.
alpha.console	If TRUE prints in the console, the program estimates initial value for alpha and the alpha estimate via the EM algorithm; if FALSE, it does not.

Remarks:

1. A common choice of frailty distribution is a gamma distribution with shape and scale parameters set equal to an unknown parameter α. The common marginal survival function may be expressed as

$$F(t) = [\alpha/(\alpha + \Lambda_0(t))]^\alpha \tag{6.1}$$

The parameter α controls the degree of association between interoccurrence times within a unit. It may be shown that the estimation of α and α_0 can be obtained via maximization of the marginal likelihood function and the EM algorithm.

To obtain a good convergence, first α is estimated. This estimation is used as an initial value in the EM procedure, and it is carried out by maximization of the profile likelihood for α. In this case, the arguments of the function mlefrailty. fit(), called alpha.min and alpha.max, are the boundaries of this maximization. The maximum is obtained using the golden section search method.

2. *Value:* If the convergence of the EM algorithm is not obtained, the initial value of α can be used as an alpha.min argument and recalculated.

n	Number of units or subjects observed.
m	Vector of number of recurrences in each subject (length n).
failed	Vector of number of recurrences in each subject (length n*m). Vector ordered (e.g., times of first unit, times of second unit, ..., times of n-unit).
censored	Vector of times of censorship for each subject (length n).
numdistinct	Number of distinct failure times.
distinct	Vector of distinct failure times.
status 0	0 if the estimation can be provided; 1 if not, depending on whether alpha could be estimated.
alpha	Parameter of gamma frailty model.
lambda	Estimates of the hazard probabilities at distinct failure times.
survfunc	Vector of survival estimated in distinct times.
tvals	Copy of argument.
MLEattvals	Vector of survival estimated in tvals times.

The following R code segment may be used to compute a cohort study based on the available dataset:

```
> install.packages("survrec")
> library(survrec)
Loading required package: boot
Attaching package: 'boot'
The following object(s) are masked from 'package:lattice': melanoma
The following object(s) are masked from 'package:survival': aml
> ls("package:survrec")
[1] "is.Survr"        "mlefrailty.fit"  "psh.fit"    "q.search"
[5] "surv.search"     "survdiffr"       "survfitr"   "Survr"
[9] "wc.fit"
> data(MMC)
> attach(MMC)
The following object(s) are masked from 'colon':
id, time
The following object(s) are masked from 'bladder (position 15)':
event, id
The following object(s) are masked from 'bladder (position 16)'':
event, id
The following object(s) are masked from 'lung':
time
> MMC # Displaying data of 99 case subjects.
```

	id	time	Event	group
1	1	112	1	Males
2	1	145	1	Males
3	1	39	1	Males
97	19	66	1	Females
98	19	100	1	Females
99	19	4	0	Females

```
>
> fit <- mlefrailty.fit(Survr(MMC$id,MMC$time,MMC$event))
Needs to Determine a Seed Value for Alpha
Seed Alpha: 20.02853
Alpha estimate= 10.17623
> fit
> plot(fit)
```

(a) What are the functions of this R code segment used in analyzing the dataset MMC?
(b) Run the preceding code segment in an R environment.
(c) Describe the results.

REFERENCES

Doll, R., Peto, R., Boreham, J., & Sutherland, I. (2004). Mortality in relation to smoking: 50 years' observations on male British doctors. *British Medical Journal, 328,* 1519–1528.

Everitt, B. S., & Hothorn, T. (2006). *A handbook of statistical analysis using R (HSAUR).* Boca Raton, FL: Chapman & Hall/CRC.

Handysides, A. R., & Landless, P. N. (2012, February). Diseases of choice. *Adventist World—NAD, 8*(2), 19.

Tammemagi, C. M., Neslund-Dudas, C., Simoff, M., & Kvale, P. (2004). Smoking and lung cancer survival: The role of comorbidity and treatment. *Chest, 125*(1), 27–37.

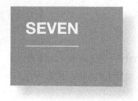

SEVEN

Randomized Trials, Phase Development, Confounding in Survival Analysis, and Logistic Regressions

7.1 RANDOMIZED TRIALS (STANLEY, 2007)[1]

A **randomized trial (RT)** or **randomized controlled trial (RCT)** is a specific type of scientific experiment, and it is the preferred design for a clinical trial in epidemiology. RTs are used to test the efficacy of various types of interventions within a case-subject population. They may also provide an opportunity to gather useful information about adverse effects, such as drug reactions.

The key distinguishing feature of the usual RT is that study case subjects, *after* assessment of eligibility and recruitment, but *before* the intervention to be studied begins, are randomly allocated to receive one or the other of the alternative treatments under the study. Random allocation in real trials is complex, but conceptually, the process is like tossing a coin. *After randomization, the two groups of subjects are followed in exactly the same way*; the only differences between the care they receive (e.g., in terms of procedures, tests, outpatient visits, follow-up calls, etc.) should be those intrinsic to the treatments being compared. The most important advantage of proper randomization is that it minimizes allocation bias in the assignment of treatments, thereby balancing both known and unknown prognostic factors.

Classifications of RTs by Study Design

One way to classify RTs is by study design, in which the four major categories are:

Parallel group—in which each participant is randomly assigned to a group and all the participants in the group receive (or do not receive) an intervention.

Crossover—in which, over time, each participant receives (or does not receive) an intervention in a random sequence.

Cluster—in which preexisting groups of participants (e.g., cities, social associations) are randomly selected to receive (or not receive) an intervention.

Factorial—in which each participant is randomly assigned to a group that receives (or does not receive) a particular combination of interventions. For example:

- Group A receives Vitamin X and Vitamin Y.
- Group B receives Vitamin X and Placebo Y.

- Group C receives Placebo X and Vitamin Y.
- Group D receives Placebo X and Placebo Y.

An analysis of the 616 RTs indexed in *PubMed* during December 2006 found that 78% were parallel-group trials, 16% were crossover, 2% were split-body, 2% were cluster, and 2% were factorial.[1]

RTs may also be classified by *efficacy* (the effectiveness of the test) or by *hypothesis* (superiority vs. noninferiority vs. equivalence, according to the corresponding statistical significance).

Randomization

The following are all advantages of proper randomization in an RT:

- It eliminates bias in treatment assignment, specifically selection bias and confounding.
- It facilitates blinding (masking) of the identity of treatments from investigators, participants, and assessors.
- It permits the use of probability theory to express the likelihood that any difference in outcome between treatment groups merely indicates chance.

In randomizing case subjects, one may choose from two processes:

1. Choose a *randomization procedure* to generate an unpredictable sequence of allocations; this may be a simple random assignment of patients to any of the groups at equal probabilities.
2. Choose *allocation concealment*, which refers to the stringent precautions taken to ensure that the group assignments of case subjects are not revealed before they are definitively allocated to their respective groups.

Nonrandom "systematic" methods of group assignment, such as alternating subjects between one group and the other, can cause limitless contamination possibilities and a breach of allocation concealment.

RANDOMIZATION PROCEDURES

An ideal randomization procedure achieves the following goals:

- *Equal group sizes.* This ensures adequate statistical power, especially in subgroup analyses.
- *Low selection bias.* The procedure should not allow an investigator to predict the next subject's group assignment by examining which group has been assigned the fewest subjects up to that point.
- *Low probability of confounding.* This implies a balance in covariates across groups.

No single randomization procedure can meet all these goals in every circumstance, so, for a given investigation, epidemiologists should choose a procedure based on its merits and the nature of the investigation.

SIMPLE RANDOMIZATION

Simple randomization is a commonly used intuitive procedure, similar to repeated fair coin tossing; it is also known as *complete* or *unrestricted* randomization. It is **robust** against both selection and accidental biases. Its main drawback is the possibility of imbalanced group sizes in small RTs. It is recommended only for RTs with more than 200 subjects.

RESTRICTED RANDOMIZATION

To balance group sizes in smaller RTs, some form of *restricted randomization* is recommended. Some major types of restricted randomization used in RT are:

- **Permuted-block randomization**, in which a block size and allocation ratio (number of subjects in one group versus the other group) are specified, and subjects are allocated randomly within each block. For example, a block size of 16 and an allocation ratio of 3:1 would lead to random assignment of 12 subjects to one group and 4 to the other. This type of randomization can be combined with stratified randomization (e.g., by center in a multicenter trial) to ensure good balance of participant characteristics in each group. A special case of permuted-block randomization is *random allocation*, in which the entire sample is treated as one block. A disadvantage of permuted-block randomization is that even if the block sizes are large and randomly varied, the procedure may still fall prey to selection bias. Another disadvantage is that proper analysis of data from permuted-block RCTs requires stratification by blocks.
- **Adaptive biased-coin randomization**, in which the probability of being assigned to a group decreases if the group is overrepresented and increases if the group is underrepresented. The methods are thought to be less affected by selection bias than permuted-block randomization.

RANDOMIZED TRIALS WITH BLINDING

An RT may be *blinded* (or *masked*) by restricting the procedures used to those that prevent study case subjects, caregivers, outcome assessors, and all others participating or involved in the study from knowing which intervention was received. However, unlike allocation concealment, blinding sometimes may be inappropriate or impossible to perform in an RT. For example, if an RT involves a treatment in which active participation of the case subject is necessary (e.g., physical therapy), participants cannot be blinded to the intervention.

Historically, blinded RT have been classified as single-blind, double-blind, or triple-blind. Currently, it is preferred that these additional categories be avoided; since 2010, authors and editors reporting blinded RT have been directed to discuss it as follows: "If blinding is used, then the report should identify who [was] blinded after assignment to interventions (e.g., participants, care providers, those assessing outcomes) and how the blinding was undertaken" (Blanchard, 2012; Moreira, Araujo, & Machado, 2012; Sigler & Stemhagen, 2011).

RCTs without blinding are referred to as *unblinded* or open. In 2008, a study concluded that the results of unblinded RTs tended to be biased toward beneficial effects

treatments for multiple sclerosis, unblinded neurologists (but not the blinded neurologists) felt that the treatments were beneficial. In practice, although the participants and providers involved in an RT are often unblinded, it is desirable and often possible to blind the assessor or obtain an objective source to evaluate outcomes.

Biostatistical Analysis of Data from RTs

The types of statistical methods used in RTs depend on the characteristics of the data.

- For **dichotomous (binary) outcome data**, logistic regression and other methods may be used (e.g., to predict sustained virological responses after receipt of treatment for hepatitis C).
- For **continuous outcome data**, analysis of covariance may be used to test the effects of predictor variables (e.g., for changes in blood lipid levels after receipt of treatment for acute coronary syndrome).
- For **time-to-event outcome data** that may be censored, survival analysis is appropriate (e.g., Kaplan–Meier [K–M] estimators and Cox proportional hazards models for time to coronary heart disease [CHD] after receipt of hormone replacement therapy in menopause).

Biostatistics for RTs in the R Environment

At the CRAN website, support for randomized clinical trials is available in terms of project design, monitoring, and analysis. To access these sources from the R environment:

Select the Help/CRAN home page
Select the "Search/An R site search" option, and enter "Randomized Clinical Trials"

This selection calls up many available sources, including the following.

(1) CRAN Task View: Clinical Trial Design, Monitoring, and Analysis (score: 3)
   Author: Unknown
   Date: Wed, 25 Apr 2012 02:57:32
   CRAN Task View: Clinical Trial Design, Monitoring, and Analysis CRAN packages
   Related links: ClinicalTrials task view information maintainer: Ed Zhang
   Contact: Ed.Zhang.jr@gmail.com
   Version: 201

From http://finzi.psych.upenn.edu/views/ClinicalTrials.html (23,531 bytes), one may select the appropriate methodologic supports for the biostatistics of RTs, including project design, monitoring, and analysis. CRAN packages are available in the following areas of RT:

- Design and monitoring

- Analysis for specific designs
- Analysis in general
- Meta-analysis

The following examples are typical.

■ **Example 7.1:** RTs' project design using package samplesize: Determination of sample size

The CRAN package samplesize computes the sample size for the Student's *t*-test, with equal and nonequal variances; and for the Wilcoxon–Mann–Whitney test for categorical data, with and without ties.

For sample size for an independent Student's *t*-test with unequal group size, use the function n.indep.t.test.eq(), with default parameters:

n.indep.t.test.neq(power = 0.8, alpha = 0.95, mean.diff = 0.8,
                          sd.est = 0.83, k = 0.5)

controlled by the following variable parameters as arguments:

power   required power 1-beta
alpha   required Level I-error 1-alpha
mean.diff   required minimum difference between group means
sd.est   standard deviation in groups
k   n_2 = n_1*k
n_1   sample size of group 1
n_2   sample size of group 2
N   total sample size: N=n_1 + n_2

The following R code segment may be used to compute sample sizes for a randomized clinical trial using this CRAN package:

```
> install.packages("samplesize")
> library(samplesize)
> ls("package:samplesize")
[1] "n.indep.t.test.eq"      "n.indep.t.test.neq"      "n.paired.t.test"
[4] "n.welch.test"           "n.wilcox.ord"
> n.indep.t.test.eq(power = 0.8, alpha = 0.95, mean.diff = 0.8,
+                   sd.est = 0.83) # For two samples of equal size:
[1] "sample.size:"   "29"
> # Going for a test with a high biostatistical power, say, power = 0.95
> n.indep.t.test.eq(power = 0.95, alpha = 0.95, mean.diff = 0.8,
+                   sd.est = 0.83)
[1] "sample.size:"   "49"
> # And for two samples of unequal size
> n.indep.t.test.neq(power = 0.8, alpha = 0.95, mean.diff = 0.8,
+ sd.est = 0.83) # At 0.8 power
[1] "sample.size:"   "32"              "sample.size n.1:"   "21.3"
```

```
> n.indep.t.test.neq(power = 0.95, alpha = 0.95, mean.diff = 0.8,
+ sd.est = 0.83) # And at 0.95 power
[1] "sample.size:"    "55"              "sample.size n.1:" "36.7"
[5] "sample.size n.2:" "18.3"
```

Remark:
For higher biostatistical power, larger samples are needed.

Review Questions for Section 7.1

1. (a) What is an RT in the context of an epidemiologic investigation?
   (b) What are the advantages of RT in a study such as a clinical trial?
2. (a) What is restricted randomization?
   (b) Explain the following terms: permuted-block randomization, adaptive biased-coin randomization.
3. In the biostatistical analysis of data from RTs, three characteristics of the data are expected. Name them and briefly explain each characteristic.
4. CRAN packages are available to analyze data from RTs. In which five areas of RTs are these packages applicable?

Exercises for Section 7.1

1. For worked Example 7.1,
   (a) Explain the function of each line of the R code segment for the computation.
   (b) Rerun this code segment in the R environment.
2. In the CRAN package CRTSize, the function n4means() may be used to provide sample size estimation information. For instance, it can compute the number of case subjects needed for a cluster RT with continuous outcome. The following R code segment is used where the outcome is continuous (e.g., blood pressure or weight). Note that if the results suggest that a small number of clusters is required, an iterative procedure will include the t distribution instead of the normal critical value for alpha, iterating until convergence. For this function n4means(), the following specification applies:

Description:
This function provides detailed sample-size estimation information to determine the number of subjects that must be enrolled in a cluster RT to compare two means.

Usage:
n4means(delta, sigma, m, ICC, alpha=0.05, power=0.8, AR=1, two.tailed=TRUE, digits=3)

Arguments:

delta	The minimum detectable difference between population means.
sigma	The standard error of the outcome.
m	The anticipated average (or actual) cluster size.
ICC	The anticipated value of the intraclass correlation coefficient, p.
AR	The allocation ratio: AR=1 implies an equal number of subjects per

that more subjects will be enrolled in the control group (e.g., in the case of a costly intervention), and AR < 1 implies that more subjects will be enrolled in the treatment group (rarely used).

alpha	The desired Type I error rate.
power	The desired level of power, recall power = 1 – Type II error.
two.tailed	Logical value. If TRUE, calculations are based on a two-tailed Type I error; if FALSE, a one-sided calculation is performed.
digits	Number of digits to round calculations.

Value:

nE	The minimum number of subjects required in the experimental group.
nC	The minimum number of subjects required in the control group.
delta	The minimum detectable difference between population means.
sigma	The standard error of the outcome.
alpha	The desired Type I error rate.
power	The desired level of power, recall power = 1 – Type II error.
AR	The allocation ratio.

The following R code segment is available to undertake the computation:

```
> install.packages("CRTSize")
> library(CRTSize)
> ls("package:CRTSize")
```

[1] "fixedMetaAnalMD"	"fixedMetaAnalRROR"
[3] "n4incidence"	"n4means"
[5] "n4meansEB"	"n4meansMeta"
[7] "n4props"	"n4propsEB"
[9] "n4propsMeta"	"print.fixedMetaAnalMD"
[11] "print.fixedMetaAnalRROR"	"print.n4incidence"
[13] "print.n4means"	"print.n4meansEB"
[15] "print.n4meansMeta"	"print.n4props"
[17] "print.n4propsEB"	"print.n4propsMeta"
[19] "summary.fixedMetaAnalMD"	"summary.fixedMetaAnalRROR"
[21] "summary.n4incidence"	"summary.n4means"
[23] "summary.n4meansEB"	"summary.n4meansMeta"
[25] "summary.n4props"	"summary.n4propsEB"
[27] "summary.n4propsMeta"	

```
> n4means(delta=10, sigma=1, m=25, ICC=0.05,
+           alpha=0.05, power=0.80);
> # Outputting:
```

The required sample size is a minimum of 1 cluster of size 25 in the Experi-

(a) Explain the function of each line of the R code segment for this computation.

(b) Rerun this code segment in the R environment.

(c) Recalculate the estimation of cluster sizes for a biostatistical power of 0.90.

(d) Comment on the results.

3. The CRAN package randomSurvivalForest describes random survival forests for right-censored and competing risks survival data (Gerds, Cai, & Schumacher, 2008; Graf, Schmoor, Sauerbrei, & Schumacher, 1999).

The outputs of the function plot.ensemble() in this package are ensemble survival curves and ensemble estimates of mortality.

This approach is applicable to competing risk analyses, but the plots are nonevent specific. For event-specific curves, and for a more comprehensive analysis, use competing.risk in such cases.

The following R code segment is available to undertake the computation, using the dataset veteran in the CRAN package survival:

```
> install.packages("randomSurvivalForest")
> library(randomSurvivalForest)
```
randomSurvivalForest 3.6.3
Type rsf.news() to see new features, changes, and bug fixes.
```
> ls(package:randomSurvivalForest) # Listing the contents:
```

[1]	"competing.risk"	"find.interaction"	"impute.rsf"
[4]	"max.subtree"	"plot.ensemble"	"plot.error"
[7]	"plot.proximity"	"plot.rsf"	"plot.variable"
[10]	"pmml2rsf"	"predict.rsf"	"print.rsf"
[13]	"randomSurvivalForest"	"rsf"	"rsf.news"
[16]	"rsf2pmml"	"rsf2rfz"	"varSel"
[19]	"vimp"		

Warning message:
In ls(package:randomSurvivalForest) :
'package:randomSurvivalForest' converted to character string
```
> install.packages("survival")
> library(survival)
```
Loading required package: splines
```
> ls("package:survival") # Listing the contents:
```

[1]	"aareg"	"aml"	"attrassign"
[4]	"basehaz"	"bladder"	"bladder1"
[7]	"bladder2"	"cancer"	"cch"
[10]	"cgd"	"clogit"	"cluster"
[13]	"colon"	"cox.zph"	"coxph"
[16]	"coxph.control"	"coxph.detail"	"coxph.fit"
[19]	"dsurvreg"	"format.Surv"	"frailty"
[22]	"frailty.gamma"	"frailty.gaussian"	"frailty.t"

[28] "is.na.Surv"   "is.ratetable"   "is.Surv"
[31] "jasa"   "jasa1"   "kidney"
[34] "labels.survreg"   "leukemia"   "logan"
[37] "lung"   "match.ratetable"   "mgus"
[40] "mgus1"   "mgus2"   "nwtco"
[43] "ovarian"   "pbc"   "pbcseq"
[46] "pspline"   "psurvreg"   "pyears"
[49] "qsurvreg"   "ratetable"   "ratetableDate"
[52] "rats"   "ridge"   "stanford2"
[55] "strata"   "Surv"   "survConcordance"
[58] "survdiff"   "survexp"   "survexp.mn"
[61] "survexp.us"   "survexp.usr"   "survfit"
[64] "survfitcoxph.fit"   "survobrien"   "survreg"
[67] "survreg.control"   "survreg.distributions"   "survreg.fit"
[70] "survregDtest"   "survSplit"   "tcut"
[73] "tobin"   "tt"   "untangle.specials"
[76] "veteran"

```
> data(veteran, package = "randomSurvivalForest")
> v.out <- rsf(Surv(time, status) ~ ., veteran, ntree = 1000)
> data(veteran, package = "randomSurvivalForest")
> v.out <- rsf(Surv(time, status) ~ ., veteran, ntree = 1000)
> plot.ensemble(v.out)
> # Outputting: Figure 7.1: randomSurvivalForest-1
```

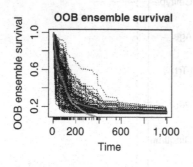

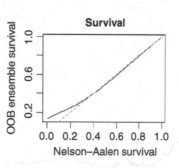

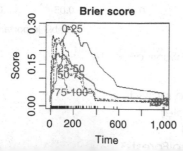

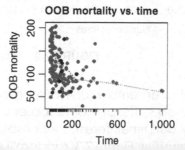

Four plots are produced (*from top to bottom, left to right*):

(1) Ensemble survival function for each individual. The thick red line is overall ensemble survival; the thick green line is the Nelson–Aalen estimator.
(2) Comparison of the population ensemble survival function to the Nelson–Aalen estimator.
(3) Brier score (0 = perfect, 1 = poor, and 0.25 = guessing) stratified by ensemble mortality. Based on the method described in Gerds et al. (2008), in which the censoring distribution is estimated using the K–M estimator. Stratification is into four groups corresponding to the 0–25, 25–50, 50–75, and 75–100 percentile values of mortality. The red line is the overall (nonstratified) Brier score.
(4) Plot of mortality versus observed time. Points in blue correspond to events; points in black are censored observations.

> plot(v.out) # *Outputting:* Figure 7.2: randomSurvivalForest-2

	Importance	Relative Imp
karno	0.1410	1.0000
celltype	0.0405	0.2871
trt	0.0036	0.0257
age	0.0001	0.0008
prior	−0.0018	−0.0128
diagtime	−0.0019	−0.0136

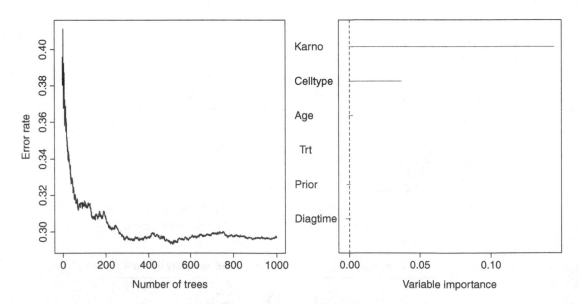

FIGURE 7.2 randomSurvivalForest-2.

```
>
> # plot of ensemble survival for a single individual
> surv.ensb <- t(exp(-v.out$oob.ensemble))
> plot(v.out$timeInterest, surv.ensb[, 1])
> # Outputting: Figure 7.3: randomSurvivalForest-3
```

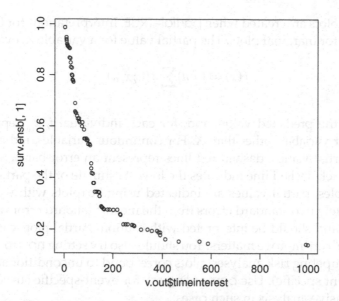

FIGURE 7.3 randomSurvivalForest-3: plot of ensemble survival for a single individual.

(a) Explain the function of each line of the R code segment for this computation.
(b) Rerun this code segment in the R environment.
(c) Recalculate the estimation of cluster sizes for another dataset from the CRAN package survival. Comment on the results.

4. To obtain the survival effects of variables, the R function plot.variable(), in the CRAN package randomSurvivalForest (rSF), may be used to create plots of ensemble mortality, predicted survival, or predicted survival time against a given x variable. Marginal and partial plots may also be created. Either mortality, relative frequency of mortality, predicted survival, or predicted survival times is plotted on the vertical axis (y-value) against x variables on the horizontal axis.

■ The choice of x variables can be specified using predictor names.
■ The choice of y-value is controlled by type.
There are four different choices:
(1) 'mort' is ensemble mortality.
(2) 'rel.freq' is standardized mortality.
(3) 'surv' is predicted survival at a given time point.
(4) 'time' is the predicted survival time.

For continuous variables, points are colored with blue, corresponding to events, and black, to censored observations. Ensemble mortality should be interpreted in terms of the total number of deaths. For example, if i has a mortality value of 100, then if all individuals were the same as i, the expected number of deaths would be 100. If type="rel.freq", then mortality values are divided by an adjusted sample size, defined as the maximum of the sample size and the maximum mortality value. Standardized mortality values do not indicate total deaths, but rather

Partial plots are created when partial=TRUE. Interpretations for these are different from those for marginal plots. The partial value for a variable X, evaluated at X = x, is

$$f(x) = (1/n)\sum_{i=1}^{n} f(x; x_{i,0})$$

where f is the predicted value; and, for each individual i, $x_{i,o}$ represents the value for all other variables other than X. For continuous variables, red points are used to indicate partial values; dashed red lines represent an error bar of +/− two standard errors. A black dashed line indicates the lowest estimate of the partial values. For discrete variables, partial values are indicated using boxplots with whiskers extending approximately two standard errors from the mean. Standard errors are provided only as a guide and should be interpreted with caution. Partial plots can be slow. Setting type="time" can improve matters. You should also try setting npts to a smaller number.

For competing risk analyses, plots correspond to unconditional values (i.e., they are nonevent specific). Use competing.risk for event-specific curves and for a more comprehensive analysis in such cases.

The usage formula for this function is

```
plot.variable(x, plots.per.page = 4, granule = 5, sorted = TRUE,
              type = c("mort", "rel.freq", "surv", "time")[1],
              partial = FALSE, predictorNames = NULL,
              npred = NULL, npts = 25, subset = NULL,
              percentile = 50, ...)
```

in which the arguments are

x   An object of class (rsf, grow) or (rsf, predict).
plots.per.page   Integer value controlling page layout.
granule   Integer value controlling whether a plot for a specific variable should be given as a boxplot or a scatter plot. Larger values coerce boxplots.
sorted   Should variables be sorted by importance values (applies only if importance values are available)?
type   Select the type of value to be plotted on the vertical axis.
partial   Should partial plots be created?
predictorNames   Character vector of x variables to be plotted. Default is all.
npred   Number of variables to be plotted. Default is all.
npts   Maximum number of points used when generating partial plots for continuous variables.
subset   Indexes indicating which rows of the predictor matrix are to be used. (Note: This applies to the processed predictor matrix, predictors of the object.) Default is to use all rows.
percentile   Percentile of follow-up time used for plotting predicted survival.
...   Further arguments passed to or from other methods.

The following R code segment is available to undertake the computation using the dataset veteran in the CRAN package survival:

```
> install.packages("randomSurvivalForest")
```

```
> ls(package:randomSurvivalForest)
>
> install.packages("survival")
> library(survival)
> ls("package:survival")
>
> # Some examples applied to veteran data.
> data(veteran, package = "randomSurvivalForest")
> v.out <- rsf(Surv(time,status) ~ ., veteran, nsplit = 10,
+              ntree = 1000)
>
> plot.variable(v.out, plots.per.page = 3)
```

Warning message:
In bxp(list(stats = c(28.3583161744737, 56.5401467687752, 78.2666123470398):
some notches went outside hinges ('box'): maybe set notch=FALSE))

```
> # Outputting: Figure 7.4: rSF-1
>
> plot.variable(v.out, plots.per.page = 2,
+               predictorNames = c("trt", "karno", "age"))
> # Outputting: Figure 7.5: rSF-2
> plot.variable(v.out, type = "surv", npred = 1, percentile = 50)
> # Outputting: Figure 7.6: rSF-3
> plot.variable(v.out, type = "rel.freq", partial = TRUE,
+   plots.per.page = 2, npred=3)
> # Outputting: Figure 7.7: rSF-4
```

    (a)   Explain the function of each line of the R code segment for this computation.
    (b)   Rerun this code segment in the R environment.
    (c)   Recalculate the estimation of cluster sizes for another dataset from the CRAN package survival. Comment on the results.

5. Repeat the computation as in Exercise 4, but this time, use the dataset pbc, as follows:

```
>
> install.packages("randomSurvivalForest")
> library(randomSurvivalForest)
> ls(package:randomSurvivalForest)
>
> install.packages("survival")
> library(survival)
> ls("package:survival")
>
> # Fast partial plots using 'time' type.
> # Top 8 predictors from PBC data
> data(pbc, package = "randomSurvivalForest")
> pbc.out <- rsf(Surv(days,status) ~ ., pbc, ntree=1000,nsplit=3)
> plot.variable(pbc.out, type = "time", partial = TRUE, npred=8)
```

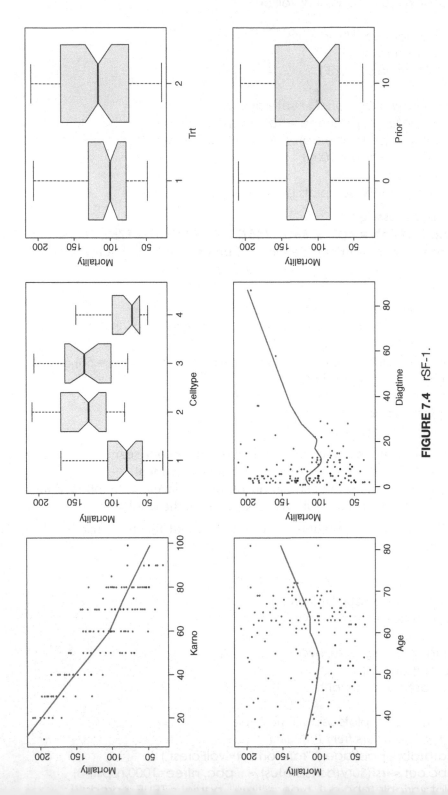

FIGURE 7.4 rSF-1.

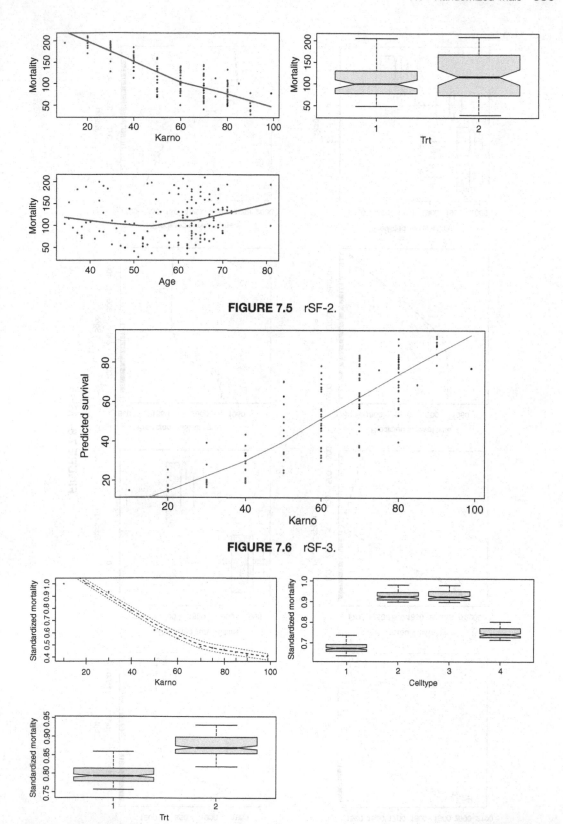

FIGURE 7.5 rSF-2.

FIGURE 7.6 rSF-3.

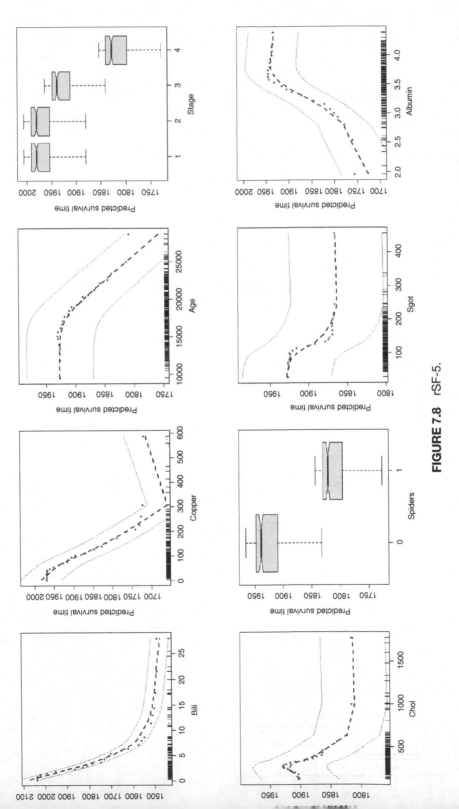

FIGURE 7.8 rSF-5.

(a) Explain the function of each line of the R code segment for this computation.
(b) Rerun this code segment in the R environment.
(c) Rerun this code segment in the R environment, but use the following output command:

```
> plot.variable(pbc.out, type = "time", partial = TRUE, npred=16)
```

to output Figure 7.9: rSF-6. Comment on the results.

7.2 PHASE DEVELOPMENT (CALVERT & PLUMMER, 2008; SIGLER & STEMHAGEN, 2011)

In the United States, as well as in many other countries around the world, the process of developing a new drug to meet a particular health need consists of many definitive stages or phases. Typically, these developmental phases are as summarized in Table 7.1.

In all phases, improper or inadequate study sample size is a common clinical trial design flaw.

Phase 0 or Preclinical Phase

During this initial phase, the drug is generally being tested in vitro (cells, test tubes) or in vivo (animals). The developer applies for governmental permission to enter into clinical testing. The procedure for applying for permission will depend on the country. For example, in the United States, an Investigational New Drug (IND) application must be granted before clinical trials can begin.

The term **preclinical** encompasses all studies undertaken before clinical trials are started. This includes **research programs**, from which the most promising compounds are selected for further development.

The concept of a phase 0 trial is relatively new. There is now a slowly increasing trend toward basing early clinical trial designs on pharmacokinetic and pharmacodynamic endpoints that have been developed in preclinical investigations. In general, trial designs use pharmacodynamic endpoints and targeted agents.

TABLE 7.1 Phases of Drug Development

PHASE OR STAGE	OBJECTIVES
Phase 0 or preclinical	Animal toxicology studies
Phase I	Clinical pharmacology studies
Phase II	Dose–response studies
Phase III	Determination of efficacy and safety

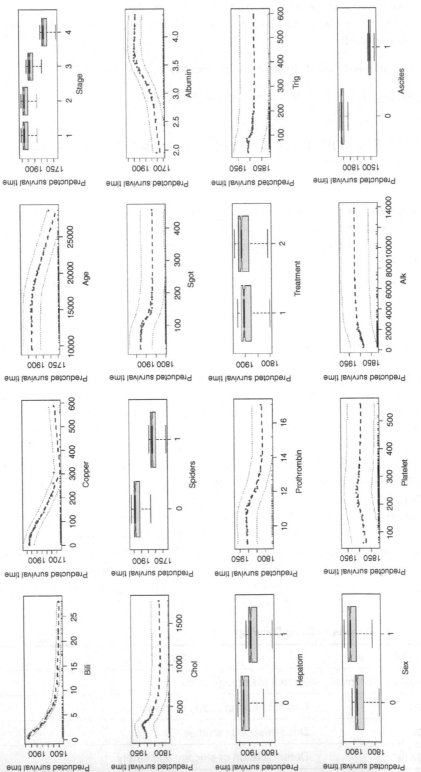

FIGURE 7.9 rSF-6.

Phase I

The objectives of Phase I include basic determinations of safety and efficacy and the initial discovery and description of the pharmacokinetics. In this phase, the first trials of a new therapy or medication are undertaken, usually conducted using healthy male volunteers. Case subjects (patients) may be evaluated instead of volunteers in Phase I trials in order to treat immediately life-threatening and serious conditions for which no comparable or satisfactory alternative therapy is available (in the United States, this is called *Treatment IND status*). Also, expanded access programs allow the use of case subjects for whom standard therapy is ineffective or contraindicated; if such persons are ineligible to enter the trials, they may receive investigational drugs in parallel with controlled trials.

Phase II

This phase seeks to provide a measure of efficacy in addition to short-term tolerability. Phase II studies are conducted in case subjects who have the disease or condition that the drug is intended to treat. Moreover, Phase II study objectives include determining the minimum dose that is maximally effective or that is sufficiently effective without undue toxicity.

In some trials, using research and development insight, a Phase II program may combine some Phase I and Phase II trials:

■ Phase IIA—Pilot or feasibility trials
■ Phase IIB—Well-controlled, pivotal trials

Phase III

The purpose in Phase III is to confirm efficacy and monitor adverse reactions from long-term use. In Phase III studies, a drug is tested under conditions more closely resembling those under which the drug would be used if approved for marketing. The goal is to gather the additional information about efficacy and tolerability that is necessary for evaluating the overall risk–benefit relationship of the drug and to provide an adequate basis for physician labeling.

Approval/disapproval decisions are based on the results of adequate and well-controlled (pivotal) studies. To be considered *pivotal*, a study must meet at least the following four Food and Drug Administration (FDA)–defined criteria:

■ Be controlled using placebo or a standard therapy.
■ Have a double-blind design when such a design is practical and ethical.
■ Be randomized.
■ Be of adequate size.

Pharmacoepidemiology: A Branch of Epidemiology

Pharmacoepidemiology is the study of the uses and effects, both adverse and benefi-

is the Anti-Epileptic Drug (AED) Pregnancy Registry, an observational cohort study or registry of women who become pregnant while on AEDs. The registry records birth outcomes and investigates whether adverse birth outcomes vary with use of specific AEDs. Because the information is primarily collected prospectively, this study is a prospective cohort study.

A **prospective cohort study** follows, over time, a group of similar case subjects (*cohorts*) who differ with respect to certain factors under study, to determine how these factors affect rates of a certain outcome. For example, one might follow a cohort of young (under 30 years of age) truck drivers whose smoking habits vary, to test the hypothesis that the 20-year incidence rate of lung cancer will be highest among heavy smokers, followed by moderate smokers, and then nonsmokers. Prospective studies are important for research on the etiology of diseases and disorders in humans because, for ethical reasons, people cannot be deliberately exposed to suspected risk factors in controlled experiments. Prospective cohort studies are typically ranked higher in the hierarchy of evidence than retrospective cohort studies.

A **retrospective cohort study** generally looks back at events that already have taken place. In medicine, *retrospective study* usually refers to reviewing (looking back at) a patient's medical history or lifestyle.

One of the advantages of prospective cohort studies is they can help determine risk factors for being infected with a new disease. This is possible because they consist of longitudinal observations over time, and the collection of results is done at regular time intervals, minimizing recall error.[2]

Pharmacoepidemiologists must make appropriate comparisons between treated and untreated patients. Among the challenges include **channeling bias**, where groups treated by Drug x versus Drug y are different in ways that predict outcome. This error is a constant consideration that has driven the development of approaches such as propensity scores to minimize channeling bias.

Some Basic Tests in Epidemiologic Phase Development

In this section, worked examples of computational procedures using R illustrate:

- Testing for the presence of a specific response in drug treatments
- Testing for the cross-classification of data
- Estimation of pharmacokinetic parameters

■ **Example 7.2:** Test for the presence of bacteria after drug treatments

Between 1999 and 2000, in a health investigation in the Northern Territory of Australia, tests were undertaken to assess the effects of a drug on 50 children with a history of otitis media. These case subjects were randomized either to take the drug or to take a placebo, and also to receive active encouragement to comply with the drug regimen. The presence of *Haemophilus influenzae* was checked at weeks 0, 2, 4, 6, and 11. (A total of 30 of the checks were missing and are not included in the data frame.)

This data frame, called bacteria, has 220 rows and the following 6 columns:

Y   Presence or absence: a factor with levels n and y.
ap   Active/placebo: a factor with levels a and p.
hilo   High/low compliance: a factor with levels hi and lo.
week   Numeric: week of test.
ID   Case-subject ID: a factor.
Trt   A factor with levels placebo, drug, and drug+, a recording of ap and hilo.

The following R code segment may be used to perform the analysis:

```
> install.packages("MASS")
> library(MASS)
> ls("package:MASS")
```

[1] "abbey"	"accdeaths"	"addterm"
[4] "Aids2"	"Animals"	"anorexia"
[7] "area"	"as.fractions"	"bacteria"
[10] "bandwidth.nrd"	"bcv"	"beav1"
[13] "beav2"	"biopsy"	"birthwt"
[16] "Boston"	"boxcox"	"cabbages"
[19] "caith"	"Cars93"	"cats"

[163] "waders"	"whiteside"	"width.SJ"
[166] "write.matrix"	"wtloss"	

```
> install.packages("survival")
> library(survival)
```
Loading required package: splines
```
>
> data(bacteria)
> attach(bacteria)
```
The following object(s) are masked _by_ '.GlobalEnv': y
```
> bacteria
```

	y	ap	hilo	week	ID	trt
1	y	p	hi	0	X01	placebo
2	y	p	hi	2	X01	placebo
3	y	p	hi	4	X01	placebo
4	y	p	hi	11	X01	placebo
5	y	a	hi	0	X02	drug+
219	n	a	hi	6	Z26	drug+

```
>
> contrasts(bacteria$trt) <- structure(contr.sdif(3),
+ dimnames = list(NULL, c("drug", "encourage")))
> ## fixed effects analyses
> summary(glm(y ~ trt * week, binomial, data = bacteria))
```

Call: glm(formula = y ~ trt * week, family = binomial, data = bacteria)

Deviance Residuals:

Min	1Q	Median	3Q	Max
−2.2144	0.4245	0.5373	0.6750	1.0697

Coefficients:

	Estimate Std.	Error	z value	Pr(>|z|)
(Intercept)	1.97548	0.30053	6.573	4.92e-11 ***
Trtdrug	−0.99848	0.69490	−1.437	0.15075
Trtencourage	0.83865	0.73482	1.141	0.25374
Week	−0.11814	0.04460	−2.649	0.00807 **
trtdrug:week	−0.01722	0.10570	−0.163	0.87061
trtencourage:week	−0.07043	0.10964	−0.642	0.52060 ---

Signif. codes: 0 '*' 0.001 '**' 0.01 '*' 0.05 '.' 0.1 ' ' 1**

(Dispersion parameter for binomial family taken to be 1) Null deviance: 217.38 on 219 degrees of freedom Residual deviance: 203.12 on 214 degrees of freedom AIC: 215.12 Number of Fisher Scoring iterations: 4

```
> summary(glm(y ~ trt + week, binomial, data = bacteria))
```
Call: glm(formula = y ~ trt + week, family = binomial, data = bacteria)

Deviance Residuals:

Min	1Q	Median	3Q	Max
−2.2899	0.3885	0.5400	0.7027	1.1077

Coefficients:

	Estimate Std.	Error	z value	Pr(>|z|)
(Intercept)	1.96018	0.29705	6.599	4.15e-11 ***
trtdrug	−1.10667	0.42519	−2.603	0.00925 **
trtencourage	0.45502	0.42766	1.064	0.28735
week	−0.11577	0.04414	−2.623	0.00872 **---

Signif. codes: 0 '*' 0.001 '**' 0.01 '*' 0.05 '.' 0.1 ' ' 1**

(Dispersion parameter for binomial family taken to be 1) Null deviance: 217.38 on 219 degrees of freedom Residual deviance: 203.81 on 216 degrees of free-

```
> summary(glm(y ~ trt + I(week > 2), binomial, data = + bacteria))
```
Call: glm(formula = y ~ trt + I(week > 2), family = binomial, data = bacteria)

Deviance Residuals:

Min	1Q	Median	3Q	Max
−2.4043	0.3381	0.5754	0.6237	1.0051

Coefficients:

	Estimate Std.	Error	z value	Pr(>|z|)
(Intercept)	2.2479	0.3560	6.315	2.71e-10 ***
trtdrug	−1.1187	0.4288	−2.609	0.00909 **
trtencourage	0.4815	0.4330	1.112	0.26614
I(week > 2)TRUE	−1.2949	0.4104	−3.155	0.00160 **---

Signif. codes: 0 '***' 0.001 '**' 0.01 '*' 0.05 '.' 0.1 ' ' 1

(Dispersion parameter for binomial family taken to be 1) Null deviance: 217.38 on 219 degrees of freedom Residual deviance: 199.18 on 216 degrees of freedom AIC: 207.18 Number of Fisher Scoring iterations: 5

```
> # conditional random-effects analysis
> library(survival)
> bacteria$Time <- rep(1, nrow(bacteria))
> coxph(Surv(Time, unclass(y)) ~ week + strata(ID), + data = bacteria, method =
    "exact")
```

Call: coxph(formula = Surv(Time, unclass(y)) ~ week + strata(ID), data = bacteria, method = "exact")

	Coef	exp(coef)	se(coef)	z	p
week	−0.163	0.85	0.0547	−2.97	0.003

Likelihood ratio test=9.85 on 1 df, p=0.0017 n= 220, number of events= 177

```
>
> coxph(Surv(Time, unclass(y)) ~ factor(week) + strata(ID), + data = bacteria,
    method = "exact")
```
Call: coxph(formula = Surv(Time, unclass(y)) ~ factor(week) + strata(ID), data = bacteria, method = "exact")

	coef	exp(coef)	se(coef)	z	p
factor(week)2	0.198	1.219	0.724	0.274	0.780
factor(week)4	−1.421	0.242	0.667	−2.131	0.033
factor(week)6	−1.661	0.190	0.682	−2.434	0.015
factor(week)11	−1.675	0.187	0.678	−2.471	0.013

```
> coxph(Surv(Time, unclass(y)) ~ I(week > 2) + strata(ID),
+    data = bacteria, method = "exact")
```

Call: coxph(formula = Surv(Time, unclass(y)) ~ I(week > 2) + strata(ID), data =
bacteria, method = "exact")

	coef	exp(coef)	se(coef)	z	p
I(week > 2)TRUE	−1.67	0.188	0.482	−3.47	0.00053

Likelihood ratio test=15.2 on 1 df, p=9.93e-05 n= 220, number of events= 177

```
>
> # PQL glmm analysis
> library(nlme)
> summary(glmmPQL(y ~ trt + I(week > 2), random = ~ 1 | ID,
+    family = binomial, data = bacteria))
```

iteration 1
iteration 2
iteration 3
iteration 4
iteration 5
iteration 6
Linear mixed-effects model fit by maximum likelihood

Data: bacteria

AIC	BIC	logLik
NA	NA	NA

Random effects:
Formula: ~1 | ID

	(Intercept)	Residual
StdDev:	1.410637	0.7800511

Variance function:
Structure: fixed weights
Formula: ~invwt
Fixed effects: y ~ trt + I(week > 2)

	Value	Std.Error	DF	t-value	p-value
(Intercept)	2.7447864	0.3784193	169	7.253294	0.0000
trtdrug	−1.2473553	0.6440635	47	−1.936696	0.0588
trtencourage	0.4930279	0.6699339	47	0.735935	0.4654
I(week > 2)TRUE	−1.6072570	0.3583379	169	−4.485311	0.0000

Correlation:

	(Intr)	trtdrg	trtncr
trtdrug	0.009		
trtencourage	0.036	−0.518	

Standardized Within-Group Residuals:

Min	Q1	Med	Q3	Max
-5.1985361	0.1572336	0.3513075	0.4949482	1.7448845

Number of Observations: 220
Number of Groups: 50
>

Review Questions for Section 7.2

1. (a) Name an area in epidemiology in which process development is usually under-taken in several phases.
   (b) In such a process, what are the usual developmental phases? Briefly describe each phase.
2. (a) Contrast a prospective cohort study with a retrospective cohort study, giving an example of each.
   (b) What is pharmacoepidemiology? If a cohort study is undertaken in this area of epidemiology, is it prospective or retrospective? Why?
3. Describe, and give examples of, some testing procedures likely to be used in a typical epidemiologic phase development?
4. For epidemiologic phase development, access the CRAN package MASS and select two R functions for testing the presence of a specific response in drug treat-ment. Demonstrate their usage by suitable worked examples.
5. For epidemiologic phase development, access the CRAN package PK and select two R functions for estimating pharmacokinetic parameters in process phase devel-opment. Demonstrate their usage by suitable illustrative examples.

Exercises for Section 7.2

1. CRAN offers a number of packages, designed for pharmacokinetics data analysis, that are suitable for phase development support. These are:
   (a) PK, PKfit, PKtools, and nlmeODE. PK supports basic pharmacokinetic func-tions and uses noncompartmental analysis methods; the other three mainly support modeling methods.
   (b) The packages MASS and drc, which support the analysis of dose responses.
   (c) The package lattice, for trellis graphics.
      For a given task in phase development analysis, one may search for a suitable R function appropriate for the task by starting within the R environment as follows:
      (i) Starting from the "Help" option, select "CRAN home page" from the drop-down menu. You will be taken to the CRAN page.
      (ii) On the CRAN page, among the left-side options, select "Search." You will be taken to the CRAN search page.
      (iii) On the CRAN search page, select "R site search"; you will be taken to the CRAN R site search page.
      (iv) Finally, enter the subject of interest into the "Query" box and select

(d) If the phase development task at hand is to test for a particular biochemical substance in each case subject after a certain drug treatment, use the preceding steps to find an R function in CRAN that is suitable for the task.

(e) Compare the result with the choice in Example 7.2.

2. Besides CRAN, there are other source platforms for biostatistical software that uses R; two of them are Bioconductor and PBSmodelling. They may be accessed from the following sources:

(i) For Bioconductor

  ■ Start from the Internet website http://bioconductor.org
  ■ Select "Install."
  ■ Select "Software" from the table of software releases.

(ii) For PBSmodelling (Schnute, Couture-Beil, Haigh, & Kronlund, 2011)

The R package PBSmodelling contains software to facilitate the design, testing, and operation of computer models. The initials *PBS* refer to the Pacific Biological Station, a major fisheries laboratory on Canada's Pacific Coast in Nanaimo, British Columbia. Initially designed for fisheries scientists, this package has broad potential application in many scientific fields. PBSmodelling focuses particularly on tools that make it easy to construct and edit a customized graphical user interface appropriate for a particular application. (The package is also available from CRAN.)

Repeat Exercise 1, using an appropriate R function from Bioconductor.

3. Repeat Exercise 1, using an appropriate R function from PBSmodelling.

4. In the CRAN package PKtools (Blanchard, 2012), which supports computations for WinBUGS, NONMEM V, NLME, and others, the R function diagtrplot() creates a trellis plot of the observed concentrations and predicted values versus time by subject. Its usage format is

diagtrplot(x,level,xvarlab,yvarlab,pages,...)

for which the arguments are

x   Variable identifying the clustering variable.
level   Level of mixed model (p—population, i—individual).
xvarlab   Label for x variable.
yvarlab   Label for y variable.
pages   Number of pages to print; "1" prints first-page additional arguments to be passed to lower-level functions.

The following R code segment illustrates an application of this package:

```
> install.packages("PKtools")
> library(PKtools)
Loading required package: lattice
Loading required package: nlme
Loading required package: R2HTML
Loading required package: xtable
> library(PKtools)
```

```
[1]   "AICcomp"        "bugs"       "coVar.id"          "desc"     "diagplot"
[6]   "diagtrplot"  "HTMLtools"      "indEst"  "Ionecpmt"  "obvsprplot"
[11]  "paramEst"          "pk"  "PKtools.AIC"   "residplot"     "RunNLME"
[16]     "RunNM"       "RunWB"    "sonecpmt"           "tex"       "trplot"

> library(nlme)
> data(Theoph)
> Theoph <- Theoph[Theoph$Time!=0,]
> id <- as.numeric(as.character(Theoph$Subject))
> dose <- Theoph$Dose
> time <- Theoph$Time
> conc <- round(sqrt(Theoph$conc),4)
> Theo <- data.frame(cbind(id,dose,time,conc))
> names(Theo) <- c("id","dose","time","conc")
> wt.v <- Theoph$Wt
> data <- list(pkvar = Theo, cov = wt.v)
> nameData <- list(covnames = c("wt"),
+                   yvarlab = "Sqrt(Theop. Conc.) (mg/L)",
+                   xvarlab = "Time since dose (hrs)",
+                   reparams = c("Cl"),
+                   params = c("Ka","V", "Cl"),
+                   tparams = c("log(Ka)","log(V)","log(CL)"))
> model.def <- list(fixed.model=lKa+lV+lCl~1,
+                    random.model=lCl~1,
+                    start.lst=c(lKa=.3,lV=-.6,lCl=-3),
+                    form=conc~sonecpmt(dose, time,
+                         lV, lKa, lCl),
+                    control=nlmeControl(returnObject=FALSE))
> MM<-RunNLME(inputStructure=model.def,data=data,
+             nameData=nameData)
> diagtrplot(x=MM,level="p", xvarlab=nameData$xvarlab,
+            yvarlab=nameData$xvarlab, pages=1)
> # Outputting: Figure 7.10.
```

  (a) Explain the function of each line of the R code segment for this computation.
  (b) Rerun this code segment in the R environment.
  (c) Compare and comment on the R code: predicted values versus observed values of this dataset.

5. R computations for pharmacokinetics of indomethacin.

  The CRAN package nlmeODE (Tornoe, 2012) (nonlinear mixed-effects modeling using ordinary differential equations) actually combines two packages: nlme and Odesolve, for mixed-effects modeling using differential equations. The following R code segment models the pharmacokinetics of indomethacin using this CRAN package:

```
> install packages("nlmeODE")
```
package odesolve successfully unpacked and MD5 sums checked

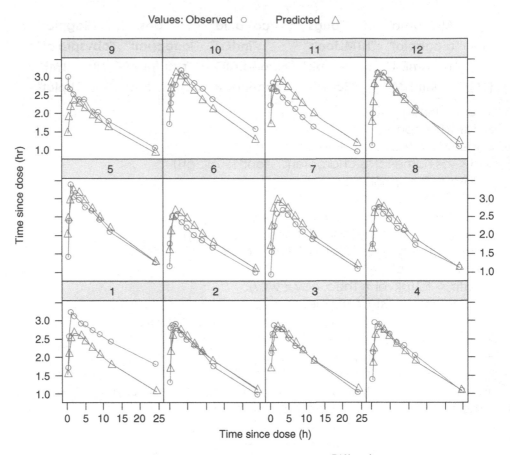

FIGURE 7.10 Using CRAN package PKtools.

```
> library(nlmeODE)
Loading required package: odesolve
odesolve is deprecated! Use the solvers in deSolve instead.
odesolve will be removed from CRAN by the end of 2012.
Loading required package: nlme
Loading required package: lattice

> ls("package:nlmeODE")
[1] "nlmeODE"
>


####################################
### Pharmacokinetics of Indomethacin ###
####################################


> data(Indometh)
> Indometh # Outputting the data frame Indometh for inspection:
```

Grouped Data: conc ~ time | Subject

	Subject	time	Conc
1	1	0.25	1.50
2	1	0.50	0.94
3	1	0.75	0.78
4	1	1.00	0.48
5	1	1.25	0.37
64	6	5.00	0.13
65	6	6.00	0.10
66	6	8.00	0.09

```
>
> TwoComp <- list(DiffEq=list(
+ dy1dt = ~ -(k12+k10)*y1+k21*y2,
+ dy2dt = ~ -k21*y2 + k12*y1),
+ ObsEq=list(
+ c1 = ~ y1,
+ c2 = ~ 0),
+ States=c("y1","y2"),
+ Parms=c("k12","k21","k10","start"),
+ Init=list("start",0))
> IndomethModel <- nlmeODE(TwoComp,Indometh)
> Indometh.nlme <- nlme(conc ~
+ IndomethModel(k12,k21,k10,start,time,Subject),
+ data = Indometh, fixed=k12+k21+k10+start~1,
+ random = pdDiag(start+k12+k10~1),
+ start=c(k12=-0.05,k21=-0.15,k10=-0.10,start=0.70),
+ control=list(msVerbose=TRUE),
+ verbose=TRUE)
```

```
0:  -12.615270:-0.785113  -1.41611  -0.440966
1:  -12.615270:-0.785095  -1.41627  -0.440425
2:  -12.615270:-0.785095  -1.41627  -0.440425
```

**Iteration 1
LME step: Loglik: 57.22393, nlm iterations: 2 reStruct parameters:

Subject1	Subject2	Subject3
-0.7850948	-1.4162729	-0.4404247

PNLS step: RSS = 0.4128427

fixed effects: -0.0331751   -0.115947   -0.111574   -0.717857

iterations: 7
Convergence:

fixed	reStruct
0.5071548	0.2703262

```
0: -11.974429:  -0.766570  -1.43832  -0.347128
1: -11.974429:  -0.766340  -1.43872  -0.345577
2: -11.974429:  -0.766497  -1.43869  -0.345660
3: -11.974430:  -0.766594  -1.43863  -0.346103
4: -11.974430:  -0.766487  -1.43861  -0.346124
5: -11.974430:  -0.766513  -1.43851  -0.346167
6: -11.974430:  -0.766544  -1.43859  -0.346197
7: -11.974430:  -0.766527  -1.43858  -0.346173
8: -11.974430:  -0.766529  -1.43857  -0.346176
```

**Iteration 2
LME step: Loglik: 56.58309, nlm iterations: 8 reStruct parameters:

Subject1	Subject2	Subject3
-0.7665286	-1.4385742	-0.3461758

PNLS step: RSS = 0.4128658
fixed effects:-0.0331751 -0.115947 -0.111574 0.717857 iterations: 1
Convergence:

Fixed	reStruct
0.000000000	0.002752387

```
0: -11.974430:  -0.766529  -1.43857  -0.346176
1: -11.974430:  -0.766529  -1.43857  -0.346176
```

**Iteration 3
LME step: Loglik: 56.58309, nlm iterations: 1 reStruct parameters:

Subject1	Subject2	Subject3
-0.7665286	-1.4385745	-0.3461757

PNLS step: RSS = 0.4128658 fixed effects:-0.0331751 -0.115947 -0.111574 0.717857
iterations: 1
Convergence:

fixed	reStruct
0.00000e+00	3.03061e-08

```
> plot(augPred(Indometh.nlme,level=0:1))
```

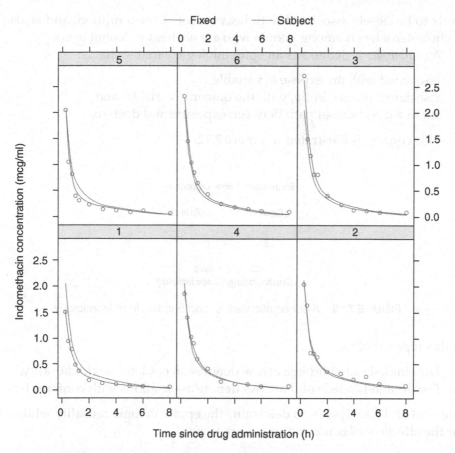

FIGURE 7.11 Pharmacokinetics of indomethacin by nlmeODE.

(a) Explain the function of each line of the R code segment for this computation.
(b) Rerun this code segment in the R environment, replacing the last command of the code segment with the following:

> plot(augPred(Indometh.nlme))

and then rerun the entire code segment. Comment on the new resulting plot.

7.3 CONFOUNDING IN SURVIVAL ANALYSIS

In survival analysis (see Chapter 5, Section 5.2), as well as in most epidemiologic investigations, one must be concerned with how to characterize the association between two variables (usually an outcome in response to an exposure) (Children's Mercy Hospital, 2000). A typical example is wanting to test whether the total cholesterol level (the outcome) of a case subject is associated with alcohol consumption (the exposure). However, previous research data appear to indicate that the case subject's smoking status has a profound effect on this relationship. In this situation, epidemiologists may consider the smoking status of the case subject to be a poten-

tends to be closely associated with heavy alcohol consumption, and is also related to cholesterol levels among people who are *not* heavy alcohol users.

A *confounder* is defined as an epidemiologic variable that is:

■ associated with the exposure variable,
■ associated, *independently*, with the outcome variable, and
■ not in a direct causal path between exposure and disease.

This concept is illustrated in Figure 7.12.

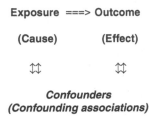

FIGURE 7.12   A schematic view of confounding in epidemiology.

In this representation:

■ The single-headed broken arrow denotes an epidemiologic causality.
■ The double-headed solid arrows denote associations with confounders.

The goal of the analysis is to determine the epidemiologic causality while adjusting for the effects of *all* confounding associations.

Biostatistical Approaches for Controlling Confounding

In epidemiologic investigations, confounding may be controlled by using experimental controls or combined experimental and analytical controls.

EXPERIMENTAL CONTROLS OF CONFOUNDING

Ways to modify an epidemiologic study design to actively exclude or control confounding variables include[3]:

■ **Case–control studies**. This approach assigns confounders to both groups—cases and controls—equally. For example, when studying the cause of myocardial infarct, the age of the case subjects may be considered a probable confounding variable. Suppose the investigator attempts to match each 59-year-old infarct patient with a healthy 59-year-old "control" person. (In case–control studies, the variables matched most often are age and gender.)
  Drawback: Case–control studies are feasible only when it is easy to find controls; that is, persons for whom all known potential confounding factors are the same as for the case subject. For example, a case–control study investigator

is trying to find the cause of a given disease in a person who is (a) 39 years old, (b) Chinese American, (c) from North Dakota, (d) a dedicated tennis player, (e) a vegan or a vegetarian, and (f) working as a firefighter. A theoretically perfect control would be a person who, in addition to *not* having the disease being investigated, also matches all six of these characteristics and has no diseases that the case subject does not also have. Obviously, finding such a control (let alone enough of them to make a control group) would be a real challenge!

■ **Cohort studies**. This approach makes close matching more practical by controlling admission of certain age groups or a certain gender into the study population, thus creating a cohort of people who share similar characteristics and making all cohorts comparable regarding the possible confounding variable. For example, if age and gender are thought to be confounders, only males 30 to 40 years of age would be admitted to a cohort study that intends to assess the myocardial infarct risk in cohorts that are either physically active or inactive.

Drawback: In cohort studies, the overexclusion of input data may lead biostatisticians to define too narrowly the set of similarly situated persons for whom they can claim the study to be useful; other persons to whom the causal relationship does in fact apply may lose the opportunity to benefit from the study's recommendations. Similarly, overstratification of input data within a study may reduce the sample size in a given stratum to the point where generalizations drawn from observations of the members of that stratum alone may not be statistically significant.

■ **Double blinding**. This approach conceals the experiment group membership of the participants from the trial population *and* the observers. When participants are prevented from knowing whether or not they are receiving treatment, any likely placebo effects should be the same for the control and treatment groups. When the observers are prevented from knowing the participants' membership, there should be no bias from researchers treating the groups differently or from interpreting the outcomes differently.

■ **Randomized controlled trial (RCT)**. In this approach, the study population is divided randomly in order to reduce the chances of self-selection by participants or bias by the study designers. Before the experiment starts, the testers will assign the members of the participant pool to their groups (control, intervention, and parallel), using a randomization process such as the use of a random number generator. For example, in a study on the effects of exercise, the conclusions would be less valid if participants were given a choice as to whether they wanted to belong to the control group (which would not exercise) or the intervention group (which would take part in an exercise program). The study would then capture other variables besides exercise, such as pre-experiment health levels and motivation to adopt healthful activities. The experimenter may choose case subjects who are more likely to show the results that the study hopes to find or may interpret subjective results (more energetic, more positive attitude) in a way favorable to the experimenter's preferences.

■ **Stratification**. To explain stratification, let us return to the previous example in which the investigation is examining the causes of myocardial infarct. Physical activity is thought to reduce the occurrence of myocardial infarct,

then stratified by age group; this means that the association between activity and infarct will be analyzed per age group. If the different age groups (or age strata) yield very different **risk ratios**, age must be viewed as a confounding variable. Some statistical tools, among them Mantel–Haenszel (M–H) methods, can account for stratification of datasets (see Example 7.3).

Of these five approaches to exclude or control confounding, the first four have been discussed previously (see Sections 6.1 and 6.2 in Chapter 6, and Section 7.1). The last approach, stratification, is discussed later in this section.

COMBINED EXPERIMENTAL AND ANALYTICAL CONTROL OF CONFOUNDING (FITZMAURICE, 2004)[4]

Generally, two approaches are used to constrain and curb confounding, and to adjust the data analysis for the effects of confounding: analysis by stratification or the use of regression modeling. Both approaches are discussed and illustrated in this subsection.

ADJUSTMENT OF CONFOUNDING BY STRATIFICATION. Stratification is an established and effective way to adjust for confounding in the analysis of cause-and-effect (exposure-and-outcome) experimental data. Consider the following hypothetical dataset from an investigation into the association between taking vitamin E supplements and the risk of the occurrence of CHDs, shown in Figure 7.13.

		CHD	
		Present	**Absent**
	Yes:	60	601
Vitamin E			
Supplement	**No:**	78	461

FIGURE 7.13 Association between vitamin E supplementation and the risk of CHD (hypothetical data frame).

This dataset has been taken from 1,200 case subjects between the ages of 40 and 45 years who were CHD-free at the start of the study; they were followed for 20 years. Over the 20-year follow-up period, those who developed CHD were identified. The case subjects were classified according to their use of vitamin E supplements (the "exposure" variable).

Analysis of the data shown in Figure 7.13 indicates that:

O1 = The odds of CHD for those who used vitamin E supplements are 60/601
   = 0.100 (rounded); and

O2 = The odds of CHD for those who did *not* use vitamin E supplements are 78/461
   = 0.169 (rounded).

[4] Dealing with confounding in the analysis. Retrieved from www.iarc.fr/en/publications/pdfs-

This apparent association may be expressed in terms of the odds ratio (OR):

$$OR = O1/O2 = 0.100/0.169 = 0.592$$

This estimated OR may imply that the odds of developing CHD are reduced by almost 50%; that is, the odds of developing CHD are nearly halved by taking vitamin E supplementation. However, a potential problem with this analysis and conclusion is that *these two groups may differ in ways other than their use of vitamin E supplements.*

Suppose that we would prefer to consider the associated risk factors. Then

R1 = The risk of CHD for those who used vitamin E supplements is 60/(60 + 601)
    = 60/661 = 0.091

and

R2 = The risk for those who did not use vitamin E supplements is 78/(78 + 461)
    = 78/539 = 0.145

giving a risk ratio of

$$RR = R1/R2 = 0.091/0.145 = 0.628$$

and implying a substantially lower risk, in substantial agreement with the previous result.

As an example of confounding, the case subjects who used vitamin E supplements may be much less likely to smoke, in which case there must be some concern that the association observed in Figure 7.13 is due, at least in part, to the **confounding** effects of smoking (smoking is a well-established and major risk factor for CHD). To deal with this possibility, one may **stratify** (classify into groups with similar and definitive characteristics) the data in Figure 7.13 according to whether a case subject is a smoker. See Figure 7.14.

Smokers:

CHD

		Present	Absent
	Yes:	13	48
Vitamin E			
Supplement	No:	59	240

Nonsmokers:

CHD

		Present	Absent
	Yes:	47	553
Vitamin E			
Supplement	No:	19	221

FIGURE 7.14 The results stratified by smoking history: association between vitamin E

From these stratified data, the odds of succumbing to CHD among the class who use vitamin E supplementation, relative to the class who do not, may now be calculated separately for smokers and for nonsmokers.

For the smokers, the estimated OR is

$$OR \text{ (Smokers)} = (13/48)/(59/240) = 0.271/0.246 = 1.097$$

For the nonsmokers, the estimated OR is

$$OR \text{ (Nonsmokers)} = (47/533)/(19/221) = 0.088/0.086 = 1.023$$

These results seem to indicate that, after controlling for the effects of smoking history, there is little or no evidence of an association between vitamin E supplementation and the risk of suffering CHD.

It should not escape attention that this apparently paradoxical result is due to the fact that the vitamin E supplementation group contains significantly fewer smokers: 360 (= 13 + 48 + 59 + 240), which is only 30% of the total case-subject population of 1,200. Thus, 70% of the total test population are nonsmokers, who had a lower risk of succumbing to CHD.

The foregoing additional analysis, based on the stratified data in Figure 7.14, demonstrates an effective technique for adjusting the effects of confounding in the initial analysis. In this approach, known as **stratification**, the confounding effect is controlled via stratification on levels of the potential confounder (which, in this example, is smoking history of the case subjects). In particular, confounding is controlled when the association of interest is included within distinct groups, or *strata*, made up of subjects who are otherwise homogeneous relative to the confounding variable.

At this point, it should be apparent that one factor that may have an important bearing on the analysis is the sample sizes, as well as the relative sample sizes of the various strata within the total population. This issue may be addressed using the MH method of stratification.

THE MH METHOD OF STRATIFICATION. The MH method of stratification computes a pooled summary measure of association by taking a weighted average of the stratum-specific estimates, using weights proportional to the sample size within each stratum. These weights are inversely proportional to the variances of the stratum-specific estimates of the OR, thus giving greater weight to the more precise estimates.

Consider the pooled estimate of the OR. Let there be K stratification levels, with each level taking a separate stratifying variable: $K = 2$ for the dataset in Figure 7.14. The data may then be summarized in terms of K 2x2 contingency tables. In each table, the four internal cells contain frequency counts of the number of case subjects having a particular combination of the two variables. Figure 7.15 shows such a generic table in which the rows correspond to an exposure (in this instance, vitamin E supplementation), and the columns correspond to disease status (in this instance, presence or absence of CHD).

DISEASE

	Present	Absent
Yes:	a_k	b_k
Exposure (Cause)		
No:	c_k	d_k

FIGURE 7.15 Stratum-specific 2x2 contingency table for MH analysis.

The MH formula for the pooled estimate of the OR, derived from a series of 2x2 contingency tables, is

$$OR_{MH} = \{\textstyle\sum_{k=1}^{K}(a_k\,d_k)/n_k\}/\{\textstyle\sum_{k=1}^{K}(b_k\,c_k)/n_k\} \tag{7.1}$$

where n_k is the total number of observations in the kth table ($n_k = a_k + b_k + c_k + d_k$) and the summation in Equation (7.1) is taken over the K levels of the stratification variable. For example, the MH pooled estimate of the OR based on the data from the two contingency tables in Figure 7.14 is calculated as follows:

$$
\begin{aligned}
ORMH &= \{(13 \times 240)/360 + (47 \times 221)/840\}/\{(48 \times 59)/360 + (553 \times 19)/840\} \\
&= (7.333 + 12.365)/(7.867 + 12.508) \\
&= 19.698/20.375 \\
&= 0.967
\end{aligned}
$$

As expected for these data, the pooled estimate of the OR is about 1.0, indicating that there is *no evidence of association* between vitamin E supplementation and the risk of succumbing to CHD, after controlling for the effects of smoking history.

Moreover, a confidence interval (CI) for the adjusted OR may be calculated. The limits of the 95% CI for the adjusted OR are in the range of [0.14, 6.33], which includes the null value of 1.0 for the OR. This approximate 95% CI for the ln OR_{MH} is estimated:

$$
\begin{aligned}
95\% \text{ CI } (\ln OR_{MH}) &= (\ln 0.95) \pm 1.96 \times 0.967 \\
&= -0.05 \pm 1.96 \times 0.967 \\
&= -0.05 \pm 1.895 \\
&= -1.945 \text{ to } 1.845
\end{aligned}
$$

An approximate 95% CI for the OR_{MH} may be obtained by taking antilogarithms:

$$
\begin{aligned}
95\% \text{ CI } [OR_{MH}] &= [e^{1.945}, e^{1.845}] \\
&= [0.14, 6.33]
\end{aligned}
$$

The last result may be obtained via computations using the following R code segment:

```
> exp(-1.945)
[1] 0.1429872
> exp(1.845)
[1] 6.3281
```

Remarks:

1. When assessing the evidence for an association between two variables, the effect of confounders (measured or otherwise) must always be considered. If unadjusted, confounding may lead to unacceptable conclusions: a causal effect may be suggested where none exists, or a true effect may be hidden. Each erroneous conclusion may lead to an incorrect interpretation or diagnosis.
2. Because of these error possibilities, confounding that cannot be controlled for in the study design should be adjusted in the analysis. The MH procedure, especially when performed by computer, provides a weighted average of the unconfounded, stratum-specific estimates of association.
3. When there are many potential confounders, resulting in strata with too few subjects to make meaningful comparisons, stratification may be much less attractive.
4. This leads to an alternative approach for adjusting for confounding in the analysis: examine the exposure effect in a **regression model** for the dependence of disease outcome on the exposure of interest and any potential confounders. This approach is discussed in the next subsection.

ADJUSTMENT OF CONFOUNDING BY REGRESSION MODELING (McNamee, 2005). As an introduction to regression analysis, consider the case of two variables measured on continuous scales, with the object of investigating the influence of one variable on another. Here, regression analysis is used to begin the application of confounder control.

■ **Example 7.3:** Adjusting confounding by regression modeling

Step 1: Starting with a simple basic model

In a given population, the investigators consider 160 nonsmoking case subjects. Variable are age and the decline with age in the forced expiratory volume (FEV) in 1 second (FEV). The data on both variables, age and FEV, have been gathered from a cross-plot of the data, as shown in Figure 7.16.

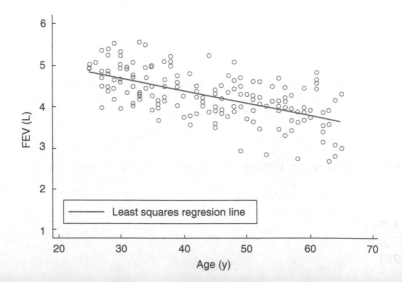

Based on this data, a model of the relationship in the population may be proposed, where the model is specified by a model form or model equations. If a linear relationship is considered, the model would have the general form:

$$\text{Model 1:} \quad \text{FEV} = a + b(\text{Age}) + r \qquad (7.2)$$

The three unknown quantities in this model—a, b, and r—may be estimated in the analysis.

Recall that in analytical or coordinate geometry, the general equation for a straight line in the X–Y plane is

$$y = m_1 x + b_1 \qquad (7.3)$$

where m_1 is the slope or gradient of the straight line, and b_1 is the ordinate (y-value) of the intercept of the straight line with the y-axis: $b = y$ (at $x = 0$).

The model in which r is ignored (by setting $r = 0$) is a description of the relationship between "age" and the mean "FEV" among people of a given age. r is a random component assumed to vary from person to person. Inclusion of this term in the model allows recognition of the fact that people of the same age are not all the same, and thus their individual FEV values will vary about the mean for that age. Random variation is unpredictable, but it may be described by a statistical distribution. With continuous variables such as FEV, the random component is often assumed to have a normal distribution with a mean of zero.

Statistical methods may then be used to estimate the regression coefficients, a and b, and $s(r)$, the standard deviation of r, from a data sample. Thus, in the least squares estimation method, the rationale is to choose values for a and b that minimize $s(r)$ in the dataset. Application of this method to the data in Figure 7.16 gives estimates of:

$a = 5.58$ L
$b = -0.03$ L/y of age, and
$s(r) = 0.46$ L

Hence, the "fitted" model is

$$\text{FEV} = 5.58 - 0.039(\text{Age}) + r \qquad (7.4)$$

Table 7.2 presents a typical output from a biostatistical computer program that fits Model 1 to the data, including 95% CI for a and b, and p values for tests of significance. In each test, the null hypothesis is that the true value of the coefficient is zero. Thus, if $b = 0$, then age would have no effect on FEV. In this case, both the significance test and the 95% CI suggest that $b < 0$.

TABLE 7.2 Typical Computer Output From Fitting Model 1 to the Data Estimation of Model 1 Coefficients (From Data in Figure 7.16)

FEV	COEFFICIENT	STD ERROR	T STATISTIC	PROBABILITY	95% CI
Age	$b = -0.0301$	0.0032	-9.52	< 0.001	-0.0363 to -0.0238
Constant	$a = 5.5803$	0.1440	38.75	< 0.001	5.2960 to 5.8647

Remarks:

1. In Example 7.3, Model 1 is a linear model, which assumes that the mean FEV declines by a fixed amount, −0.0301 liters (30.1 milliliters), per year in age.
2. Note that linearity was *assumed*, not proven, and that the biostatistical analysis simply estimated the coefficients of an assumed linear model.
3. Additional postestimation regression diagnostic methods (such as the analysis of residuals and various quantitative measures for identifying influential observations) are available to assess the goodness of fit. Thus, one may take the modeling to a higher level, as illustrated in the next worked example.

Step 2: Extending the basic model with additional dependent variables: Further adjusting confounding by regression modeling

It is thought that, for each case subject, the body height and the smoking history (the number of cigarettes smoked per day) may affect the FEV. Modifying Regression Model 1, Equation (7.2), to include these additional variables, and *assuming that each dependent variable has a linear relationship with FEV, and that the joint effect of the three dependent variables (factors) is the sum of their separate effects*, one may write:

$$\text{Model 2:} \quad \text{FEV} = a + b(\text{Age}) + c(\text{Height}) + d(\text{Cigarettes}) + r \tag{7.5}$$

With this model and the same dataset, a standard statistical analysis would produce estimates of the coefficients a, b, c, and d, and $s(r)$; the 95% CIs; and the null hypothesis test for each coefficient.

One may postulate that because FEV measures volumes, it should be expected that FEV will vary as the *cube* of height $(\text{Height})^3$, and this should be factored in for Model 2, to give Model 3:

$$\text{Model 3:} \quad \text{FEV} = a + b(\text{Age}) + c(\text{Height})^3 + d(\text{Cigarettes}) + e(\text{Group}) + r \tag{7.6}$$

However, regression analysis may help which model form is more suitable, linear or cubic.

One may also consider if the magnitude of the effect of smoking should vary with age; this interactional effect is known as **effect modification**. To that end, one might postulate an additional product term combining Age and Cigarettes. This would modify Model 2 to give Model 4:

$$\text{Model 4:} \quad \text{FEV} = a + b(\text{Age}) + c(\text{Height})^3 + d(\text{Cigarettes}) \\ + e(\text{Age})(\text{Cigarettes}) + f(\text{Group}) + r \tag{7.7}$$

Again, this will be followed by analysis to evaluate the coefficients: $a, \ldots, f, r$. Clearly, one must decide how far this process should be taken.

Another general method available is the generalized additive model (GAM) (Hastie & Tibshirani, 1990; Wood, 2006), which takes the following form:

$$\text{Model 5:} \quad \text{GAM:} \quad g(E[\text{FEV}]) = a_0 + f_1(\text{Age}) + f_2(\text{Height}) + f_3(\text{Cigarettes}) + \\ f_4(\text{Group}) + f_m(x_m) \tag{7.8}$$

This model specifies a distribution (such as a normal distribution or a binomial distribution) and a **link function** g relating the expected value of the distribution to the m

The functions $f_i(x_i)$ may be fitted using parametric or nonparametric means, thus providing the potential for better fits to data than other methods. However, the method is very general.

Using Regression Modeling for Controlling Confounding

In this approach to control confounding, the objective of the regression modeling is to discover the effect of the exposure on the disease, while controlling or adjusting for the others. The steps in the process are as follows:

1. Begin with a model equation in which the right side includes the terms representing the exposure and the potential confounders.
2. Next, enter the variable with the most biostatistically significant relationship to the health outcome into the model.
3. Next, a second variable is chosen from the remainder on the basis that it adds the most "significance" to the model created in the previous step.
4. Continue this process until additional variables would not increase significance in the model.

It is entirely possible, when using available biostatistical packages, that different automated procedures may result in different selections for the same dataset. As no biostatistical algorithm alone can identify all confounders, epidemiologic judgment based on subject-matter knowledge will be needed to complete the decision process. In other words, automated selection procedures should not be used to identify confounders, as these procedures may lead to inappropriate inclusions or exclusions in a model.

FURTHER MODIFICATIONS FOR CONTROLLING CONFOUNDING BY REGRESSION MODELING

A number of modifications have been developed and practiced to further control confounding by regression modeling. Some examples follow.

BY COMPARING GROUPS. When one is only able to classify the case subjects into groups such as *low*, *medium*, and *high*, the exposure is **categorical**. Such variables may be classified as predictors on the right side of a model equation. For example, consider a case with the two categories Exposed and Unexposed, based on the preceding example for FEV in two groups, in which one plans to adjust the comparison for age, height, and smoking. The dataset contains a variable "Group," which takes the value of 1 if the case subject is exposed, and 0 if the case subject is not exposed. Model 2 of Equation (7.5) can then be modified to:

$$\text{Model 6:} \quad \text{FEV} = a + b(\text{Age}) + c(\text{Height}) + d(\text{Cigarettes}) + e(\text{Group}) + r \quad (7.9)$$

in which the coefficient e is of primary interest. It represents the effect of increasing the variable Group by one unit—assuming that the model is correct and all other

(Group = 1) and unexposed (Group = 0) when Age, Height, and Cigarettes were the same for each group.

LOGISTIC REGRESSION MODELS FOR DISEASE OUTCOMES. In the same epidemiologic investigation, if the outcome measure is the absence or presence of some respiratory sickness, it calls for a dichotomous variable with corresponding values 0 (for absence of disease) and 1 (for presence of disease).

The probability p of disease is then a function of Age, Cumulative Pack-Years of Cigarette Smoking, and Exposure Concentration, for which a model may be:

$$\text{Model 7:} \quad \ln\{p/(1-p)\} = a + b(\text{Age}) + c(\text{Pack-Years}) + d(\text{Concentration}) \quad (7.10)$$

This is a **logistic regression model**. The term *logistic* represents the form of the left side of Equation (7.10). The random component is assumed to have a binomial distribution.

POISSON REGRESSION MODELS FOR DISEASE OUTCOMES. For incidence investigations in which the follow-up duration varies among the case subjects, a logistic regression model is not appropriate. In such investigations, the basic parameter of interest is the

$$\text{Incidence density rate} = \frac{\text{Number of cases of disease } Y}{\text{Person} - \text{Time of observation } T}$$

The Poisson regression model is well suited for studying these rates.

Consider an occupational cohort study with two exposure groups under scrutiny for lung cancer over many years. A suitable Poisson regression model, with predictors Age, cigarette Pack-Years, and exposure Group, may take the following form:

$$\text{Model 8:} \quad \ln(T) = a + b(\text{Age}) + c(\text{Pack-Years}) + d(\text{Group}) + r \quad (7.11)$$

Because the random component of the model is assumed to follow a Poisson distribution, this model is called a **Poisson regression model**.

Confounding and Collinearity

WHAT IS COLLINEARITY? (CHILDREN'S MERCY HOSPITAL, 2000)

In biostatistics, **collinearity** occurs when there is a *near*-perfect linear relationship among some or all of the independent variables in a regression model. (It is also known as *ill-conditioning*, *near-collinearity*, or *multicollinearity*.) This situation may result in some redundancy or overlap among these variables.

Collinearity may appear as a very high correlation between two independent variables. Another type of collinearity has several of the variables add up to something that is very close to a constant value.

Collinearity may cause a loss in biostatistical power, making interpretation more difficult. The following example shows confounding owing to simple collin-

■ **Example 7.4:** An example of collinearity[5]

This example shows that for continuous variables, confounding may occur owing to two variables being collinear with a third, as shown by the following R code segment:

```
> # Create a first dependent variable x1 (rounding off to one decimal place):
> x1 <- round(rnorm(1000, mean = 0, sd=1), 1)
> # Next, create a second dependent variable x2 (accurate to one decimal place):
> x2 <- round(rnorm(1000, mean = 5, sd=3), 1)
> # Finally, create a third independent variable x3 that is a direct function of
> # x1 and x2:
> x3 <- 5*x1 + 3*x2
> # Now, create a binary outcome variable that depends on all three variables.
> # Note that the probability of the binomial is an R function inv.logit().
> y <- rbinom(1000, 1, exp(x1 + 3*x2 -5 * x3)/(1+ exp(x1 + 3*x2 -5 * x3)))
> collinear.dat <- data.frame(x1=x1, x2=x2, x3=x3, y=y)
> pairs(collinear.dat) # Outputting: Figure 7.17.
```

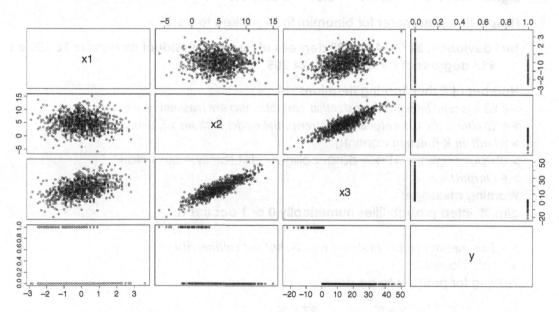

FIGURE 7.17 Confounding and collinearity: high correlation is obvious, but assessing perfect collinearity requires further analysis.

```
> # Further analysis for collinearity
> output <- glm(y ~ x1 + x2 + x3, data = collinear.dat,
+                family=binomial)
```

Warning message:
glm.fit: fitted probabilities numerically 0 or 1 occurred

```
> # Apparently R has detected collinearity; note the warning message below:
> summary(output) # Outputting:
```

Call: glm(formula = y ~ x1 + x2 + x3, family = binomial, data = collinear.dat)

Deviance Residuals:

Min	1Q	Median	3Q	Max
−2.122	0.000	0.000	0.000	1.815

Coefficients: (1 not defined because of singularities)

	Estimate	Std. Error	z value	Pr(>|z|)
(Intercept)	0.8332	1.2312	0.677	0.49858
x1	−22.2919	6.9281	−3.218	0.00129 **
x2	−12.0320	3.7462	−3.212	0.00132 **
x3	NA	NA	NA	NA

Signif. codes: 0 '*' 0.001 '**' 0.01 '*' 0.05 '.' 0.1 ' ' 1**

(Dispersion parameter for binomial family taken to be 1)

Null deviance: 517.564 on 999 degrees of freedom Residual deviance: 18.205 on 997 degrees of freedom AIC: 24.205

Number of Fisher Scoring iterations: 14

```
> # x3 has now been eliminated; other variables also are reasonably estimated.
> # To obtain the CIs automatically, rerun the model without x3, using the
> # built-in R function confint():
> output <- glm(y~x1+x2, data=collinear.dat.family = binomial)
> # Outputting:
```

Warning message:
glm.fit: fitted probabilities numerically 0 or 1 occurred

```
> # This message points to strong results, but not collinearity.
> confint(output)
```

Waiting for profiling to be done...

	2.5 %	97.5 %
(Intercept)	−1.351273	3.736777
x1	−41.218618	−12.389357
x2	−22.278406	−6.683552

There were 36 warnings (use warnings() **to see them)**

```
> # Checking a few fitted values:
> output$fitted[1:5]
```

1	2	3	4	5
9.999559e-01	2.220446e-16	2.220446e-16	2.220446e-16	2.220446e-16

Review Questions for Section 7.3

1. (a) In epidemiologic investigations, what is a confounder or confounding variable?
   (b) Give two examples of such investigations and the associated confounders.
2. Name two biostatistical approaches for controlling confounding in epidemiologic investigations, and briefly describe each approach, giving examples.
3. If confounding is not properly adjusted, what are the possible consequences for the analytical results of an epidemiologic study? Give some examples.
4. Describe the commonly available combined experimental and analytical controls of confounding, and give examples.
5. Describe the MH method of stratification, and give an example of how it is used in controlling confounding.
6. Describe the use of regression modeling for the purpose of adjusting confounding in a biostatistical investigation. Give an example.
7. Write out five possible regression models suitable for adjusting confounding in public health studies, and give examples of their use.
8. (a) What is collinearity? Give an example.
   (b) How can the function confint() be used for testing collinearity?
9. (a) In survival analysis of longitudinal data, how does confounding affect the computation?
   (b) How may confounding be adjusted in such analysis?
10. (a) In using the Cox proportional hazards regression model to fit a dataset, how are the data adjusted for confounding effects?
    (b) If the same dataset were to be analyzed using the K–M plot, how does one control the confounding effects?

Exercises for Section 7.3

1. *Survival analysis: receiver operating characteristic (ROC) curves in R.*
   The ROC curve (shown in Figure 7.18) is a tool used in prediction and classification. It shows the trade-off between sensitivity and specificity—for a range of thresholds applied to an explanatory variable—to predict a binary outcome decision. The sensitivity versus specificity relationship is usually plotted, with the area under the curve often being used as a measure of discriminatory performance: 1 = perfect and 0.5 = no better than a random guess.
   The R function survivalROC(), in the CRAN package survivalROC, creates time-dependent ROC curves from censored survival data, using the K–M or nearest-neighbor estimation (NNE) method of Heagerty, Lumley, and Pepe (2000).
   The usage formula for the function survivalROC() is

```
survivalROC(Stime, status, marker, entry = NULL, predict.time,
          cut.values = NULL, method = "NNE",
          lambda = NULL, span = NULL,
          window = "symmetric")
```

for which the arguments are

Stime   Event time or censoring time for subjects.

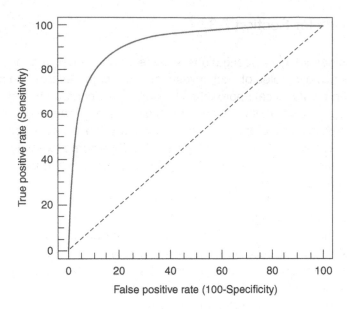

FIGURE 7.18   An ROC curve.

marker	Predictor or marker value.
entry	Entry time for the subjects.
predict.time	Time point of the ROC curve.
cut.values	Marker values to use as a cutoff for calculation of sensitivity and specificity.
method	Method for fitting joint distribution of (x, t), either of K–M or NNE; the default method is NNE.
lambda	Smoothing parameter for NNE.
span	Span for the NNE; need either lambda or span for NNE.
window	Window for NNE, either symmetric or asymmetric.

Suppose that you have censored survival data along with a baseline marker value and you would like to see how well the marker predicts the survival time for the subjects in the dataset. In particular, suppose that you have survival times in days and you want to see how well the marker predicts 1-year survival (predict. time = 365 days). The function roc.KM.calc() returns the unique marker values TP (True Positive), FP (False Positive), K–M survival estimate corresponding to the time point of interest (predict.time), and AUC [area under (ROC) curve] at the time point of interest.

The function survivalROC() returns a list of the following items:

cut.values	Unique marker values for calculation of TP and FP.
TP	True positive corresponding to the cutoffs in x.

FP	False positive corresponding to the cutoffs in x.
predict.time	Time point of interest.
Survival	K–M survival estimate at predict.time.
AUC	Area under the ROC curve at time predict.time.

Using the dataset mayo, the following R code segment is used to generate an ROC curve as in Figure 7.18, using the NNE method:

```
> install.packages("survivalROC")
> library(survivalROC)
> ls("package:survivalROC")
```

[1] "survivalROC"   "survivalROC.C"

```
> data(mayo)
```

mayo

	time	Censor	mayoscore5	mayoscore4
1	41	1	11.251850	10.629450
2	179	1	10.136070	10.185220
3	334	1	10.095740	9.422995
....				
....				
312	533	0	6.115321	6.902997

```
> nobs <- NROW(mayo)
> nobs
```

[1] 312
```
> cutoff <- 365
>
> ## MAYOSCORE 4, METHOD = NNE:
> Mayo4.1= survivalROC(Stime=mayo$time,
+ status=mayo$censor,
+ marker = mayo$mayoscore4,
+ predict.time = cutoff,span = 0.25*nobs^(-0.20) )
> plot(Mayo4.1$FP, Mayo4.1$TP, type="l", xlim=c(0,1),
+ ylim=c(0,1),
+ xlab=paste( "FP", "\n", "AUC = ",round(Mayo4.1$AUC,3)),
+ ylab="TP",main="Mayoscore 4, Method = NNE \n Year = 1")
> abline(0,1)
> # Outputting: Figure 7.19.
```

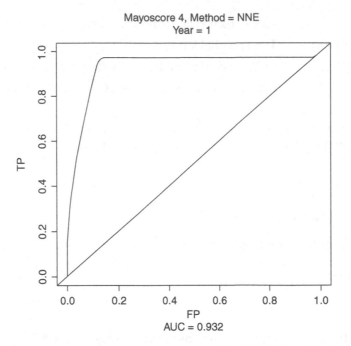

FIGURE 7.19 An ROC curve for dataset mayo using survivalROC(); method = NNE (nearest neighbor estimation).

    (a) Explain the function of each line of the R code segment for this computation.
    (b) Rerun this code segment in the R environment.
    (c) Comment on the resulting plot.

2. *Survival analysis: ROC curves in* R. Again, using the dataset mayo, the following R code segment is used to generate an ROC curve (Figure 7.20), but using the K–M method:

```
>
> ## MAYOSCORE 4, METHOD = KM:
> Mayo4.2= survivalROC(Stime=mayo$time,
+    status=mayo$censor,
+    marker = mayo$mayoscore4,
+    predict.time = cutoff, method="KM")
> plot(Mayo4.2$FP, Mayo4.2$TP, type="l", xlim=c(0,1),
+    ylim=c(0,1),
+ xlab=paste("FP", "\n", "AUC = ,round(Mayo4.2$AUC,3)),
+ ylab="TP",main="Mayoscore 4, Method = KM \n Year = 1")
> abline(0,1)
> # Outputting: Figure 7.20.
```

    (a) Explain the function of each line of the R code segment for this computation.
    (b) Rerun this code segment in the R environment.
    (c) Comment on the resulting plot.

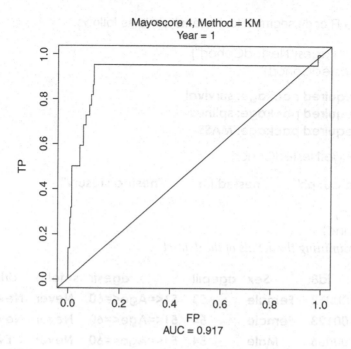

FIGURE 7.20   The ROC curve for dataset mayo using survivalROC(); method = Kaplan–Meier (K–M).

3. *Survival analysis and confounding: CRAN package* NestedCohort *for survival analysis of epidemiologic investigations nested within cohorts* (Katki & Mark, 2008, 2009).

This package contains R functions that undertake survival analysis (K–M and Cox models) for epidemiologic investigations nested within cohorts; these functions are used for estimating hazard ratios, estimating survival probabilities, and standardizing for confounders. The function NestedCohort() is particularly appropriate for evaluating survival probabilities and known risks.

In the following worked example, the observations consisted of the esophageal cancer outcome and survival time on all case subjects, along with known confounders. The main investigational interest centered on the effect of the concentrations of various metals, especially zinc, on this cancer. However, measuring the effect of the concentrations required esophageal biopsy tissue and a costly measurement technique, and it was difficult and expensive to measure concentrations on all the case subjects. Hence, the investigators measured concentration of zinc (along with copper, nickel, iron, calcium, and sulfur) on a selected sample of the cohort. This sample oversampled the cases and those with advanced baseline histologies (i.e., those most likely to become cases), as these were considered the most informative case subjects. Because of availability and cost constraints, less than 30% of the cohort could be sampled.

In this example, the function NestedCohort() provides adjusted hazard ratios, standardized survival probabilities, and population-attributable risks (PARs) for the effect of zinc on the cancer. In particular, in this example, the function nested.km() is used to estimate and fit the K–M survival curves to the nested cohort data.

The R code segment for the analysis is as follows:

```
> install.packages("NestedCohort")
> library(NestedCohort)
```

Loading required package: survival
Loading required package: splines
Loading required package: MASS

```
> ls("package:NestedCohort")
```

[1] "nested.coxph"   "nested.km"   "nested.stdsurv"

```
> data(zinc)
> attach(zinc)
> zinc # Examining the details of the dataset.:
```

	id8	Sex	agepill	agestr	smoke	drink	anyhist
1	10100012	Female	53	51<=Age<=60	Never	Never	<NA>
2	10100123	Female	54	51<=Age<=60	Never	Never	<NA>
3	10300066	Male	54	51<=Age<=60	Never	Ever	<NA>
...							
440	32500344	Female	57	51<=Age<=60	Never	Never	No Family History

	basehist	dysp1	dysp2	mildysp	moddysp
1	Normal	1	0	Worst isn't mild	Worst isn't moderate
2	Normal	1	0	Worst isn't mild	Worst isn't moderate
3	Normal	1	0	Worst isn't mild	Worst isn't moderate
...					
440	Normal	1	0	Worst isn't mild	Worst isn't moderate

	Sevdysp	ec01	futime01	zincset	pcent
1	Worst isn't severe	0	5980	Unobserved Elements	NA
2	Worst isn't severe	0	5980	Unobserved Elements	NA
3	Worst isn't severe	0	5980	Unobserved Elements	NA
440	Worst isn't severe	1	3973	Observed Elements	-0.02219326

	Scent	cacent	fecent	nicent	cucent
1	NA	NA	NA	NA	NA
2	NA	NA	NA	NA	NA
3	NA	NA	NA	NA	NA
440	0.187727832	−1.08682017	0.662201065	−0.787517392	0.811040423

	zncent	pqt	sqt	caqt	feqt	niqt	cuqt	znqt	pq1	pq2	pq3	pq4	sq1	sq2	sq3
1	NA	NA	NA	NA	NA	NA	NA	NA	NA	NA	NA	NA	NA	NA	NA
2	NA	NA	NA	NA	NA	NA	NA	NA	NA	NA	NA	NA	NA	NA	NA
3	NA	NA	NA	NA	NA	NA	NA	NA	NA	NA	NA	NA	NA	NA	NA
440	0.680324598	2	3	1	4	2	3	3	0	1	0	0	0	0	1

	sq4	caq1	caq2	caq3	caq4	feq1	feq2	feq3	feq4	niq1	niq2	niq3	niq4	cuq1	cuq2
1	NA	NA	NA	NA	NA	NA	NA	NA	NA	NA	NA	NA	NA	NA	NA
2	NA	NA	NA	NA	NA	NA	NA	NA	NA	NA	NA	NA	NA	NA	NA
3	NA	NA	NA	NA	NA	NA	NA	NA	NA	NA	NA	NA	NA	NA	NA
440	0	1	0	0	0	0	0	0	1	0	1	0	0	0	0

	cuq3	cuq4	znq1	znq2	znq3	znq4	stdagepill	znquartiles	observed
1	NA	NA	NA	NA	NA	NA	−0.1818182	<NA>	0
2	NA	NA	NA	NA	NA	NA	0.0000000	<NA>	0
3	NA	NA	NA	NA	NA	NA	0.0000000	<NA>	0
440	1	0	0	0	1	0	0.5454545	Q3	1

```
> str(zinc)
'data.frame' :  431 obs. of 61 variables:
$ id8      :  int 10100012 10100123 10300066 10400038 10400106 10400245
             10500252 10500267 10800011 10800049 ...
$ sex      :  Factor w/ 2 levels "Female","Male": 1 1 2 2 2 1 1 1 2 2 ...
$ agepill  :  int 53 54 54 44 44 43 49 48 41 61 ...
$ agestr   :  Factor w/ 3 levels "Age<=50","51<=Age<=60",..: 2 2 2 1 1 1 1 1 1 3
             ...
$ smoke    :  Factor w/ 2 levels "Never","Ever": 1 1 1 1 1 1 1 1 1 2 ...
$ drink    :  Factor w/ 2 levels "Never","Ever": 1 1 2 2 1 1 1 1 2 2 ...
$ anyhist  :  Factor w/ 2 levels "No Family History",..: NA NA NA NA NA NA NA
             NA NA NA ...
```

```
$ basehist  :  Factor w/ 7 levels "Normal","Esophagitis",..: 1 1 1 1 3 2 1 1 1 1 ...
$ dysp1     :  int 1 1 1 1 3 2 1 1 1 1 ...
$ dysp2     :  int 0 0 0 0 1 0 0 0 0 0 ...
$ mildysp   :  Factor w/ 2 levels "Worst isn't mild",..: 1 1 1 1 2 1 1 1 1 1 ...
$ moddysp   :  Factor w/ 2 levels "Worst isn't moderate",..: 1 1 1 1 1 1 1 1 1 1 ...
$ sevdysp   :  Factor w/ 2 levels "Worst isn't severe",..: 1 1 1 1 1 1 1 1 1 1 ...
$ ec01      :  num 0 0 0 0 0 0 0 0 0 0 ...
$ futime01  :  int 5980 5980 5980 5980 5980 3404 5980 5980 5980 5980 ...
$ zincset   :  Factor w/ 2 levels "Unobserved Elements",..: 1 1 1 1 1 1 1 1 1 1 ...

$ pcent     :  num NA NA NA NA NA NA NA NA NA NA ...
$ scent     :  num NA NA NA NA NA NA NA NA NA NA ...
$ cacent    :  num NA NA NA NA NA NA NA NA NA NA ...
$ fecent    :  num NA NA NA NA NA NA NA NA NA NA ...
$ nicent    :  num NA NA NA NA NA NA NA NA NA NA ...
$ cucent    :  num NA NA NA NA NA NA NA NA NA NA ...
$ zncent    :  num NA NA NA NA NA NA NA NA NA NA ...
$ pqt       :  int NA NA NA NA NA NA NA NA NA NA ...
$ sqt       :  int NA NA NA NA NA NA NA NA NA NA ...
$ caqt      :  int NA NA NA NA NA NA NA NA NA NA ...
$ feqt      :  int NA NA NA NA NA NA NA NA NA NA ...
$ niqt      :  int NA NA NA NA NA NA NA NA NA NA ...
$ cuqt      :  int NA NA NA NA NA NA NA NA NA NA ...
$ znqt      :  int NA NA NA NA NA NA NA NA NA NA ...
$ pq1       :  int NA NA NA NA NA NA NA NA NA NA ...
$ pq2       :  int NA NA NA NA NA NA NA NA NA NA ...
$ pq3       :  int NA NA NA NA NA NA NA NA NA NA ...
$ pq4       :  int NA NA NA NA NA NA NA NA NA NA ...
$ sq1       :  int NA NA NA NA NA NA NA NA NA NA ...
$ sq2       :  int NA NA NA NA NA NA NA NA NA NA ...
$ sq3       :  int NA NA NA NA NA NA NA NA NA NA ...
$ sq4       :  int NA NA NA NA NA NA NA NA NA NA ...
$ caq1      :  int NA NA NA NA NA NA NA NA NA NA ...
$ caq2      :  int NA NA NA NA NA NA NA NA NA NA ...
$ caq3      :  int NA NA NA NA NA NA NA NA NA NA ...
$ caq4      :  int NA NA NA NA NA NA NA NA NA NA ...
$ feq1      :  int NA NA NA NA NA NA NA NA NA NA ...
$ feq2      :  int NA NA NA NA NA NA NA NA NA NA ...
$ feq3      :  int NA NA NA NA NA NA NA NA NA NA ...
$ feq4      :  int NA NA NA NA NA NA NA NA NA NA ...
$ niq1      :  int NA NA NA NA NA NA NA NA NA NA ...
$ niq2      :  int NA NA NA NA NA NA NA NA NA NA ...
$ niq3      :  int NA NA NA NA NA NA NA NA NA NA ...
$ niq4      :  int NA NA NA NA NA NA NA NA NA NA ...
$ cuq1      :  int NA NA NA NA NA NA NA NA NA NA ...
$ cuq2      :  int NA NA NA NA NA NA NA NA NA NA ...
```

```
$ cuq3        :  int NA NA NA NA NA NA NA NA NA NA ...
$ cuq4        :  int NA NA NA NA NA NA NA NA NA NA ...
$ znq1        :  int NA NA NA NA NA NA NA NA NA NA ...
$ znq2        :  int NA NA NA NA NA NA NA NA NA NA ...
$ znq3        :  int NA NA NA NA NA NA NA NA NA NA ...
$ znq4        :  int NA NA NA NA NA NA NA NA NA NA ...
$ stdagepill  :  num -0.182 0 0 -1.818 -1.818 ...
$ znquartiles :  Factor w/ 4 levels "Q1","Q2","Q3",..: NA NA NA NA NA NA NA NA
                 NA NA ...
$ observed    :  num 0 0 0 0 0 0 0 0 0 0 ...


>
> mod <- nested.km(survfitformula =
+                     "Surv(futime01,ec01==1)~znquartiles",
+ samplingmod = "ec01*basehist", exposureofinterest = "Q4",
+ data = zinc)
```

Risk Differences vs. znquartiles=Q4 by time 5980

	Risk Difference	StdErr	95% CI Left	95% CI Right
Q4 - Q1	0.2817534	0.10416236	0.07759516	0.4859116
Q4 - Q2	0.0555103	0.07565667	−0.09277677	0.2037974
Q4 - Q3	0.1068147	0.08073547	−0.05142680	0.2650562

```
> summary(mod)
```

**Call: survfit(formula = as.formula(survfitformula), data = data,
weights = 1/p.i.h.a.t.,**
    na.action = na.omit, type = "fl")

308 observations deleted due to missingness
        znquartiles=Q1

Time	n.risk	n.event	survival	std.err	lower 95% CI	upper 95% CI
1037	59.8	1.42	0.977	0.0235	0.840	0.997
4143	44.4	1.42	0.946	0.0388	0.789	0.987
5189	41.1	1.37	0.915	0.0514	0.736	0.975

....

....

| 5893 | 59.8 | 1.57 | 0.633 | 0.0862 | 0.441 | 0.775 |

znquartiles=Q2

Time	n.risk	n.event	survival	std.err	lower 95% CI	upper 95% CI
1038	116.9	1.57	0.987	0.0133	0.909	0.998
1064	115.3	4.51	0.949	0.0260	0.864	0.981
1070	110.8	2.33	0.929	0.0324	0.830	0.971
....						
4139	63.5	1.37	0.859	0.0520	0.718	0.933

znquartiles=Q3

time	n.risk	n.event	survival	std.err	lower 95% CI	upper 95% CI
318	125.1	1.20	0.990	0.00948	0.934	0.999
733	123.9	1.20	0.981	0.01340	0.926	0.995
1001	122.7	1.37	0.970	0.01759	0.907	0.991
....						
5351	64.6	1.42	0.808	0.05800	0.662	0.896

znquartiles=Q4

Time	n.risk	n.event	survival	std.err	lower 95% CI	upper 95% CI
1037	59.8	1.42	0.977	0.0235	0.840	0.997
4143	44.4	1.42	0.946	0.0388	0.789	0.987
5189	41.1	1.37	0.915	0.0514	0.736	0.975

```
> plot(mod, ymin = 0.6, xlab = "Time in days",
+        ylab = "Survival probabilities",
+        main = "Survival Analysis by Quartile of Zinc",
+        lty = 1:4)
> legend(1000,0.7, c("Q1", "Q2", "Q3", "Q4"), lty=1:4)
> # Outputting: Figure 7.21.
```

(a) Explain the function of each line of the R code segment for this computation.
(b) Rerun this code segment in the R environment.
(c) Comment on the resulting plot (Figure 7.21).
(d) In this analysis, how is confounding adjusted?

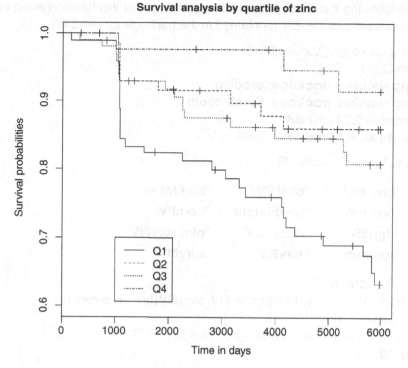

FIGURE 7.21 K–M survival analysis curves for cancer survival by each quartile of zinc, standardized for confounders.

4. *Survival analysis: The CRAN package* survivalBIV *(bivariate distribution function)* (Moreira et al, 2012).

The CRAN package survivalBIV estimates the bivariate distribution function for sequentially ordered events under univariate censoring. This package contains a number of R functions designed for special applications in survival analysis. Some of these applications are illustrated here.

(a) A conditional Kaplan–Meier (CK–M) estimator: bivCKM(). This function provides estimates for the bivariate distribution function for the CK–M estimator, and has a usage formula of the form:

bivCKM(object, t1, t2, conf = FALSE, n.boot = 1000,
conf.level = 0.95, method.boot = "percentile")

with the following arguments:

object	An object of class survBIV.
t1	The first time for obtaining estimates for the bivariate distribution function; if missing, 0 will be used.
t2	The second time for obtaining estimates for the bivariate distribution function; if missing, the maximum of time2 will be used.
Conf	Provides point-wise confidence bands; defaults to FALSE.
n.boot	The number of bootstrap samples; defaults to 1,000 samples.
conf.level	Level of confidence; defaults to 0.95 (corresponding to 95%).
method.boot	Method used to compute bootstrap CIs. Possible options are "per-

The following R code segment illustrates the use of this function when applied to the dataset bladderBIV (contained in the package survivalBIV):

```
> install.packages("survivalBIV")
> library(survivalBIV)
Loading required package: prodlim
Loading required package: KernSmooth
KernSmooth 2.23 loaded
Copyright M. P. Wand 1997-2009

> ls("package:survivalBIV")
```

[1]	"bivCKM"	"bivIPCW"	"bivKMPW"
[4]	"bivKMW"	"bladderBIV"	"corrBIV"
[7]	"dgpBIV"	"is.survBIV"	"plot.survBIV"
[10]	"summary"	"survBIV"	"survBIV"

```
> data("bladderBIV")
> bladderBIV_obj <- with(bladderBIV, survBIV(time1, event1,
+ time2, event2))
> bivCKM(object = bladderBIV_obj, t1 = 5, t2 = 20)
0.1920702
> #or
> bladderBIV_obj <- survBIV(bladderBIV$time1,
+              bladderBIV$event1, bladderBIV$time2,
+              bladderBIV$event2)
> bivCKM(object = bladderBIV_obj, t1 = 5, t2 = 20, conf = TRUE,
+ conf.level = 0.9)
```

	5%	95%
0.1920702	0.1185156	0.2657545

(a) Explain the function of each line of the R code segment for this computation.
(b) Rerun this code segment in the R environment.
(c) Comment on the results.
(d) Another R function in this package is bivIPCW(), which provides estimates for the bivariate distribution function for the inverse probability of censoring weighted (IPCW) estimator. The following R code segment applies this function to the same dataset bladderBIV:

```
> data("bladderBIV")
> bladderBIV_obj <- with(bladderBIV, survBIV(time1, event1,
+                 time2, event2))
> bivIPCW(object = bladderBIV_obj, t1 = 5, t2 = 20,
+         method.cens = "prodlim")
```

Run this R code segment, and comment on the result:

0.1868247

```
> #or
> bladderBIV_obj <- survBIV(bladderBIV$time1,
+     bladderBIV$event1, bladderBIV$time2,
+     bladderBIV$event2)
> bivIPCW(object = bladderBIV_obj, t1 = 5, t2 = 20,
+           conf = TRUE, conf.level = 0.9,
+ method.boot = "basic")
```

	5%	95%
0.1866335	0.1105516	0.2646384

```
> data("bladderBIV")
> bladderBIV_obj <- with(bladderBIV, survBIV(time1, event1,
+                   time2, event2))
> bivKMPW(object = bladderBIV_obj, t1 = 5, t2 = 20)
```
0.1897386
```
> #or
> bladderBIV_obj <- survBIV(bladderBIV$time1,
+                 bladderBIV$event1, bladderBIV$time2,
+                 bladderBIV$event2)
> bivKMPW(object = bladderBIV_obj, t1 = 5, t2 = 20,
+           conf = TRUE, conf.level = 0.9)
```

	5%	95%
0.1897386	0.1202276	0.2619701

```
> data("bladderBIV")
> bladderBIV_obj <- with(bladderBIV, survBIV(time1, event1,
+                   time2, event2))
> bivKMW(object = bladderBIV_obj, t1 = 5, t2 = 20)
```
0.1921058
```
> # or
> bladderBIV_obj <- survBIV(bladderBIV$time1,
+                 bladderBIV$event1, bladderBIV$time2,
+                 bladderBIV$event2)
> bivKMW(object = bladderBIV_obj, t1 = 5, t2 = 20,
+           conf = TRUE, conf.level = 0.9)
```

	5%	95%
0.1921058	0.1180276	0.2656078

```
> # Example for the bivariate exponential distribution:
> dgpBIV(n = 100, corr = 1, dist = "exponential",
+           model.cens = "uniform",
+ cens.par = 3, dist.par = c(1, 1), to.data.frame = TRUE)
```

	time1	event1	time2	event2
1	0.0005895626	1	0.75564858	1
2	0.6982030278	1	0.23072713	1
3	0.0558737679	1	0.85410701	1
4	0.6485372734	1	0.52543358	0
5	0.6713170423	0	0.00000000	0
6	0.8790889907	1	0.03043959	1
7	0.6068865498	1	0.10316399	1
8	0.0975181995	1	0.95176635	1
9	0.7997097191	0	0.00000000	0
10	0.2697271148	0	0.00000000	0
11	0.4367546837	0	0.00000000	0
12	0.2809143670	1	1.17781751	0
13	1.2135338530	1	0.10468994	1
14	1.4306760170	1	0.56626825	0
15	0.1780562948	0	0.00000000	0
16	0.3228512866	1	0.99409678	0
17	0.3177933234	1	0.99625677	0
18	0.2284733959	1	0.23741045	0
19	0.5274914715	1	0.30927187	1
20	0.2926479652	1	0.87673844	1
21	0.5181994882	1	0.84130949	1
22	1.6557341524	1	0.84904600	0
23	0.2561566898	1	0.02706028	1
24	1.0438891871	1	0.69471175	0
25	0.1166925130	0	0.00000000	0
26	0.2389276870	1	0.93371568	1
27	0.9899928542	1	1.72177471	0
28	0.2674041729	1	0.04035089	1
29	0.0177538705	0	0.00000000	0
30	0.7928811121	1	0.11645234	1
31	0.4532970815	1	0.81096417	1
32	0.9278468457	0	0.00000000	0
33	0.3206757427	1	0.27408256	1
34	0.2955963112	1	0.25176147	0
35	0.4530449047	1	0.12346276	1
36	1.9161922988	0	0.00000000	0
37	0.8300401610	0	0.00000000	0
38	0.2012448817	1	0.25938102	1

39	0.3447902738	1	0.02007339	1
40	0.9947645486	1	0.45997132	0
41	0.2069979079	1	0.28359194	1
42	0.5122642969	0	0.00000000	0
43	0.6378745642	1	0.06128698	1
44	1.9400842474	0	0.00000000	0
45	0.6603214571	0	0.00000000	0
46	0.6634516153	0	0.00000000	0
47	0.1856409729	1	0.23703461	1
48	0.9697090527	0	0.00000000	0
49	0.3939246334	1	0.12125044	0
50	0.0515332760	1	0.07251975	1
51	2.0156175639	0	0.00000000	0
52	1.2559016843	1	0.04350289	0
53	1.3967063204	1	0.18671369	1
54	0.9279630573	1	0.08916433	0
55	0.8164238634	1	0.05462287	1
56	0.0245129673	0	0.00000000	0
57	0.5157781137	1	0.26861503	1
58	0.3728056342	1	0.07303738	1
59	0.6157245501	1	0.41411110	0
60	0.4798975375	1	0.36525051	1
61	0.7601117366	0	0.00000000	0
62	0.4095801464	1	0.87768139	1
63	0.6044178131	1	0.04452789	0
64	0.0403524034	0	0.00000000	0
65	0.8983658056	0	0.00000000	0
66	0.4816842741	1	0.09519841	0
67	0.0310373344	1	0.36791676	1
68	0.9049734917	1	0.26968932	1
69	1.0606460375	1	1.37214910	1
70	0.1874751560	1	0.54789536	1
71	0.2055806991	1	0.94832239	1
72	1.8742257392	0	0.00000000	0
73	2.5159698048	1	0.26259136	1
74	2.6107399651	1	0.01456952	0
75	0.6080606624	0	0.00000000	0
76	2.2104980203	0	0.00000000	0
77	0.6885901640		0.00000000	

78	0.1329671829	0	0.00000000	0
79	0.1822175515	1	0.13577832	1
80	0.6162270399	1	0.31167067	1
81	1.1962075245	0	0.00000000	0
82	1.0517517613	1	0.30542583	0
83	0.2711551202	1	0.93749705	0
84	0.4736238314	1	0.42495908	1
85	0.1668557518	0	0.00000000	0
86	0.4283004184	1	0.13572692	1
87	1.4244481432	1	0.25146951	1
88	0.2768717642	1	0.27988718	1
89	0.0087164905	1	0.03962044	1
90	2.4277168578	0	0.00000000	0
91	0.2097113177	0	0.00000000	0
92	0.0021386391	1	0.16532315	1
93	0.6734751035	1	1.46594482	0
94	1.8577060935	0	0.00000000	0
95	0.1409383491	0	0.00000000	0
96	0.7416686579	1	0.83971735	1
97	2.0469178744	0	0.00000000	0
98	0.5584133468	1	0.58440127	0
99	2.0667516228	1	0.07517950	1
100	0.2160539478	0	0.00000000	0

```
> # Example for the bivariate Weibull distribution:
> dgpBIV(n = 100, corr = 1, dist = "weibull", model.cens =
+ "exponential",
+ cens.par = 0.08, dist.par = c(2, 7, 2, 7))
```

$data

	time1	event1	time2	event2	Stime
1	1.388147729	0	0.0000000	0	1.388147729
2	0.743709478	0	0.0000000	0	0.743709478
3	4.311593760	1	2.2516124	0	6.563206116
4	4.470056068	0	0.0000000	0	4.470056068
5	5.997286522	0	0.0000000	0	5.997286522
6	0.005249357	0	0.0000000	0	0.005249357
7	2.609313119	0	0.0000000	0	2.609313119
8	7.146119245	1	0.3176864	0	7.463805680
9	6.447898338	1	5.9024270	1	12.350325305

10	4.169294109	1	4.2948521	1	8.464146250
11	8.247212600	1	4.7068117	0	12.954024341
12	3.595728674	1	6.0022950	1	9.598023643
13	10.117623649	1	3.7784823	0	13.896105950
14	8.209468634	0	0.0000000	0	8.209468634
15	7.006549462	1	9.0528632	1	16.059412663
16	6.835012301	1	2.7363197	0	9.571331956
17	8.472035429	1	3.5261148	0	11.998150183
18	2.849277534	1	8.8820817	1	11.731359253
19	3.051419189	1	6.6459485	1	9.697367718
20	6.553231439	1	0.7711965	1	7.324427896
21	11.004396078	1	6.2054960	1	17.209892032
22	2.567791299	1	7.7498997	0	10.317690996
23	4.204659119	1	10.1619853	1	14.366644423
24	7.360276219	0	0.0000000	0	7.360276219
25	2.734720899	0	0.0000000	0	2.734720899
26	2.904995325	1	6.7961131	1	9.701108398
27	11.153064089	1	1.6165403	1	12.769604432
28	6.035556386	1	1.7032070	1	7.738763414
29	7.222186275	1	7.4833385	1	14.705524741
30	5.468072242	0	0.0000000	0	5.468072242
31	12.965649468	1	3.1403897	1	16.106039130
32	3.061703269	1	0.7260095	0	3.787712725
33	3.751140080	1	9.1630566	0	12.914196669
34	1.680568964	1	3.8075400	0	5.488108939
35	4.353856486	1	6.9240779	1	11.277934414
36	0.572074048	0	0.0000000	0	0.572074048
37	6.673796084	1	5.2544671	1	11.928263191
38	7.689879433	1	7.5970093	1	15.286888712
39	10.583878851	1	2.0478638	0	12.631742695
40	4.089472140	0	0.0000000	0	4.089472140
41	11.093751137	1	0.9952871	0	12.089038279
42	0.756349065	0	0.0000000	0	0.756349065
43	2.838233864	0	0.0000000	0	2.838233864
44	5.285847816	0	0.0000000	0	5.285847816
45	5.899664003	1	5.8729714	1	11.772635387
46	5.924026349	1	1.2014802	1	7.125506594
47	2.294302556	1	5.7817984	1	8.076100916
48	7.228772283	1	0.8181344	0	

49	6.849679163	1	4.2819505	1	11.131629712
50	6.960093893	1	6.7772215	0	13.737315346
51	3.703865355	1	13.3599371	1	17.063802422
52	2.978508038	0	0.0000000	0	2.978508038
53	0.632452127	0	0.0000000	0	0.632452127
54	4.437267513	0	0.0000000	0	4.437267513
55	11.433835033	0	0.0000000	0	11.433835033
56	0.026654385	0	0.0000000	0	0.026654385
57	4.366620830	1	4.6884216	1	9.055042468
58	2.086997694	0	0.0000000	0	2.086997694
59	4.386038504	1	4.1407420	0	8.526780544
60	0.166223885	0	0.0000000	0	0.166223885
61	5.881654616	1	4.8989473	1	10.780601869
62	4.387691111	0	0.0000000	0	4.387691111
63	3.327461537	0	0.0000000	0	3.327461537
64	5.439083596	1	5.9484436	1	11.387527240
65	3.043832240	0	0.0000000	0	3.043832240
66	3.866050823	0	0.0000000	0	3.866050823
67	9.206512038	1	1.9021350	1	11.108647010
68	2.077167493	0	0.0000000	0	2.077167493
69	1.169742962	0	0.0000000	0	1.169742962
70	7.836676569	0	0.0000000	0	7.836676569
71	3.094922049	1	7.5165716	1	10.611493699
72	5.456891474	1	3.0843889	0	8.541280357
73	6.777679345	1	1.6365333	1	8.414212682
74	4.037906132	1	6.6897972	1	10.727703306
75	0.513964477	0	0.0000000	0	0.513964477
76	6.690673682	1	1.0181006	1	7.708774302
77	13.279659553	1	13.3269520	1	26.606611569
78	3.841746730	1	4.1038628	1	7.945609505
79	1.444641809	0	0.0000000	0	1.444641809
80	2.937351998	1	2.8168339	0	5.754185881
81	1.223288129	1	6.1965012	1	7.419789348
82	1.275968027	0	0.0000000	0	1.275968027
83	3.611468174	0	0.0000000	0	3.611468174
84	6.549168425	1	1.3645790	1	7.913747386
85	7.801177148	1	3.5133309	1	11.314508024
86	6.137463114	1	16.4784673	1	22.615930434
87	7.844500803	0	0.0000000	0	7.846500803

88	3.163988848	1	9.5916571	1	12.755645964
89	2.120092746	1	6.5040954	1	8.624188137
90	0.664639455	0	0.0000000	0	0.664639455
91	3.582123312	0	0.0000000	0	3.582123312
92	0.886321417	0	0.0000000	0	0.886321417
93	6.554446964	1	0.3444679	0	6.898914900
94	5.485892578	1	2.4127827	1	7.898675250
95	0.434836076	0	0.0000000	0	0.434836076
96	3.084640881	1	3.4676929	0	6.552333769
97	7.621512087	1	12.4836850	1	20.105197113
98	3.049349878	0	0.0000000	0	3.049349878
99	7.862905945	1	9.2293236	1	17.092229502
100	0.869275234	0	0.0000000	0	0.869275234

```
attr(,"class")
[1] "survBIV"


>
```

5. *Plot methods for a survBIV object.*
   The following R code segments provide the plots for the bivariate distribution
   function and marginal distribution, such as those in Exercise 4:

```
> install.packages("survivalBIV")
> library(survivalBIV)
```

Loading required package: prodlim
Loading required package: KernSmooth
KernSmooth 2.23 loaded
Copyright M. P. Wand 1997-2009

```
> ls("package:survivalBIV")
```

[1]	"bivC"	"bivIPCW"	"bivKMPW"
[4]	"bivKMW"	"bladderBIV"	"corrBIV"
[7]	"dgpBIV"	"is.survBIV"	"plot.survBIV"
[10]	"summary"	"survBIV"	"survBIV"

```
> data("bladderBIV")
> bladderBIV_obj <- with(bladderBIV, survBIV(time1, event1,
+                        time2, event2))
>
> op <- par(mfrow = c(2, 2))
> plot(bladderBIV_obj, plot.marginal = TRUE, method = "CKM")
```
Waiting to confirm page change...
```
> plot(bladderBIV_obj, plot.marginal = TRUE, method = "IPCW")
```

```
> plot(bladderBIV_obj, plot.marginal = TRUE, method = "KMW")
> par(op)
> # Outputting: Figure 7.22 survivalBIV-1.
```

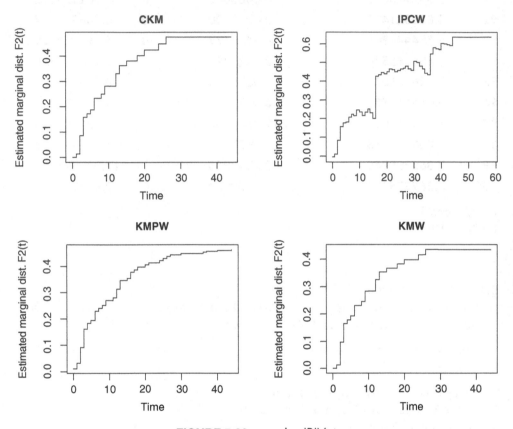

FIGURE 7.22   survivalBIV-1.

```
> plot(bladderBIV_obj, plot.marginal = TRUE,
+ plot.bivariate = TRUE, method = "CKM")
```

Waiting to confirm page change...
```
> # Outputting: Figure 7.23 survivalBIV-CKM-1.
```

Waiting to confirm page change...
```
> # Outputting: Figure 7.24 survivalBIV-CKM-2.
```

Waiting to confirm page change...
```
> # Outputting: Figure 7.25 survivalBIV-CKM-3.
```

```
> plot(bladderBIV_obj, plot.bivariate = TRUE, method = "IPCW")
```

Waiting to confirm page change...
> # *Outputting:* Figure 7.26 survivalBIV-IPCW-**1**.

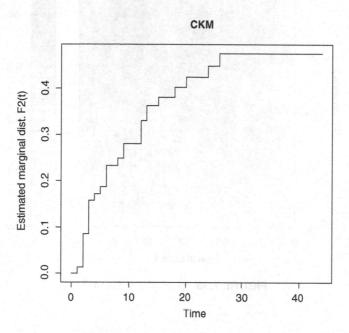

FIGURE 7.23 survivalBIV-CKM-1.

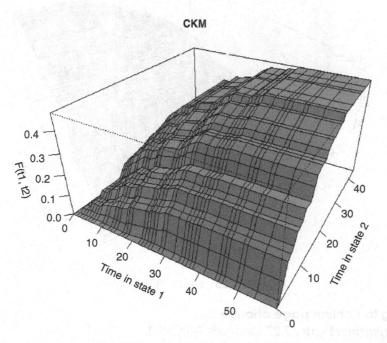

FIGURE 7.24 survivalBIV-CKM-2.

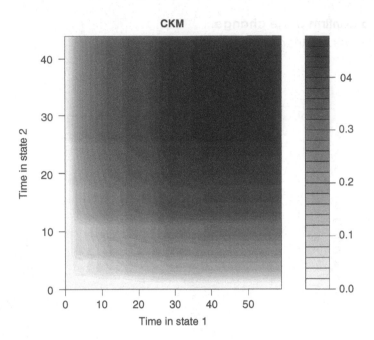

FIGURE 7.25 survivalBIV-CKM-3.

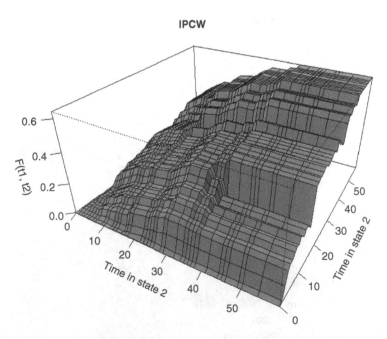

FIGURE 7.26 survivalBIV-IPCW-1.

Waiting to confirm page change...
> # *Outputting:* Figure 7.27 survivalBIV-IPCW-**2**.

> plot(bladderBIV_obj, plot.persp = TRUE, method = "KMPW")

> # *Outputting:* Figure 7.28 survivalBIV-KMPW.

> plot(bladderBIV_obj, plot.contour = TRUE, method = "KMW")

Waiting to confirm page change...
> # *Outputting:* Figure 7.29 survivalBIV-KMW.

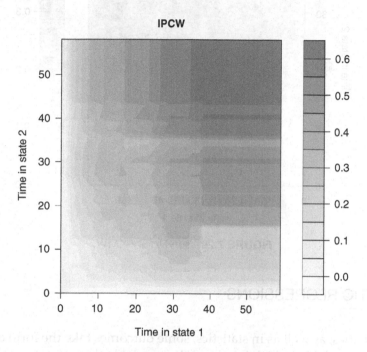

FIGURE 7.27 survivalBIV-IPCW-2.

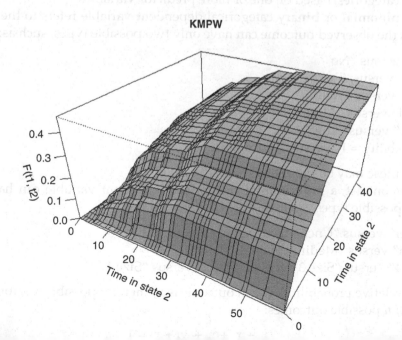

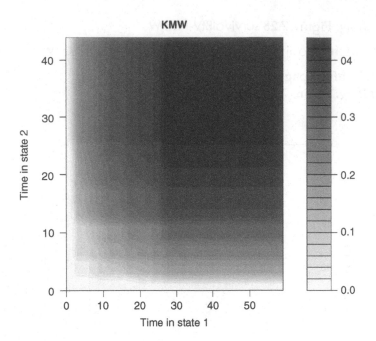

FIGURE 7.29   survivalBIV-KMW.

7.4   LOGISTIC REGRESSIONS

In biostatistics, as well as in statistics, some outcomes take the form of a **categorical dependent variable**, which is a dependent variable that can take on a limited number of categories, based on one or more predictor variables.

A **binomial** or **binary** categorical dependent variable refers to the instance in which the observed outcome can have only two possible types, such as:

"Yes" versus "No"
"Pass" versus "Fail"
"Sick" versus "Well"
"Dead" versus "Alive"
"High" versus "Low"
"Probability = 1" versus "Probability = 0"

All of these may be represented by "1" versus "0."

In contrast, a **multinomial** categorical dependent variable can have three or more possible types, such as:

"Better" versus "Unchanged" versus "Worse"
"High" versus "Medium" versus "Low"
"Size 4" versus "Size 3" versus "Size 2" versus "Size 1"

If the relative probability of each outcome is x_i, then for possibility I, for the general case of n possible outcomes:

$$x_1 + x_2 + x_3 + \ldots + x_n = 1$$

To model the categorical dependent variables that have limited ranges, one approach is to use a **logistic regression model analysis** (Everitt & Hothorn, 2006; Daniel, 2005; Dalgaard, 2002). Chapter 3 presented linear regression analysis involving one, two, or several variables in Section 3.5.

For a **univariate system**, the simple linear regression model may be expressed by the equation:

$$y = \beta_0 + \beta_{1x} + e \qquad (7.12A)$$

in which

x is the value *independent* variable X,
y is an arbitrary observed value of the continuous *dependent* variable Y,
β_0 and β_1 are the coefficients of the linear regression, and
e is the error term.

In a linear regression, when the observed value of Y is $\mu_{y|x}$ (the mean of a subset of Y values for a given value of X), the quantity e (the difference between the observed Y and the regression line) is zero. Equation (7.12) may thus be written as follows:

$$\mu_{y|x} = \beta_0 + \beta_{1x} \qquad (7.13A)$$

or

$$E(y \mid x) = \beta_0 + \beta_{1x} \qquad (7.14A)$$

In general, the right side of Equations (7.12A), (7.13A), and (7.14A) may have *any value between negative infinity and positive infinity.*

Inappropriateness of the Simple Linear Regression When y Is a Categorical Dependent Variable

When y is a dichotomous variable (a simple categorical dependent variable having only two possible outcomes; e.g., "1" or "0"), the simple linear regression model just discussed is *not* appropriate because the mean (the expected value of Y) is the probability that $Y = 1$ and is therefore limited to the range of 0 to 1, inclusive. This contradicts the property shared by Equations (7.12A), (7.13A), and (7.14A); namely, that the right side may take any value.

The Logistic Regression Model

In this model, one may let p be the probability that $Y = 1$:

$$p = P(Y = 1) \qquad (7.15)$$

The ratio $p/(1 - p)$ may be considered as follows:

(the probability of a Success for y)/(1 – the probability of a Success for y)
= (the probability of a Success for y)/(the probability of a Failure for y)
= the odds, π, of the Response 0 taking the value of 1

Thus, the ratio $p/1-p)$ can assume values between negative infinity $(-\infty)$ and positive infinity $(+\infty)$, as is required by the right side of Equations (7.12), (7.13), and (7.14). Hence, one may rewrite it as

$$\log[p/(1-p)] = \beta_0 + \beta_{1x} \qquad (7.16A)$$

This is known as the **logistic regression model**. The transformation of $\mu_{y|x}$ (i.e., p) to $\log[p/(1-p)]$ is known as the **logit transformation**. Equation (7.16A) may also be written as

$$p = \exp(\beta_0 + \beta_1 x)/[1 + \exp(\beta_0 + \beta_1 x)], \qquad (7.17A)$$

in which exp is the inverse of the natural logarithm $\log_e$ or ln.

The Logit

The logit of the probability p is the log of the odds π of the response taking the value of 1:

$$\text{logit}(\pi) = \log[\pi/(1-\pi)] \qquad (7.18)$$

This logistic regression model is commonly used in biostatistics, epidemiology, and the health sciences, particularly when a categorical dependent variable is investigated. In epidemiologic analysis, it is commonly applied in attempts to model the probability (or the risk) that a case subject will acquire a particular disease during some specific duration in which the subject is exposed to conditions known to be associated with that disease.

For a **multivariate system**, the resultant equations corresponding to Equations (7.12A), (7.13A), (7.14A), (7.16A), and (7.17A) are, respectively:

$$y = \beta_0 + \beta_1 x_1 + \beta_2 x_2 + \beta_3 x_3 + \cdots + \beta_n x + e \qquad (7.12B)$$

$$\mu_{y|x} = \beta_0 + \beta_1 x_1 + \beta_2 x_2 + \beta_3 x_3 + \cdots + \beta_n x_n \qquad (7.13B)$$

$$E(y|x) = \beta_0 + \beta_1 x + \beta_2 x_2 + \beta_3 x_3 + \cdots + \beta_n x_n \qquad (7.14B)$$

$$\log[p/(1-p)] = \beta_0 + \beta_1 x + \beta_2 x_2 + \beta_3 x_3 + \cdots + \beta_n x_n \qquad (7.16B)$$

$$p = \exp(\beta_0 + \beta_1 x + \beta_2 x_2 + \beta_3 x_3 + \cdots + \beta_n x_n)/$$
$$[1 + \exp(\beta_0 + \beta_1 x + \beta_2 x_2 + \beta_3 x_3 + \cdots + \beta_n x_n] \qquad (7.17B)$$

Logistic Regression Analysis

This class of analysis is usually performed using biostatistical models belonging to the class of generalized linear models (see Chapter 3, Section 3.5, on univariate, bivariate, and multivariate data analysis). These models are generally characterized by the following elements:

1. a response distribution, such as the binomial and Poisson distributions, and
2. a link function that transfers the mean value to a scale where the relationship to other variables may be expressed as additive and linear. For logistic regression

For example, in the analysis of count data, the multiplicative Poisson model may be used, in which case the link function is log λ, where λ is the mean of the observed Poisson distribution.

All these models may be treated by the same algorithm, permitting the analyst to define suitable link functions.

Generalized Linear Models in R

This topic was presented in Chapter 3, Section 3.5 (which discussed univariate, bivariate, and multivariate data analysis), where it was shown that, in R, generalized linear models are applied using the function glm(), which is similar to the familiar function lm(). These two functions are also very similar in application, in that both functions use the same model formulas and extractor functions (such as summary(), etc.). However, the function glm() requires a designated generalized linear model, which may be achieved using the family argument within the function glm().

The following worked example illustrates practical logistic regressional modeling in biostatistical applications in epidemiology and public health.

■ **Example 7.5:** Logistic regression for predicting a binary-valued clinical variable using a *binomial* regression link

The data package faraway contains 124 sets of results of clinical investigations of a large number of case subjects regarding certain metabolic syndromes (such as diabetes). Within this package is a dataset named pima containing the records of certain health conditions of 768 case subjects (each including the diagnosis of diabetes) and their corresponding body mass index (BMI) bmi.

(a) Using logistic regression, show that a diagnosis of diabetes in a case subject is significantly linked to that case subject's BMI.
(b) Estimate the probability for someone whose BMI is 35 to have diabetes.
(c) For someone in the 95% percentile probability of having diabetes, estimate the probability for that person to have a BMI of 35.

Solutions:
The following R code segment undertakes the computations for this example. First, call up the package faraway, and then examine the dataset pima:

R **version 2.15.2 (2012-10-26) -- "Trick or Treat"**
Copyright (C) 2012 The R **Foundation for Statistical Computing**
ISBN 3-900051-07-0
Platform: i386-w64-mingw32/i386 (32-bit)

R **is free software and comes with ABSOLUTELY NO WARRANTY.**
You are welcome to redistribute it under certain conditions.
Type 'license()' or 'licence()' for distribution details.

Natural language support but running in an English locale
R **is a collaborative project with many contributors.**
Type 'contributors()' for more information and 'citation()' on how to cite R **or** R

Type 'demo()' for some demos, 'help()' for on-line help, or 'help.start()' for an HTML browser interface to help.
Type 'q()' to quit R.

[Previously saved workspace restored]

First, examine the data file under investigation:

```
>
> install.packages("faraway")
```
Installing package(s) into 'C:/Users/bertchan/Documents/R/win-library/2.15' (as 'lib' is unspecified)
--- Please select a CRAN mirror for use in this session ---
trying URL 'http://cran.stat.ucla.edu/bin/windows/contrib/2.15/faraway_1.0.5.zip'

Content type 'application/zip' length 593494 bytes (579 Kb)
opened URL
downloaded 579 Kb

package 'faraway' successfully unpacked and MD5 sums checked

The downloaded binary packages are in
C:\Users\bertchan\AppData\Local\Temp\RtmpwPV84x\downloaded_packages

```
> library(faraway)
> ls("package:faraway")
```

[1] "aatemp"	"abrasion"	"aflatoxin"	"africa"	"alfalfa"
[6] "amlxray"	"babyfood"	"beetle"	"bliss"	"breaking"
[11] "broccoli"	"cathedral"	"chicago"	"chiczip"	"chmiss"

....

[71] "nes96"	"oatvar"	"odor"	"ohio"	"orings"
[76] "ozone"	"parstum"	"peanut"	"penicillin"	"pima"
[81] "pipeline"	"pneumo"	"potuse"	"prostate"	"prplot"

....

[121] "wavesolder"	"wbca"	"weldstrength"	"wheat"

```
> pima
```

	pregnant	Glucose	diastolic	triceps	insulin	bmi	diabetes	age	test
1	6	148	72	35	0	33.6	0.627	50	1
2	1	85	66	29	0	26.6	0.351	31	0
3	8	183	64	0	0	23.3	0.672	32	1
....									
767	1	126	60	0	0	30.1	0.349	47	1
768	1	93	70	31	0	30.4	0.315	23	0

```
 [1] 0 0 1 0 0 0 0 1 1 0 0 0 0 0 0 0 1 0 1 0 1 1 0
     0 1 0 1 0 0 1 0 0 0 0 0 0 0 0 0 0 1 0 1 0 1 1 0
     0 0 0 0 0 1 0 1 0 0 0 0 0 0 0 1 0 1 0 1 0
     0 1 0 0 0 1 0 0 0 0 0 1 0 1 0 0 1 0 1 0
     0 0 0 1 0 1 0 0 0 0 0 0 1 0 0 1 0 0 1 0
     1 0 0 0 1 1 0 0 0 0 0 0 0 0 1 0 0 0 1 0
     0 0 0 0 0 1 0 0 0 0 0 0 1 0 0 0 0 1 1 0
     0 1 0 0 0 1 0 0 0 1 0 0 0 1 0 1 0 1 0 0 0
     0 0 0 0 0 0 0 0 1 0 0 1 0 0 1 0 0 0 1 0
     0 1 0 0 1 0 0 0 1 1 1 0 0 0 1 0 1 0 0 1
     1 0 1 0 0 0 0 0 0 0 0 0 0 1 1 0 0 1
     1 0 1 0 0 0 1 1 0 0 0 0 1 0 1 0 0 0 0
     1 1 0 0 0 1 0 1 0 1 0 1 0 1 0 0 0 0 0
     1 0 0 0 0 1 0 0 0 0 1 0 0 0 1 0 0 1 0
     1 0 0 0 0 1 0 0 0 0 0 0 0 0 0 1 0 0 0
     0 0 0 1 0 1 0 0 0 1 0 0 1 0 0 0 0 0 1
     0 0 0 1 0 0 0 0 0 0 0 0 0 0 0 0 0 0
     1 1 1 0 0 0 0 0 0 0 0 0 0 1 1 0 1 0 1 1
     0 0 0 1 0 0 0 0 1 0 1 1 0 0 0 0 0 0 0
     1 0 0 1 0 1 0 0 1 1 0 0 0 0 0 0 0 0 1
     1 0 0 0 0 0 0 0 0 0 0 0 0 0 0 0 0 0 1
     1 0 1 1 0 0 0 1 0 1 0 0 0 0 0 1 0 0 0
     1 0 0 1 0 1 0 1 0 0 0 0 0 0 0 0 0 0 1
     0 0 0 0 0 1 0 0 1 0 0 0 1 0 1 0 1 0 1
     1 0 0 0 0 0 1 0 0 0 1 0 0 0 1 0 1 0 0
     0 0 1 0 1 0 1 0 1 0 0 0 0 0 0 0 0 1 0
     1 1 0 0 0 0 0 0 0 0 0 0 0 0 0 1 1 1 1
     1 1 0 0 0 0 0 0 0 0 0 0 0 0 0 0 0 1 0
     0 0 0 0 0 1 1 0 1 0 0 1 1 0 0 0 0 0 0 1
     1 1 0 0 1 0 0 0 1 0 0 0 1 1 0 1 0 1 1
     0 0 0 1 0 0 0 0 1 0 0 0 0 0 1 0 0 1 1
     1 0 1 1 1 1 0 0 1 1 0 0 1 1 0 0 0 0 0
     0 0 0 1 0 0 0 0 0 0 1 0 0 0 0 0 0 1
     1 1 0 0 0 1 0 1 1 0 0 1 0 0 0 0 0 0
     0 1 0 0 0 0 1 0 0 0 1 0 0 0 0 0 1 1 0
     1 1 0 0 0 1 0 1 0 1 0 0 1 0 0 0 0 0 0
```

[1] [38] [75] [112] [149] [186] [223] [260] [297] [334] [371] [408] [445] [482] [519] [556] [593] [630] [667] [704] [741]

(a) Correlating the dataset pima by a logistic regression function lr(), with bmi as the variable, and using a generalized linear model glm() with a binomial function binomial() as the link function:

```
> lr <- glm(f ~ bmi, family = binomial, data = pima)
```

To examine the critical computed results, call:

```
> summary(lr)
> # Outputting:
```

Call:
glm(formula = f ~ bmi, family = binomial, data = pima)

Deviance Residuals:

Min	1Q	Median	3Q	Max
−1.9209	−0.9178	−0.6838	1.2351	2.7244

Coefficients:

	Estimate	Std. Error	z value	Pr(>|z|)
(Intercept)	−3.68641	0.40896	−9.014	< 2e-16 ***
bmi	0.09353	0.01205	7.761	8.45e-15 ***

Signif. codes: 0 '***' 0.001 '**' 0.01 '*' 0.05 '.' 0.1 ' ' 1

(Dispersion parameter for binomial family taken to be 1)

Null deviance: 993.48 on 767 degrees of freedom
Residual deviance: 920.71 on 766 degrees of freedom
AIC: 924.71

Number of Fisher Scoring iterations: 4

Clearly, the bmi variable in the dataset is significant.

(b) To estimate the probability for someone whose BMI is 35 to have diabetes, you may use the logistic regression model to compute the probability that a case subject with an average BMI of 35 will test positive for a diagnosis of diabetes:

```
> predict(lr, type = "response", newdata = newdata)
> # Outputting:
     1
0.39823
```

Thus, according to this model, the calculated probability is 39.8%, or nearly 40%, or 2 out of 5.

(c) For someone in the 95% percentile probability of suffering from diabetes, estimate the probability of this case; that is, for a case subject whose BMI is 35.

```
> newdata1 <- data.frame(bmi = 35)
```

> predict(lr, type = "response", newdata = newdata1)
> # *Outputting:*
  95%
0.6144066

Thus, according to this model's calculated probability, a case subject with a BMI of 35 would have a probability of 61.4% (or approximately 2/3, or 2 out of 3) of being in the 95th percentile of those having a diagnosis of diabetes.

Review Questions for Section 7.4

1. In logistic regression, is it advisable to use additive models for probabilities? Why or why not?
2. In logistic regression modeling, there are no error terms, and no variance parameters as in the normal distribution. Why?
3. In logistic regression, can the parameters of the model be estimated by the method of maximum likelihood? Why or why not?
4. In logistic regression, the link function, which transfers the mean value to a scale where the relations to other variables can be described, is linear and additive. Show that this may be achieved using the following link function:

$$\log p = \log \{p/(1 - p)\}$$

5. In generalized linear models, the function predict() may be used to establish the probability of occurrence of certain events. Given a set of data of outcomes observed under a set of independent variable conditions, outline a procedure for using the function predict() to establish a predicted probability curve for any one of given independent variables.
6. (a) When should the logistic regression model be used?
   (b) Define the terms *odds* and *odds ratio*. Give examples of each.
7. Suggest an example in epidemiology in which logistic regression analysis is appropriate:
   (a) when the independent variable is continuous
   (b) when the independent variable is discrete
8. If p = probability and o = odds, then

$$o = [p/(1 - p)]$$

and thus

$$p = [o/(1 + o)]$$

(a) What are the upper and lower limits for p? For o?
(b) What advantages does the use of p have? Why?
(c) What advantages does the use of o have? Why?

9. In a system with n covariates, the corresponding logistic regression model may be expressed as

$$\log(\text{odds}) = \beta_0 + \beta_1 x_1 + \beta_2 x_2 + \beta_3 x_3 + \dots + \beta_n x_n + e.$$

β_1 may be considered as follows: A unit increase in x_1, with x_2, x_3, ..., x_n held fixed, increases the log odds of success by β_1, or increases the odds of success by a factor of $\exp(\beta_1)$.

   Write an expression for the "odds" when the dependences on the covariates are nonlinear.

10. For a given outcome, if the probability of
    (a) "success" in the presence of Condition A is p_1, and
    (b) "failure" in the absence of Condition A is p_2,

    what is the meaning of the ratio p_1/p_2? Explain and give examples.

Exercises for Section 7.4

1. Logistic regression models are often used to compute a survival curve for longitudinal censored data. The following R code segment computes an estimate of a survival curve for censored data using either the K–M or the Fleming–Harrington method for computing the predicted survivor function. For competing risks data, it computes the cumulative incidence curve. This calls the survival package's survfit. formula function with a different default value for conf.type (log–log basis). Moreover, attributes of the event time variable are saved.

   Usage:
   survfit(formula, data, ...)

   Arguments:

formula	A formula object, which must have a Surv object as the response on the left of the ~ operator and, if needed, terms separated by + operators on the right. One of the terms may be a strata object. For a single survival curve, the right side should be ~ 1.
data	A data frame in which to interpret the variables named in the formula, subset and weights arguments.
...	See survfit.formula
Details	See survfit.formula for details.
Value	An object of class "survfit". See survfit.object for details.
	Methods defined for survfit objects are print, plot, lines, and points.

   See also:
   survfit.cph for survival curves from Cox models; print, plot, lines, coxph, Surv, strata.

   Authors:
   Thomas Lumley (tlumley@u.washington.edu); and Terry Therneau

■ **Examples:**

```
require(survival)
# fit a Kaplan-Meier curve and plot it:
fit <- survfit(Surv(time, status) ~ x, data = aml)
plot(fit, lty = 2:3)
legend(100, .8, c("Maintained", "Nonmaintained"), lty = 2:3)

# fit a Cox proportional hazards model and plot the
# predicted survival for a 60-year-old:
fit <- coxph(Surv(futime, fustat) ~ age, data = ovarian)
plot(survfit(fit, newdata=data.frame(age=60)),
     xscale=365.25, xlab = "Years", ylab="Survival")

# Here is the dataset from Turnbull.
# There are no interval censored subjects, only left-censored (status=3),
# right-censored (status 0), and observed events (status 1).


Time
1 2 3 4
Type of observation
death 12 6 2 3
losses 3 2 0 3
late entry 2 4 2 5

tdata <- data.frame(time =c(1,1,1,2,2,2,3,3,3,4,4,4),
                    status=rep(c(1,0,2),4),
                    n =c(12,3,2,6,2,4,2,0,2,3,3,5))
fit <- survfit(Surv(time, time, status, type='interval') ~1,
          data=tdata, weights=n)


# Time to progression/death for patients with monoclonal gammopathy:
Competing risk curves (cumulative incidence)
fit1 <- survfit(Surv(stop, event=='progression') ~1, data=mgus1,
                subset=(start==0))
fit2 <- survfit(Surv(stop, status) ~1, data=mgus1,
                subset=(start==0), etype=event)
# competing risks;
# CI curves are always plotted from 0 upward, rather than 1 down:
plot(fit2, fun='event', xscale=365.25, xmax=7300,
        mark.time=FALSE,col=2:3, xlab="Years post diagnosis
        of MGUS")
lines(fit1, fun='event', xscale=365.25, xmax=7300,
        mark.time=FALSE,conf.int=FALSE)
text(10, .4, "Competing Risk: death", col=3)
text(16, .15,"Competing Risk: progression", col=2)
text(15, .30,"KM:prog")
```

The following R code segment undertakes the execution of this exercise:

```
>
> install.packages("rms")
```

Installing package(s) into 'C:/Users/bertchan/Documents/R/win-library/2.14'
(as 'lib' is unspecified)
--- Please select a CRAN mirror for use in this session ---
trying URL 'http://cran.stat.ucla.edu/bin/windows/contrib/2.14/rms_3.6-3.zip'
Content type 'application/zip' length 933733 bytes (911 Kb)
opened URL
downloaded 911 Kb

package 'rms' successfully unpacked and MD5 sums checked

The downloaded packages are in

C:\Users\bertchan\AppData\Local\Temp\RtmpyAfTbf\downloaded
_packages

```
> library(rms)
```

Loading required package: Hmisc
Loading required package: survival
Loading required package: splines
Hmisc library by Frank E Harrell Jr

Type library(help='Hmisc'), ?Overview, or ?Hmisc.Overview')
to see overall documentation.

NOTE:Hmisc no longer redefines [.factor to drop unused levels
when subsetting. To get the old behavior of Hmisc type
dropUnusedLevels().

Attaching package: 'Hmisc'

The following object(s) are masked from 'package:survival':
 untangle.specials
The following object(s) are masked from 'package:base':
 format.pval, round.POSIXt, trunc.POSIXt, units

Attaching package: 'rms'
The following object(s) are masked from 'package:survival':
 Surv

```
> ls("package:rms")
```

[1]	"%ia%"
[2]	".rms"
[3]	".Surv"
[4]	"AIC.rms"
[5]	"anova.rms"

[205] "Survival"

```
>
> require(survival)
> # fit a Kaplan-Meier and plot it:
> fit <- survfit(Surv(time, status) ~ x, data = aml)
> plot(fit, lty = 2:3)
> legend(100, .8, c("Maintained", "Nonmaintained"), lty = 2:3)
> # Outputting: Figure 7.30.
```

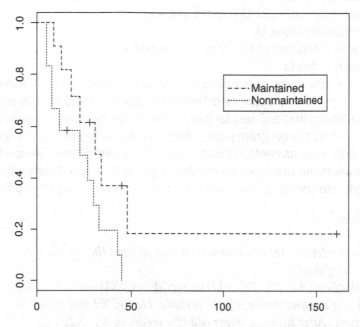

FIGURE 7.30 Logistic regression, K–M survival plot.

(a) Note the ordinate (vertical axis) of the survival plot. In what way does this plot resemble a probability plot?

(b) Note the abscissa (horizontal axis) of the survival plot. What are the units for this axis?

(c) What other features of this survival plot are characteristic of a typical logistic regression plot?

(d) Do the two survival graphs on the survival plot intersect? Why or why not?

(e) In the survival plot, the "Maintained" plot is always above the "Nonmaintained" plot. Why?

2. *Validation of Predicted Probabilities Using Logistic Regression: The Function* val. prob()

The function val.prob() may be used for validating predicted probabilities against binary events. Given a set of predicted probabilities p, or predicted log odds logit, and a vector of binary outcomes y that were not used in developing the predictions p or logit, the function val.prob() computes the following statistics and indexes:

(1) D_{xy} rank correlation between p and y [2(C − 0.5), C = ROC area]. In curve comparison and analysis, the ROC is a metric for comparing the diagnostic performance of two or more diagnostic tests. The diagnostic performance of a test, or the accuracy of a test, is its ability to discriminate diseased cases from normal cases. When one considers the results of a particular test in two populations, one population with a disease and the other population without the disease, one will rarely observe a perfect separation between the two groups; the distribution of the test results will most likely overlap.

(2) R-squared index.

(3) Discrimination index D (logistic model).

(4) Unreliability index U.

(5) χ^2 with 2 degrees of freedom, and its *p*-value.

(6) Quality index Q.

(7) Brier score (average squared difference in p and y), its intercept, and its slope.

(8) E_{max} = maximum absolute difference in predicted and calibrated probabilities.

(9) The Spiegelhalter Z-test for calibration accuracy, and its two-tailed p-value. If pl = TRUE, the program plots a fitted logistic calibration curve and optionally a smooth nonparametric fit using lowess (p,y,iter=0) and grouped proportions versus mean predicted probability in group. If the predicted probabilities or logits are constant, the statistics are returned and no plot is produced.

■ **Examples:**

```
# Fit logistic model on 100 observations simulated from the
# actual model given by
# Prob(Y=1 given X1, X2, X3) = 1/(1+exp[-(-1 + 2X1)]),
# where X1 is a random uniform [0,1] variable. Hence, X2 and X3
# are irrelevant. After fitting a linear additive model in X1, X2,
# and X3, the coefficients are used to predict Prob(Y=1) on a
# separate sample of 100 observations. Note that data splitting is
# an inefficient validation method unless n > 20,000.
set.seed(1)
n <- 200
x1 <- runif(n)
x2 <- runif(n)
x3 <- runif(n)
logit <- 2*(x1-.5)
P <- 1/(1+exp(-logit))
y <- ifelse(runif(n)<=P, 1, 0)
d <- data.frame(x1,x2,x3,y)
f <- lrm(y ~ x1 + x2 + x3, subset=1:100)
pred.logit <- predict(f, d[101:200,])
phat <- 1/(1+exp(-pred.logit))
val.prob(phat, y[101:200], m=20, cex=.5) # subgroups of 20 obs.
# Validate predictions more stringently by stratifying on whether
# x1 is above or below the median:
```

```
v <- val.prob(phat, y[101:200], group=x1[101:200], g.group=2)
v
plot(v)
plot(v, flag=function(stats) ifelse(
stats[,'ChiSq2'] > qchisq(.95,2) |
stats[,'B ChiSq'] > qchisq(.95,1), '*', ' ') )
```
 # Starts rows of statistics in plot corresponding to significant
 # miscalibration at the 0.05 level instead of the default, 0.01:
```
plot(val.prob(phat, y[101:200], group=x1[101:200], g.group=2),
col=1:3) # 3 colors (1 for overall)
```
 # Weighted calibration curves
 # plot(val.prob(pred, y, group=age, weights=freqs))

 # Fit logistic model on 100 observations simulated from the
 # actual model given by
 # Prob(Y=1 given X1, X2, X3) = 1/(1+exp[-(-1 + 2X1)]),
 # where X1 is a random uniform [0,1] variable. Hence, X2 and X3
 # are irrelevant. After fitting a linear additive model in X1, X2,
 # and X3, the coefficients are used to predict Prob(Y=1) *on a*
 # separate sample of 100 observations. Note that data splitting
 # is an inefficient validation method unless n > 20,000.
```
set.seed(1)
n <- 200
x1 <- runif(n)
x2 <- runif(n)
x3 <- runif(n)
logit <- 2*(x1-.5)
P <- 1/(1+exp(-logit))
y <- ifelse(runif(n)<=P, 1, 0)
d <- data.frame(x1,x2,x3,y)
f <- lrm(y ~ x1 + x2 + x3, subset=1:100)
pred.logit <- predict(f, d[101:200,])
phat <- 1/(1+exp(-pred.logit))
val.prob(phat, y[101:200], m=20, cex=.5) # subgroups of 20 obs.
```

The following R code segment undertakes the execution of this exercise:

 # Fit logistic model on 100 observations simulated from the
 # actual model given by
 # Prob(Y=1 given X1, X2, X3) = 1/(1+exp[-(-1 + 2X1)]),
 # where X1 is a random uniform [0,1] variable. Hence, X2 and X3
 # are irrelevant. After fitting a linear additive model in X1, X2,
 # and X3, the coefficients are used to predict Prob(Y=1) *on a*
 # separate sample of 100 observations. Note that data splitting is
 # an inefficient validation method unless n > 20,000.

```
set.seed(1)
n <- 200
x1 <- runif(n)
x2 <- runif(n)
x3 <- runif(n)
logit <- 2*(x1-.5)
P <- 1/(1+exp(-logit))
y <- ifelse(runif(n)<=P, 1, 0)
d <- data.frame(x1,x2,x3,y)
f <- lrm(y ~ x1 + x2 + x3, subset=1:100)
pred.logit <- predict(f, d[101:200,])
phat <- 1/(1+exp(-pred.logit))
val.prob(phat, y[101:200], m=20, cex=.5) # subgroups of 20 obs.
>
# Validate predictions more stringently by stratifying on whether
# x1 is above or below the median:
v <- val.prob(phat, y[101:200], group=x1[101:200], g.group=2)
v
plot(val.prob(phat, y[101:200], group=x1[101:200], g.group=2),
col=1:3) # 3 colors (1 for overall)
# Weighted calibration curves:
# plot(val.prob(pred, y, group=age, weights=freqs)) val.
>
> # Fit logistic model on 100 observations simulated from the
> # actual model given by Prob(Y=1 given X1, X2, X3) =
> # 1/(1+exp[-(-1 + 2X1)]),
> # where X1 is a random uniform [0,1] variable. Hence, X2 and
> # X3 are irrelevant. After fitting a linear additive model in X1,
> # X2, and X3, the coefficients are used to predict Prob(Y=1) on
> # a separate sample of 100 observations. Note that data
> # splitting is an inefficient validation method unless n > 20,000.
> set.seed(1)
> n <- 200
x1 <- runif(n)
> x2 <- runif(n)
> x3 <- runif(n)
> logit <- 2*(x1-.5)
> P <- 1/(1+exp(-logit))
> y <- ifelse(runif(n)<=P, 1, 0)
> d <- data.frame(x1,x2,x3,y)
> f <- lrm(y ~ x1 + x2 + x3, subset=1:100)
> pred.logit <- predict(f, d[101:200,])
> phat <- 1/(1+exp(-pred.logit))
> val.prob(phat, y[101:200], m=20, cex=.5) # subgroups of 20
> obs
```

> # *Outputting:*

Dxy	C (ROC)	R2	D	D:Chi-sq	D:p
0.320528211	0.660264106	0.094994525	0.063901031	7.390103054	0.006558373

U	U:Chi-sq	U:p	Q	Brier	Intercept
−0.019128530	0.087146981	0.957362194	0.083029561	0.231896346	0.052287214

Slope	Emax	S:z	S:p	Eavg
0.956517813	0.019247505	0.144009939	0.885492622	0.025838218

> # *Validate predictions more stringently by stratifying on*
> # *whether x1 is above or below the median:*
> v <- val.prob(phat, y[101:200], group=x1[101:200],
+   g.group=2)
> v
> # *Outputting:*

	n	Pavg	Obs	ChiSq	ChiSq2	Eavg	Eavg/P90	Med OR	C	B
[0.0131,0.526)	50	0.364	0.36	0.004	0.149	0.046	0.170	1.228	0.637	0.220
[0.5260,0.993]	50	0.590	0.62	0.195	1.902	0.058	0.213	1.083	0.514	0.244
Overall	100	0.477	0.49	0.073	0.088	0.026	0.065	1.084	0.660	0.232

	B ChiSq	B cal
[0.0131,0.526)	0.073	0.212
[0.5260,0.993]	0.327	0.230
Overall	0.021	0.230

Quantiles of Predicted Probabilities

	0.01	0.025	0.05	0.1	0.25	0.5	0.75	0.9	0.95	0.975
[0.0131,0.526)	0.213	0.222	0.242	0.270	0.301	0.364	0.407	0.471	0.516	0.531
[0.5260,0.993]	0.397	0.411	0.444	0.488	0.535	0.601	0.650	0.668	0.715	0.748
Overall	0.216	0.243	0.271	0.292	0.365	0.479	0.598	0.654	0.668	0.714

	0.99
[0.0131,0.526)	0.545
[0.5260,0.993]	0.764
Overall	0.750

> plot(v)
> # *Outputting:*

Group [0.0131,0.526) [0.5260,0.993] Overall
n 50 50 100
Pavg 0.364 0.590 0.477
Obs 0.36 0.62 0.49
ChiSq 0.0 0.2 0.1

ChiSq2 0.1 1.9 0.1
Eavg 0.046 0.058 0.026
Eavg/P90 0.170 0.213 0.065
Med OR 1.228 1.083 1.084
C 0.637 0.514 0.660
B 0.220 0.244 0.232
B ChiSq 0.1 0.3 0.0
B cal 0.212 0.230 0.230

```
> # Outputting: Figure 7.31
> # Stars rows of statistics in plot corresponding to significant
> # miscalibration at the 0.05 level instead of the default, 0.01:
> plot(val.prob(phat, y[101:200], group=x1[101:200],
+                           g.group=2),
+                           col=1:3) # 3 colors (1 for overall)
```

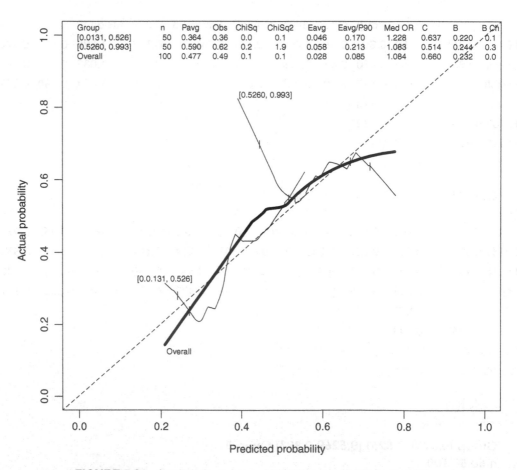

FIGURE 7.31 Logistic regression: Validating predicted probabilities.

```
> # Outputting:
```

Group [0.0131,0.526) [0.5260,0.993] Overall

Pavg 0.364 0.590 0.477
Obs 0.36 0.62 0.49
ChiSq 0.0 0.2 0.1
ChiSq2 0.1 1.9 0.1
Eavg 0.046 0.058 0.026
Eavg/P90 0.170 0.213 0.065
Med OR 1.228 1.083 1.084
C 0.637 0.514 0.660
B 0.220 0.244 0.232
B ChiSq 0.1 0.3 0.0
B cal 0.212 0.230 0.230

> # *Outputting:* Figure 7.32.

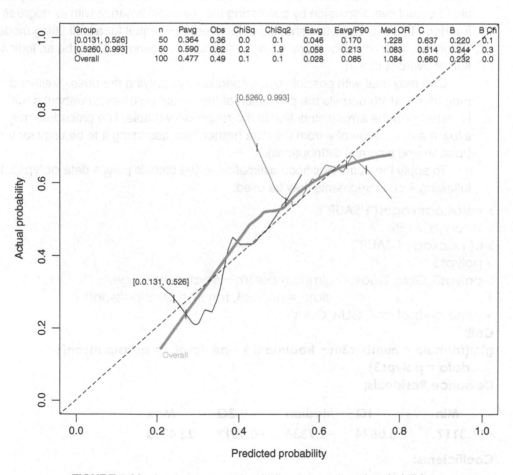

Group	n	Pavg	Obs	ChiSq	ChiSq2	Eavg	Eavg/P90	Med OR	C	B	B Ch
[0.0131, 0.526]	50	0.364	0.36	0.0	0.1	0.046	0.170	1.228	0.637	0.220	0.1
[0.5260, 0.993]	50	0.590	0.62	0.2	1.9	0.058	0.213	1.083	0.514	0.244	0.3
Overall	100	0.477	0.49	0.1	0.1	0.028	0.085	1.084	0.660	0.232	0.0

FIGURE 7.32 Logistic regression: Validating predicted probabilities.

(a) The statement of this exercise indicated that eight criteria are computed by this methodology of using logistic regression to validate predicted probabilities. Review each of these eight criteria (start by searching the Internet for "*D* rank

(b) Rank these eight criteria, starting with the most effective criterion, and give reasons for your ranking.

(c) In Figures 7.30 and 7.31, if the predicted probabilities were the same as the actual probabilities, then the predicted data points/lines would all be on the diagonal (45-degree) line. Comment on the accuracy of the computed predicted probabilities.

(d) In both plots, it appears that the predictions are more accurate around the middle section, where the probability is at about 0.5. Comment on this feature of the logistic regression model as a predictive tool.

(e) Provide a rationale for application of the logistic regression model as a statistical tool for prediction of successes (and failures) in applied probability problems in biostatistics and epidemiology.

3. *Quasi-likelihood estimation.*

In fitting generalized models with Poisson or binomial error distributions, it is possible to detect overdispersion by comparing the residual deviance with its degrees of freedom. The two quantities should be approximately equal for a well-fitting model. When the deviance is far larger than the degrees of freedom, it may be an indication of overdispersion.

One may deal with possible overdispersion by applying the quasi-likelihood procedure, which permits the estimation of the model parameters without a full knowledge of the error distribution of the response variable. The procedure may allow the calculation of φ from the data (rather than assuming it to be unity for the Poisson and binomial distributions).

To apply the quasi-likelihood estimation to the colonic polyps data polyps3, the following R code segments may be used:

```
> install.packages("HSAUR")
> library(HSAUR)
> ls("package:HSAUR")
> polyps3
> polyps3_GLM_Quasi <- glm(number3m ~ treatment + age,
+                          data = polyps3, family = quasipoisson() )
> summary(polyps3_GLM_Quasi)
Call:
glm(formula = number3m ~ treatment + age, family = quasipoisson(),
    data = polyps3)
Deviance Residuals:
```

Min	1Q	Median	3Q	Max
−11.3117	−5.0824	−2.7838	−0.4611	22.4333

Coefficients:

	Estimate	Std. Error	t value	Pr(>|t|)
(Intercept)	5.72284	1.16148	4.927	9.36e-05 ***
Treatmentactive	−1.19595	0.74361	−1.608	0.124
Age	−0.07243	0.05145	−1.408	0.175

(Dispersion parameter for quasipoisson family taken to be 91.14169)

   Null deviance: 1603.1 on 21 degrees of freedom
Residual deviance: 1191.6 on 19 degrees of freedom AIC: NA

Number of Fisher Scoring iterations: 6
>

   (a) Compare the regression coefficients for both explanatory variables: treatment
       and age.
       (i) What are their values?
       (ii) Is each value significant?
   (b) Compare the estimated standard errors for both explanatory variables:
              treatment (0.74316) and age (0.05145)
       with the previously calculated values for simple Poisson distribution:
              treatment (0.077891) and age (0.005389).
   (c) It is evident that the dispersions for the quasi-likelihood case are much larger.
       Why?
   (d) One explanation suggested for such overdispersion in the data is that colonic
       polyps may occur in clusters (i.e., they do not occur independently). Comment
       on this suggestion.
4. *The functions* predict() *and* predict.glm().
   A useful biostatistical tool, based on logistic regression, is the function predict(),
   which has several variations, including the function predict.glm(). These are
   documented in the CRAN package stats.
      Each of these R functions may be used to compute predictions and to estimate
   standard errors (among other things) of the predictions from a fitted generalized
   linear model object.

Usage:

```
predict(object, newdata = NULL,
        type = c("link", "response", "terms"),
        se.fit = FALSE, dispersion = NULL, terms = NULL,
        na.action = na.pass, ...)
```

Arguments:

object	A fitted object of class inheriting from "glm".
newdata	Optionally, a data frame in which to look for variables with which to predict.
type	The type of prediction required. The default is on the scale of the linear predictors; the alternative "response" is on the scale of the response variable.
se.fit	A logical switch indicating if standard errors are required.
dispersion	The dispersion of the generalized linear model fit to be assumed in computing the standard errors. If omitted, the result returned by

terms   With type="terms", by default all terms are returned. A character vector specifies which terms are to be returned.

na.action   The function determining what should be done with missing values in newdata. The default is to predict NA.

...   Further arguments passed to or from other methods.

Value:

If se = FALSE, a vector or matrix of predictions.
If se = TRUE, a list with components.

fit   Predictions.

se.fit   Estimated standard errors.

residual.scale A scalar giving the square root of the dispersion used in computing the standard errors.

glm, SafePrediction

Examples:
```
require(graphics)
## example from Venables and Ripley (2002, pp. 190–192.)
ldose <- rep(0:5, 2)
numdead <- c(1, 4, 9, 13, 18, 20, 0, 2, 6, 10, 12, 16)
sex <- factor(rep(c("M", "F"), c(6, 6)))
SF <- cbind(numdead, numalive=20-numdead)
budworm.lg <- glm(SF ~ sex*ldose, family=binomial)
summary(budworm.lg)

plot(c(1,32), c(0,1), type = "n", xlab = "dose",
     ylab = "prob", log = "x")
text(2^ldose, numdead/20, as.character(sex))
ld <- seq(0, 5, 0.1)
lines(2^ld, predict(budworm.lg, data.frame(ldose=ld,
     sex=factor(rep("M", length(ld)), levels=levels(sex))),
     type = "response"))
lines(2^ld, predict(budworm.lg, data.frame(ldose=ld,
     sex=factor(rep("F", length(ld)), levels=levels(sex))),
     type = "response"))
```

The following R code segment undertakes the execution of this example exercise:
```
>
> require(graphics)
>
> ## example from Venables and Ripley (2002, pp. 190–192.)
> ldose <- rep(0:5, 2)
> numdead <- c(1, 4, 9, 13, 18, 20, 0, 2, 6, 10, 12, 16)
> sex <- factor(rep(c("M", "F"), c(6, 6)))
> SF <- cbind(numdead, numalive=20-numdead)
```

```
> budworm.lg <- glm(SF ~ sex*ldose, family=binomial)
> summary(budworm.lg)
Call:
glm(formula = SF ~ sex * ldose, family = binomial) Deviance Residuals:
```

Min	1Q	Median	3Q	Max
−1.39849	−0.32094	−0.07592	0.38220	1.10375

Coefficients:

	Estimate	Std. Error	z value	Pr(>|z|)
(Intercept)	−2.9935	0.5527	−5.416	6.09e-08 ***
sexM	0.1750	0.7783	0.225	0.822
ldose	0.9060	0.1671	5.422	5.89e-08 ***
sexM:ldose	0.3529	0.2700	1.307	0.191

Signif. codes: 0 '***' 0.001 '**' 0.01 '*' 0.05 '.' 0.1 ' ' 1

(Dispersion parameter for binomial family taken to be 1)

Null deviance:	124.8756	on	11	degrees of freedom
Residual deviance:	4.9937	on	8	degrees of freedom

AIC: 43.104
Number of Fisher Scoring iterations: 4

```
>
> # Preparing the graph and the labels on the two axes:
> plot(c(1,32), c(0,1), type = "n", xlab = "dose",
+                        ylab = "prob", log = "x")
> text(2^ldose, numdead/20, as.character(sex))
> ld <- seq(0, 5, 0.1)
>
> # Drawing the predict() line for males:
> lines(2^ld, predict(budworm.lg, data.frame(ldose=ld,
+   sex=factor(rep("M", length(ld)), levels=levels(sex))),
+   type = "response"))
>
># Drawing the predict() line for females:
> lines(2^ld, predict(budworm.lg, data.frame(ldose=ld,
+   sex=factor(rep("F", length(ld)), levels=levels(sex))),
+   type = "response"))
>
> # Outputting: Figure 7.33 predict()
>
```

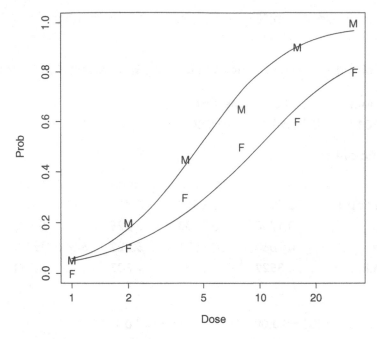

FIGURE 7.33 predict().

(a) In this program, when using the function predict(), at what stage is the linear regression function glm() introduced?

(b) What is the link function used in the model? Is this a good choice? Why or why not?

(c) How and when was the link function introduced into the model computation?

(d) Comment on the magnitudes and significances of the standard errors of the dependent variables for the regression.

(e) Suggest an effective approach for ascertaining these errors.

5. *Logistic regression in survival analysis: chronic granulomatous disease* (cgd) *infection data.*

In survival analysis, the K–M procedure is used to estimate the probability of surviving for a given duration of time. The computations consist of calculating the proportions of case subjects in a sample who survive for various durations of time. These sample proportions are then used as estimates of the probabilities of survival that one would expect to observe in the type of population represented by the test sample. In mathematical statistics, this approach is known as a *nonparametric technique,* in contrast to the common link functions (in which Poisson, binomial, or other probabilities are assumed) used in a basic logistic regression.

The cgd dataset in Fleming and Harrington (1991) is from a placebo-controlled RT of gamma interferon in chronic granulomatous disease (CGD). A total of 128 case subjects from 13 hospitals were followed for about a year. The number of case subjects per hospital ranged from 4 to 26. Each may have experienced more than one infection. The survival times (times to event) are the times between recurrent CGD infections on each patient (i.e., gap times). Censoring occurred at the last observation for all patients except one, who experienced a

Usage:
data(cgd)

Format:
The CGD dataset contains 15 columns and 203 rows. A brief description of the data columns is as follows:

Id	Patient number for 128 case subjects.
Center	Enrolling center number for 13 hospitals.
Random	Date of randomization.
Treat	Gamma-interferon treatment (rIFN-g) or placebo (Placebo).
Sex	Sex of each case subject (male, female).
Age	Age of each case subject at study entry, in years.
Height	Height of each case subject at study entry, in centimeters.
Weight	Weight of each case subject at study entry, in kilograms.
Inherit	Pattern of inheritance (autosomal recessive, X-linked).
Steroids	Using corticosteroids at times of study entry (1 = Yes, 0 = No).
Proylac	Using prophylactic antibiotics at time of study entry (1 = Yes, 0 = No).
hos.cat	A categorization of the hospital region into four groups.
Tstart	Start of each time interval.
Enum	Sequence number. For each patient, the infection records are in sequence number order.
Tstop	End of each time interval.
Status	Censoring indicator (1 = uncensored, 0 = censored).

References:
Fleming and Harrington (1991).
Therneau and Grambsch (2001).

The following R code segment undertakes the execution of this example exercise:

```
>
> install.packages("packHV")
> library(packHV)
Loading required package: WriteXLS
> ls("package:packHV")
```

```
[1]   "compare"      "convert_factor"   "convert_zero_NA"   "desc"
[5]   "hist_boxplot"  "IC_OR_glm"        "IC_RR_coxph"       c "multitable"
[9]   "plot_km"      c "plot_mm"         "plot_multi.table"  ccc"plot_reg"
```

```
> IC_OR_glm
```

(Output Omitted)

```
> cgd
```

id	center	random	treat	sex	age	height	weight
1 1	Scripps Institute	1989-06-07	rIFN-g	female	12	147.0	62.0
2 1	Scripps Institute	1989-06-07	rIFN-g	female	12	147.0	62.0
3 1	Scripps Institute	1989-06-07	rIFN-g	female	12	147.0	62.0
203 135	Scripps Institute	1989-12-29	placebo	female	3	96.0	13.1

	inherit	steroids	propylac	hos.cat	tstart	enum	tstop	status
1	autosomal	0	0	US:other	0	1	219	1
2	autosomal	0	0	US:other	219	2	373	1
3	autosomal	0	0	US:other	373	3	414	0
203	autosomal	0	1	US:other	0	1	227	0

```
>
> cgd$time=cgd$tstop-cgd$tstart
> plot_km(Surv(time,status)~sex,data=cgd,lwd=2,
+      col=c("black","red"))
> # Outputting: Figure 7.34.
```

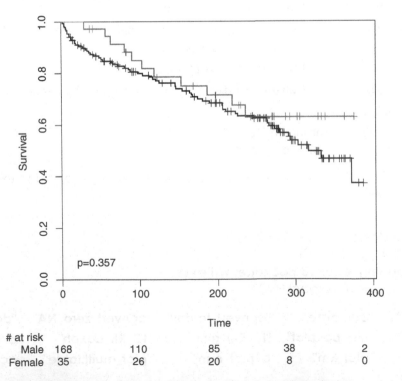

# at risk					
Male	168	110	85	38	2
Female	35	26	20	8	0

FIGURE 7.34 Logistic regression: Survival analysis of cgd data. Plots: male (lower curve) and female (upper curve).

(a) In survival analysis, what link function is used in the resultant logistic regression?

(b) Looking at Figure 7.34, what may be concluded regarding the link functions for the two populations: male and female case subjects?

(c) If the "steps" of the survival curves were to be smoothed out, what type of link functions could be expected?

(d) In Figure 7.34, the red curve (for female case subjects) lies *above* the black curve (for male case subjects). How does this characteristic reflect on the survival probabilities of these two cohorts?

(e) Since both curves show a decreasing slope with respect to time, what family of probability distribution curves may be used to model the survival process?

REFERENCES

Blanchard, M. S. (2012). CRAN package PKtools. sblanchard@coh.org

Calvert, A. H., & Plummer, R. (2008, June 15). The development of phase I cancer trial methodologies: The use of pharmacokinetic and pharmacodynamic end points sets the scene for phase 0 cancer clinical trials. *Clinical Cancer Research, 14,* 3664.

Children's Mercy Hospital. (2000). *What is collinearity?* Retrieved from "Ask Professor Mean," Category: Modeling issues; http://www.childrensmercy.org/stats/ask/collinearity.aspx

Dalgaard, P. (2002). *Introductory statistics with R* (Springer Series in Statistics and Computing). New York, NY: Springer.

Daniel, W. W. (2005). *Biostatistics: A foundation for analysis in the health sciences* (7th ed.; Wiley Series in Probability and Statistics). New York, NY: Wiley.

Everitt, B. S., & Hothorn, T. (2006). *A handbook of statistical analyses using R* (HSAUR). Boca Raton, FL: Chapman & Hall/CRC.

Fitzmaurice, G. (2004). Adjusting for confounding. *Nutrition, 20*(6), 594596. Retrieved from http://epicentre.massey.ac.nz/Portals/0/EpiCentre/Downloads/Education/227-407/Fitzmaurice_2004.pdf/

Fleming, T. R., & Harrington, D. R. (1991). *Counting processes and survival analysis.* New York, NY: Wiley.

Gerds, T. A., Cai, T., & Schumacher, M. (2008). The performance of risk prediction models. *Biometrical Journal, 4,* 457479.

Graf, E., Schmoor, C., Sauerbrei, W., & Schumacher, M. (1999). Assessment and comparison of prognostic classification schemes for survival data. *Statistics in Medicine, 18,* 25292545.

Hastie, T. J., & Tibshirani, R. J. (1990). *Generalized additive models.* Boca Raton, FL: Chapman & Hall/CRC.

Heagerty, P. J., Lumley, T., & Pepe, M. S. (2000). Time-dependent ROC curves for censored survival data and a diagnostic marker. *Biometrics, 56,* 337344.

Katki, H. A., & Mark, S. D. (2008). Survival analysis for cohorts with missing covariate information. *R-News, 8*(1), 14–19. Retrieved from http://dceg.cancer.gov/Files/RNewsNestedCohortWrapper_old.pdf

Katki, H. A., & Mark, S. D. (2009). Survival analysis of studies nested within cohorts using the NestedCohort package. CRAN (The Comprehensive R Archive Network). https://CRAN.r-project.org/

McNamee, R. (2005). Regression modelling and other methods to control confounding. *Occupational & Environmental Medicine, 62,* 500506. Retrieved from http://oem.bmj.com/content/62/7/500.full

Moreira, A., Araujo, A. A., & Machado, L. M. (2012). CRAN Package survivalBIV. Retrieved from http://cran.r-project.org/

Schnute, J. T., Couture-Beil, A., Haigh, R., & Kronlund, A. R. (2011). *PBSmodelling 2.62: User's guide*. Nanaimo, British Columbia, Canada: Fisheries and Oceans Canada, Science Branch. CRAN (The Comprehensive R Archive Network). https://CRAN.r-project.org/

Stanley, K. (2007). Statistical primer for cardiovascular research: Design of randomized controlled trials. *Circulation, 115*, 1164–1169.

Sigler, C., & Stemhagen, A. (2011). Epidemiology in drug development. Retrieved from http://www.pharmasug.org/proceedings/2011/HS/PharmaSUG-2011-HS10.pdf

Therneau, T. M., & Grambsch, P. M. (2001). Modeling survival data: Extending the Cox Model. *Statistics for Biology and Health*. New York, NY: Springer.

Tornoe, C. W. (2012). CRAN package nlmeODE. ctornoe@gmail.com

Venables, W. N., & Ripley, B. D. (2002). *Modern applied statistics with S* (4th ed., pp. 190–192). New York, NY: Springer Science & Business Media.

Wood, S. N. (2006). *Generalized additive models: An introduction with R*. Boca Raton, FL: Chapman & Hall/CRC.

Index